PSYCHOANALYSIS AND PSYCHIATRY

Psychoanalysis and Psychiatry: Partners and Competitors in the Mental Health Field offers a comprehensive overview of the many links between the two fields. There have long been connections between the two professions, but this is the first time the many points of contact have been set out clearly for practitioners from both fields.

Covering social and cultural factors, clinical practice, including diagnosis and treatment, and looking at teaching and continuing professional development, this book features contributions and exchange of ideas from an international group of clinicians from across both professions.

Psychoanalysis and Psychiatry: Partners and Competitors in the Mental Health Field will appeal to all practicing psychoanalysts and psychiatrists and anyone wanting to draw on the best of both fields in their theoretical understanding and clinical practice.

Cláudio Laks Eizirik (MD, PhD), lives in Porto Alegre, Brazil. He is a training and supervising analyst of the SPPA (Porto Alegre Psychoanalytic Society), and teaches at the Institute of Psychoanalysis, and works in private practice as psychoanalyst and psychotherapist. He is Professor Emeritus of Psychiatry at the Federal University of Rio Grande do Sul, where he teaches psychoanalysis and supervises residents of psychiatry. He was President of FEPAL (Latin American Psychoanalytic Federation) and the IPA (International Psychoanalytical Association) and is currently chair of the IPA's International New Groups Committee. Formerly he chaired the IPA Committee on Psychoanalysis and the Mental Field. He has published books, book chapters, papers, lectured widely and heavily researched his main areas of interest: psychoanalytic training, the clinical practice of psychoanalysis and psychoanalytic psychotherapy, the human life cycle, the process of ageing and the relationship between psychoanalysis and culture. He received the Sigourney Award in 2011.

Giovanni Foresti (MD, PhD), lives in Pavia, Italy. He is training and supervising analyst of the SPI (Italian Psychoanalytic Society), works in private practice as a psychoanalyst, psychiatrist and organizational consultant, and teaches at the State University of Milan (School of Specialization in Psychiatry), at the Milan Catholic University (Psychology of Organizations and Marketing) and at the SPI National Institute for Training. He is a member of OPUS, London, and part of Scientific Committee of IL NODO group, Turin. Co-chair for Europe of the Committee "Psychoanalysis and the Mental Health Field," he is now on the IPA Board as European Representative. His interests are focused on clinical issues, institutional functioning and group dynamics.

Recent titles in the Series include

Finding the Body in the Mind: Embodied Memories, Trauma, and Depression
Marianne Leuzinger-Bohleber

The Future of Psychoanalysis: The Debate about the Training Analyst System
Edited by Peter Zagermann

The Analytical Process: Journeys and Pathways
Thierry Bokanowski

Psychotic Organisation of the Personality: Psychoanalytic Keys
Antonio Perez-Sanchez

Psychoanalytic Perspectives on Virtual Intimacy and Communication in Film
Edited by Andrea Sabbadini, Ilany Kogan and Paola Golinelli

Transformational Processes in Clinical Psychoanalysis: Dreaming, Emotions and the Present Moment
Lawrence J. Brown

The Psychoanalyst and the Child: From the Consultation to Psychoanalytic Treatment
Michel Ody

Psychoanalytic Studies on Dysphoria: The False Accord in the Divine Symphony
Marion Oliner

PSYCHOANALYSIS AND PSYCHIATRY

Partners and Competitors in the Mental Health Field

Edited by Cláudio Laks Eizirik and Giovanni Foresti

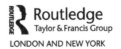

Routledge
Taylor & Francis Group

LONDON AND NEW YORK

First published 2019
by Routledge
2 Park Square, Milton Park, Abingdon, Oxon OX14 4RN

and by Routledge
52 Vanderbilt Avenue, New York, NY 10017

Routledge is an imprint of the Taylor & Francis Group, an informa business

British Library Cataloguing-in-Publication Data
A catalogue record for this book is available from the British Library

Library of Congress Cataloging-in-Publication Data

Names: Eizirik, Cláaudio Laks, editor. | Foresti, Giovanni Battista, editor.
Title: Psychoanalysis and psychiatry : partners and competitors in
    the mental health field/edited by Cláaudio Laks Eizirik and
    Giovanni Battista Foresti.
Description: New York : Routledge, 2019. | Includes bibliographical
    references and index.
Identifiers: LCCN 2018033797 (print) | LCCN 2018046062 (ebook) |
    ISBN 9780429447129 (Master) | ISBN 9780429823763 (Web PDF) |
    ISBN 9780429823756 (ePub) | ISBN 9780429823749 (Mobipocket/
    Kindle) | ISBN 9781138331723 (hardback : alk. paper) |
    ISBN 9781138331730 (pbk. : alk. paper) | ISBN 9780429447129 (ebk)
Subjects: LCSH: Psychoanalysis. | Psychiatry.
Classification: LCC BF173 (ebook) | LCC BF173 .P775269 2019 (print) |
    DDC 150.19/5—dc23
LC record available at https://lccn.loc.gov/2018033797

ISBN: 978-1-138-33172-3 (hbk)
ISBN: 978-1-138-33173-0 (pbk)
ISBN: 978-0-429-44712-9 (ebk)

Typeset in Palatino
by Apex CoVantage, LLC

CONTENTS

SERIES EDITOR'S FOREWORD

The Publications Committee of the International Psychoanalytic Association continues, with the present volume, the series Psychoanalytic Ideas and Applications.

The aim of this series is to focus on the scientific production of significant authors, whose works are outstanding contributions to the development of the psychoanalytic field and to set out relevant ideas and themes, generated during the history of psychoanalysis, that deserve to be known and discussed by present day psychoanalysts.

The relationship between psychoanalytic ideas and their applications needs to be put forward from the perspective of theory, clinical practice, and research, in order to maintain their validity for contemporary psychoanalysis.

The Publication's Committee's objective is to share these ideas with the psychoanalytic community and with professionals in other related disciplines, so as to expand their knowledge and generate a productive interchange between the text and the reader.

In this volume, Cláudio Laks Eizirik and Giovanni Foresti present the results of the work of the IPA Committee on Psychoanalysis and the Mental Health Field that has as its objective to conceive and implement actions at the interface between psychoanalysis and mental health. The editors describe many of the concerns and possibilities that were identified during the Committee's work. The reader will find a collective discussion on the responsibilities and opportunities shared by psychoanalysts and professionals in the mental health field.

This book contributes in an important fashion by describing and proposing ways to implement possible interdisciplinary and fertile dialogues. Attempts to create these type of bridges could have a positive impact, allowing members of the mental field to consider ways of facing similarities and differences in the modes of understanding mental suffering and its treatment. The editors of this book succeeded at putting together a comprehensive review of the ways in which practitioners of the two fields could increase a reciprocal understanding of their disciplines, promoting better cooperation and benefiting as a result from an interdisciplinary cross-fertilization.

Skilfully divided in three parts, this book compares different regional perspectives, reviews the methodologies developed to devise diagnostic tools and illustrates examples of integration of psychoanalysis in the realm of training and continuous education.

I have no doubt this book will be of great interest to psychoanalysts and practitioners of the mental field and specifically to those who work in institutional settings. Creating bridges between disciplines can increase an attitude of open mindedness, enriching the theoretical and clinical skills of all professionals working in the field of mental health.

Gabriela Legorreta
Series Editor
Chair, IPA Publications Committee

FOREWORD

Virginia Ungar

This book, edited by the Publications Committee of the IPA is very welcome indeed and has appeared at a very opportune moment. There is no
doubt that the world has radically changed since the inception of Psychoanalysis. Many of the social and cultural transformations witnessed
by humankind over the last one hundred years have directly affected our
practice, for example, the changes in sexuality and the concept of gender,
the emergence of new family configurations, changes in child rearing practices, technological innovations, growing social violence, and the prevalence of uncertainty in our everyday lives. I believe that everything that
takes place in our consulting rooms today should be considered within a
specific social context. In this sense, there is a connection between social
violence and uncertainty, and the increase in more severe pathologies that
we are witnessing in our practice at present. At some point, the changes in
clinical presentations could be viewed as a result of manifold social transformations that generate uncertainty and anxiety, transformations which
include the loss of job security and the weakening of the social safety net,
the decline of community organizations, and the increase in various forms
of social violence.

Another important factor is technological progress. We must look at
the new role of the mass media in children's lives. Today, the media pierce
through the entire protective shield that was provided years ago by the

family, the school, religion, or the state and are utterly transforming the space in which children forge relationships. That space used to be the family, the school, summer camp. These days, however, all these institutions have been colonized by the discourse of the media. There are no isolated spaces; the TV and the internet reach everywhere.

Children have to 'get inside' something that has already been programmed but that, at the same time, offers different options to set their violence loose, to play roles with the machine or in a network, alone or with other children. They are dealing with a different reality – virtual or information reality. Today, in 2018, we are forced to think of the fact that we, and even more so our children and grandchildren, spend many hours of the day inside this other reality, which is neither real nor fictional, neither true nor false. Furthermore, it exists in a space that is so strong and pervading that it has transformed the notions of privacy and intimacy, notions which are necessary for the psychoanalytic experience to unfold.

In the case of tweens and teens, chatting spaces sometimes constitute the place for group activities. These spaces can become a kind of autonomous organism, like a city that does not exist anywhere and is inhabited by an imaginary community of fleeting residents who come from remote and diverse places. Neither is it necessary to meet in person; they can use an electronic device.

Freud and his theories sparked one of the most revolutionary cultural events of the start of the twentieth century and we can still experience its impact. Thanks to Freud, we learned that we live in more than one world through the concept of the unconscious, that children have a sexuality, that it is possible to work through mental suffering within a therapeutic relationship in which one speaks (the talking cure), and that social and cultural phenomena are governed by mechanisms which are very similar to those experienced by individuals.

We now also know that Psychoanalysis has had an enormous effect on other fields such as Medicine – especially in Paediatrics – Education and Law. We believe that we must now strengthen this effect and this can be achieved if we psychoanalysts move outside of our consultation rooms and societies and spend time working in the community, especially in those places where young professionals are working and facing complex realities in different contexts (such as addiction, domestic violence, sexual abuse, migration, eating disorders, etc.). I am here referring to the different services offered at hospitals (psychopathology, psychiatry, paediatrics), to community centres, to the different levels of schooling, universities, etc.

This book was an initiative of the IPA Mental Health Committee and was brought about by Claudio Eizirik and Giovanni Foresti. It shows throughout its twenty-two chapters that Psychoanalysis has a lot to contribute but that, at the same time, our discipline is learning to listen to what other disciplines have to say. As a result of this, it is not now possible to think simply about the patient and their defences and resistance and nor it is possible to focus solely on the position of the analyst. Following on the great contribution made by the Barangers with their theory on the analytic field – which was then taken up by authors outside of Latin America once their works were translated – we know that what prevails is precisely that which happens *between* the analyst and the patient. Ours is a difficult moment for the 'globalised' world, where inequalities are starker than ever and intolerance to that which is different and the difficulty of accepting diversity is very evident indeed. As a result of this it is not possible now to think in a form of Psychoanalysis which does not take into account the context and the culture in which psychoanalysts work.

In the first section of the book, this issue appears right from the title: Global Trends and Local Specificities. Here, distinguished authors from the three regions of the IPA show us how the meeting point between Psychoanalysis and Psychiatry should be studied in the context of each era and each culture.

The second section turns to nosology, diagnosis and treatment and also covers the different approaches to a topic which is part of the debate and the controversies that appear at that interface between the two disciplines that is to say, the necessity to find a common language that will facilitate clinical work and even more so in clinical presentations such as those which are called 'severe mental illness'.

The third and final part of the book is dedicated to the formative dimension and contains the ideas of renowned colleagues in their countries and the rest of the world.

With respect to the place of Psychoanalysis in the training of a psychiatrist or a psychotherapist, or even of any professional who works in the field of mental health, I believe it is important that they undergo an experience of personal treatment. There is nothing that more shakes the internal balance of a young professional than working in the field of mental health and in this situation the therapeutic experience itself is invaluable.

This excellent and necessary publication leaves in the end many doors open for us to continue thinking, working and listening to each other. I believe that a confrontation between Psychoanalysis and Psychiatry is not the right path to take. Firstly, we would be erasing an essential historical fact: Psychoanalysis was born out of Psychiatry. Nor can we forget the latter's curative therapeutic dimension which Freud included in a number of his definitions of our discipline. As the editors of this present volume state, we work with human beings and with their sufferings which these days are added to by a high level of social distress and an uncertainty which leaves individuals in different states of helplessness.

Moreover, in our practice we very work in teams and we cannot work in isolation treating such a wide range of clinical challenges such as severe pathologies, addictions, eating disorders, violent contexts in their numerous forms, to name but a few of the cases where the necessity exists to work in teams.

This, however, does not negate the specificity of the task, the conceptual tools and techniques that each of the two disciplines entail in their own right, but we must never fear dilution if we are able to preserve sufficient open-mindedness, the necessary passion for the work we undertake and the transmission of that work which we carry out in order to alleviate suffering and help the individual find their desire and their own path.

Virginia Ungar, MD
President of the IPA

FOREWORD

Helen Herrman

The publication of this volume is significant and timely. The fields of psychoanalysis and psychiatry are each undergoing change and examination. The editors describe the origins of the book in the work of a committee established by the International Psychoanalytic Association in 2013 to "imagine, conceive, reflect on, plan and implement effective actions in the interface of psychoanalysis and mental health" (p. 4). The concept of the mental health field is adopted and used effectively and provides a useful starting point for all contributors to consider the best ways to collaborate in improving mental health for people and communities.

A distinguished group of editors and contributors have worked together following the extensive examinations of the committee. Leaders in the mental health field address realities of the complementary, contrasting and sometimes conflicting views across the field; and offer the basis for collaborative approaches to addressing the prominent uncertainties within our shared field.

The work is timely also in that a major project of the mental health field is understanding how to reduce inequities in mental health care within and between countries and regions across the world. The World Psychiatric Association (WPA) for example has a vision of "a world in which people live in conditions that promote mental health and have access to mental health treatment and care that meet appropriate professional and ethical standards, integrate public health principles and respect human rights" (www.wpanet.org). The WPA aims to expand the contribution of psychiatry to improved mental health worldwide, reaching people who face adversity and disadvantage. It is engaged in supporting psychiatrists and partners to optimize the use of psychiatry in building community capacity for appropriate response to mental health needs inherent in adversities and emergencies. The work is based on collaborating successfully with other organizations; and working with psychiatrists and others to use their expertise in a range of community settings.

This aim must be fulfilled without diminishing the expertise required by a well-trained psychiatrist wherever he or she works. The training curricula promoted by WPA emphasize that all psychiatrists, including those trained and working in countries with few professional resources, need to be competent in a range of psychotherapeutic approaches and understand psychodynamic principles based on the discipline of psychoanalysis. They need these capacities whether working directly with patients or through other cadres whom they train and supervise in mental health work. As noted by contributors to this book, the understanding of the patient as a person and the concept of formulating the case history and examination – along with the patient and family – are and must remain central to the work of the general psychiatrist, with many of the insights for this work derived originally from the field of psychoanalysis.

The expertise of all professionals working in the field of mental health is essential to promote good health and to offer comprehensive health care. Our patients and their families need us to work alongside them and other partners in clinical practice, teaching, research and advocacy. We have to be centrally involved in national and international debates, policies and initiatives in mental health. However, to do this we need a united voice. This book is an important contribution to understanding and progress of this enterprise. I hope it is read by many who wish to advance the mental health field.

Helen Herrman
President
World Psychiatric Association
Melbourne

ACKNOWLEDGMENTS

We are grateful to Stefano Bolognini, former IPA president, whose vision led him to establish the Committee on Psychoanalysis and the Mental Health Field, to all Members of this committee and contributors of this book, to our families and to our patients, whose constant presence and support in our lives made it possible to transform a generous idea into this contribution for understanding the complex relations between psychoanalysis and psychiatry.

CONTRIBUTORS

Editors

Cláudio Laks Eizirik, MD, PhD, lives in Porto Alegre, Brazil. He is a training and supervising analyst of the SPPA (Porto Alegre Psychoanalytic Society), and teaches at the Institute of Psychoanalysis, and works in private practice as psychoanalyst and psychotherapist. He is Professor Emeritus of Psychiatry at the Federal University of Rio Grande do Sul, where he teaches psychoanalysis and supervises residents of psychiatry. He was President of FEPAL (Latin American Psychoanalytic Federation) and the IPA (International Psychoanalytical Association) and is currently chair of the IPA's International New Groups Committee. Formerly he chaired the IPA Committee on Psychoanalysis and the Mental Field. He has published books, book chapters, papers, lectured widely and researched on his main areas of interest: psychoanalytic training, the clinical practice of psychoanalysis and psychoanalytic psychotherapy, the human life cycle, mainly the process of ageing and the relation of psychoanalysis and culture. He received the Sigourney Award in 2011.

Giovanni Foresti, MD, PhD, lives in Pavia (Italy). He is training and supervising analyst of the SPI (Italian Psychoanalytic Society), works in private practice as psychoanalyst, psychiatrist and organizational consultant, and teaches at the State University of Milan (School of Specialization in Psychatry), at the Milan Catholic University (Psychology of Organizations and Marketing) and at the SPI National Institute for Training. He is a member of OPUS, London, and part of the Scientific Committee of IL NODO group, Turin. Co-chair for Europe of the Committee "Psychoanalysis and the Mental Health Field," he is now on the IPA Board as European Representative. His interests are focused on clinical issues, institutional functioning and group dynamics.

Contributors

Antonio Andreoli, MD, is Training and Supervising Analyst of the Swiss Psychoanalytic Society and was trained in psychiatry at the University of Geneva Hospital Centre and Medical School. Former Professor and Chief of psychiatric services at the Geneva University General Hospital, he is presently in private practice.

Stefano Bolognini, MD Psychiatrist, Training and Supervising analyst of the Italian Psychoanalytical Society, Stefano Bolognini is a former President of the Bologna Psychoanalytic Center, former National Scientific Secretary and former President of the Italian Psychoanalytical Society. Honorary Member of the New York Contemporary Freudian Society and of the Los Angeles Institute and Society for Psychoanalytic Studies. For 10 years (2002–2012) he was a member of the European Editorial Board of the *International Journal of Psychoanalysis*; current chair of the *IPA Inter-Regional Encyclopedic Dictionary of Psychoanalysis* (IRED); past-President of the International Psychoanalytical Association, after having been IPA Board Representative for two mandates and member and chair of several IPA committees. Under his Presidency he organized the creation of the IPA Mental Health Field Committee and of the Sub-Committee on Addiction. He was co-founder (1992) of the SPI Serious Pathologies Committee, and for 30 years up to now Supervisor of National Health Psychiatric Services in Venice and Bologna.

Heinz Boeker, MD, was trained in Paediatric and Adolescent Psychiatry, Neural-Paediatrics, Neurology, Psychiatry and Psychotherapy/Psychoanalysis in Hamburg, Giessen and Frankfurt/Main, Germany. He has been a member of the IPA/German Psychoanalytic Association since 1992. He completed his habilitation thesis at the University of Zurich.

He is Professor of Clinical Psychiatry at the University of Zurich. Since 2009 until December 2015 he was Head of the Centre for Depressions, Anxiety Disorders and Psychotherapy at the Department for Psychiatry, Psychotherapy and Psychosomatics, University Hospital of Psychiatry Zurich. Since 2016 he has worked in a private practice in Zurich. He is associated to the University of Zurich and guest professor at the International Psychoanalytic University /IPU Berlin.

Alessandra D'Agostino, PhD, is Clinical Psychologist, Psychotherapist, Psychoanalyst in Training at the Italian Psychoanalytical Society (SPI), and Postdoctoral Research Fellow in Clinical Psychology at the University of Urbino (Italy). She has published: with M. Rossi Monti, *L'autolesionismo* (Roma, 2009); *Il suicidio* (Roma, 2012).

Anna Ferruta, PhD, Full Member and Training Analyst of the Italian Psychoanalytical Society and of the International Psychoanalytical Association. She is a member of the Monitoring and Advisory Board of the *International Journal of Psychoanalysis*, Consultant Supervisor in Psychiatric and Neurological Institutions and Foundation Member of "Mito&Realtà– Association for Therapeutic Communities."

Allen Frances, MD, is Professor Emeritus and former chair of the Department of Psychiatry at Duke University. He was chair of the DSM-IV Task Force and is author of *Saving Normal*.

Glen O. Gabbard, MD, is a training and supervising analyst at the Houston Center for Psychoanalytic Studies and winner of the Sigourney Award in 2000. He has authored or edited 28 books, including *Psychoanalysis and the Cinema*, and was the first Film Review Editor of the *International Journal of Psychoanalysis*.

Peter Hartwich, Prof. MD, Department of Psychiatry, Psychotherapy, Psychosomatics of the General Hospital of Frankfurt/M, Teaching Hospital of the University of Frankfurt.

Mads Gram Henriksen, MA, PhD, Mental Health Center Glostrup, Institute of Clinical Medicine, Faculty of Health and Medical Sciences University of Copenhagen; Department of Media, Communication and Cognition, Philosophy Section, Faculty of Humanities, University of

Copenhagen; Center for Subjectivity Research, Faculty of Humanities, University of Copenhagen.

Robert D. Hinshelwood, MD, Professor, Centre for Psychoanalytic Studies (1997–2015), and currently Professor Emeritus Department for Psychosocial and Psychoanalytic Studies, University of Essex. Previously, 1993–1997, Director of The Cassel Hospital; Visiting Professor, Committee for Social Thought, University of Chicago, 2002–2003; and Consultant Psychotherapist, Ealing Hospital, 1976–1993. He is Fellow of the British Psychoanalytical Society, and Fellow of the Royal College of Psychiatrists. Relevant publications: *What Happens in Groups* (1987); (with Wilhelm Skogstad) *Observing Organisations* (2000); *Thinking about Institutions* (2001); *Suffering Insanity* (2004); (edited with Nuno Torres) *Bion's Sources* (2013); *Research on the Couch* (2013); *Countertransference and Alive Moments* (2016); (with Kalina Stamenova) *Methods of Qualitative Research in Psychoanalytic Studies* (due October 2018).

Do-Un Jeong, MD, PhD, Professor Emeritus of the Seoul National University, is the first IPA direct member from Korea and the founding/immediate past president and training/supervising analyst of the Korean Psychoanalytic Study Group of the IPA. He is now active as CEO/Director of JD Institute, Seoul, Republic of Korea, practicing and teaching psychoanalysis.

Otto F. Kernberg, MD, FAPA, is Director of the Personality Disorders Institute at The New York Presbyterian Hospital, Westchester Division, and Professor of Psychiatry at the Weill Medical College of Cornell University. Dr. Kernberg is a Past-President of the International Psychoanalytic Association. He is also Training and Supervising Analyst of the Columbia University Center for Psychoanalytic Training and Research. He is the author of 13 books and co-author of 12 others, including: *Borderline Conditions and Pathological Narcissism Severe Personality Disorders: Psychotherapeutic Strategies, Psychodynamic Psychotherapy of Borderline Patients, Contemporary Controversies in Psychoanalytic Theory, Techniques and their Applications, The Inseparable Nature of Love and Aggression* and most recently *Psychoanalytic Education at the Crossroads* and *Resolution of Aggression and Recovery of Eroticism*.

Joachim Küchenhoff, MD, is a psychoanalyst and member of the IPA and of the Swiss and German psychoanalytic societies. He is a specialist in psychiatry, psychotherapy and psychosomatic medicine, and is Professor of Psychiatry and Psychotherapy at the University of Basel, Switzerland. He has been working as the medical director of the department of adult psychiatry in Baseland, Switzerland, since 2007. He is editor-in-chief of the SANP (Swiss Archives of Neurology, Psychiatry and Psychotherapy), president of the supervisory board at IPU (International Psychoanalytic University) Berlin and member of many other advisory boards. His latest publication is *Understanding Psychosis* (Routledge).

Levent Küey, MD, is an Associate Professor of Psychiatry, currently teaching psychopathology at Istanbul Bilgi University, Istanbul, Turkey and working in private practice. He is a member of the European Psychiatric Association Board (2015–2019); former Secretary General of the World Psychiatric Association (2008–2014); former editor of WPA News (2008–2014) and of WPA Website (2008–2014); and former member of the Editorial Board of World Psychiatry (2008–2014).

Vittorio Lingiardi, MD, is a psychiatrist and psychoanalyst. He is Full Professor of Dynamic Psychology and past Director of the Clinical Psychology Specialization Program in the Department of Dynamic and Clinical Psychology of the Faculty of Medicine and Psychology, Sapienza University of Rome, Italy. He and Nancy McWilliams comprised the Steering Committee of the new edition of the *Psychodynamic Diagnostic Manual* (*PDM-2*, 2017).

Robert Michels, MD, is the Walsh McDermott University Professor of Medicine and Psychiatry at Weill-Cornell Medical College, where he previously served as Provost, Dean, and Chairman of the Department of Psychiatry. He is former Joint Editor-in-Chief of *The International Journal of Psychoanalysis*, and a former Training and Supervising Analyst at Columbia Psychoanalytic Center.

Susana Muszkat is a psychologist and Master in social psychology by the University of São Paulo, full member and faculty of the Brazilian Society of Psychoanalysis of São Paulo (SBPSP) and IPA member; co-editor of the book series "What shall I do?" edited by Blucher publishing House. Author of the books *Violence and Masculinity* (2011), published by *Casa do Psicólogo*, and *Family Violence* (2016), by Blucher publishing house. She has a private psychoanalytic practice in São Paulo, Brazil, for individual patients, families and couples.

Andrea Narracci, MD, is psychiatrist and psychoanalyst, an ordinary member of the Italian Psychoanalytical Society (SPI-IPA), Consultant Psychiatrist at Asl Roma 1 in Rome and founder of the Italian Laboratory for Multifamiliar Psychoanalytical Groups. Among his publications are "The Multifamiliar Psychoanalysis in Italy" (in collaboration with prof. Jorge Garcia Badaracco) and "Multifamiliar Psychoanalysis as Esperanto."

Georg Northoff, is philosopher, neuroscientist and psychiatrist, holding degrees in all three disciplines. Being originally from Germany, he is now working in Ottawa/Canada where he researches the relationship between the brain and mind in its various facets. The question driving his work is: why and how can our brain construct subjective phenomena such as self, consciousness, emotions.

Mario Perini, MD, psychiatrist, working as a psychoanalyst, an organizational consultant, an executive coach, and a Balint group leader. Member, International Psychoanalytic Association and International Society for the Psychoanalytic Study of Organizations. Scientific director, IL NODO group. Adjunct Professor, Department of Psychology, Turin University. Chair, Committee on Healthcare and Welfare Institutions, Italian Psychoanalytic Society.

Humberto Lorenzo Persano, MD, PhD, psychiatrist, Professor – Mental Health and Psychiatry Department School of Medicine – University of Buenos Aires (UBA); Training and Supervising Analyst, Child and Adolescent Psychoanalyst Argentine Psychoanalytic Association (APA), Member of Health Committee IPA, Past Co Chair for Latin America Psychoanalysis and The Mental Health Field Committee IPA, Director Postgraduate in Psychiatry (UBA). Research Reviewer IPA, Fellow Member at College of *The International Journal of Psychoanalysis* (IJPA). Head of Unit on Adolescent and Youth Eating Disorders at Jose T. Borda Psychiatric Hospital Buenos Aires. Member of Argentine Psychiatrist's Association (APSA) and International Member of the American Psychiatric Association (APA).

Florence Quartier, MD, Psychiatrist-psychotherapist FMH; Former Consultant Physician, University Hospital Geneva; Psychoanalyst Full member, Psychoanalytical Swiss Society (API); Former Chair WPA Section "Psychoanalysis in Psychiatry."

Bent Rosenbaum, MD, specialist in psychiatry and has a degree of DMSci (Doctor of Medical Science). He is adjunct professor at the University of Copenhagen, Department of Psychology, and senior researcher at the Clinic for Psychotherapy, Psychiatric Centre of Copenhagen, Capital Region of Denmark. He is also training and supervising analyst in the Danish Psychoanalytic Society and has a part-time psychoanalytic practice. Previously, President for the Danish Psychiatric Association (1998–2000) and the Danish Psychoanalytic Society (2003–2011) and member of the EPF council; European co-chair of the IPA committee for New Groups (2009–2013), and member of the IPA Board 2013–2015). His primary research areas have been psychoanalytic psychotherapy for people with psychosis, severe trauma and with suicide risk.

Mario Rossi Monti is Psychiatrist, Member of the Italian Psychoanalytical Society (SPI), and Professor of Clinical Psychology (University of Urbino, Italy). He has recently published: with G. Foresti, *Esercizi di visioning. Psicoanalisi, psichiatria, istituzioni* (Roma, 2010); and *Psicopatologia del presente. Crisi della nosografia e nuove forme della clinica* (Milano, 2012).

Borut Škodlar, MD, PhD, is a psychiatrist and a psychotherapist, Head of the Center for Mental Health and Psychotherapy Unit at the University Psychiatric Clinic Ljubljana and Associate Professor at the Faculty of Medicine, University of Ljubljana. For his PhD, he worked at the Medical School, University of Ljubljana and Center for Subjectivity Research, University of Copenhagen, and later as a postdoctoral researcher at the latter. He has completed training in logotherapy and existential analysis at Süddeutsches Institut für Logotherapie in Fürstenfeldbruck, training in psychoanalytic psychotherapy (Slovenian Association of Psychotherapists) and training in group analysis (Institute for Group Analysis Ljubljana).

Marta Vigorelli, psychologist, full member and training Analyst of Italian Society of Psychoanalytic Psychotherapy and member of European Federation for Psychoanalytic Psychotherapy in the Public Sector. Adjunct Professor Psychology Department University of Milan-Bicocca. Founder and current President of Mito&Realtà, Association for Therapeutic Communities. Consultant Supervisor in Psychiatric Institutions.

Introduction

Cláudio Laks Eizirik and Giovanni Battista Foresti

Background

In the last two decades, many complex and unexpected processes have changed the relationship between psychoanalysis and the disciplines that constitute the "mental health field" (a definition that comes from community and social psychiatry which we have come to recognize as useful because of its comprehensiveness). As an overall trend, despite some specific centers or places where there still is a strong and relevant psychoanalytic influence, what we can observe is a smaller and weaker presence of psychoanalysis than in previous periods.

To understand these changes, we have to put the new data into perspective. Seldom in history have we witnessed so many countries being influenced by such powerful transformations in their overall economic structure – a phenomenon concisely referred to as "globalization." These transformations have cascaded from the industrial organizations to the health systems and the mental health institutions. Even if they have had a worldwide impact and produced an unforeseen homogenization of values and cultures, the processes of globalization haven't changed the societies so radically as is often and somewhat apocalyptically represented. The speed and the results of the changes depend upon the overall system of factors that characterize the different institutional, social and cultural realities.

1

In order to imagine, conceive, reflect on, plan and implement effective actions in the interface of psychoanalysis and mental health, the IPA established, in the administration of Stefano Bolognini, a new committee, the Committee on Psychoanalysis and the Mental Health Field, that begun its activity in July 2013. In order to fulfill its mission, the Committee considered that it should elaborate an assessment of the resources at their disposal and focus on the specific limitations present in each peculiar regional, national and/or local situation. It was consensual to the Committee that the actions to be undertaken to ameliorate the relationship between psychoanalysis and the disciplines of the mental health field, should be based on a specific analysis of the reality within which that action, or set of actions, could be realized.

The first stage of the Committee's work was the elaboration of an instrument that was sent to IPA psychoanalytic societies and that was based on several distinctions. The first distinction took into account the trends of general/global factors *versus* national/local factors. The second one distinguished the obstacles and resources that are external to the psychoanalytic institutions and the obstacles and resources that are internal to the psychoanalytic institution and the psychoanalytic movement at large. After the many answers received, and the joint reflection, the Committee was able to identify several relevant factors that are present in the current relation of psychoanalysis and the mental health field.

The major external/general factors that were identified are:

- so called "neoliberalism," deregulation and managed care (the effects of globalization in the health systems and in the mental health field: for instance, the Health Maintenance Organizations and the DRGs in the US and the split between public purchasers and public providers within the National Health System in the UK);
- new trends in psychiatric nosology (neo-Kraepelianism): operational criteria and diagnoses of disorder in different dimensions (DSM-III, IV, V and their cultural *sequelae*), upsurge of biological psychiatry, exclusively drug-oriented research and practice, the politics of "evidence-based" guidelines;
- a prevailing trend in the current culture that grants scientific and financial privileges to quick, concrete and non reflexive answers to emotional symptoms and suffering;
- positive reactions of psychoanalytically oriented thinkers and changes of the psychoanalytic movement culture: new trends in

neurobiology and neurosciences (e.g. mirror neurons); empirical and conceptual research in psychoanalysis (e.g. research on pattern of attachment and psychopathology).

The regional, national and local factors identified were:

- institutional strength and past history (prestige) of the disciplines of the mental health field;
- institutional specificities of the local health system (public *versus* private: UK *versus* US solutions, for instance);
- financial support for psychanalytic/psychotherapeutic activities (insurance, state owned or privately arranged support versus out-of-pocket payments);

The factors internal to the psychoanalytic movement and the psychoanalytic institutions were described as follows:

- strength and history of the local psychoanalytic institutions (society or societies);
- strength and history of the local psychoanalytic movement (other unorthodox components);
- prevailing attitudes of separatedness and isolation (arrogance based in the supposed ability of psychoanalysis to understand and treat beyond its concrete possibilities) or widespread trends of openness, cooperation/integration and curiosity (the local psychoanalytic culture), accepting realistic possibilities and limitations and the need for joint work with the mental health field;
- level of inner conflicts and stagnation with possible consequences in isolation and self-absorption (involutional spirals);
- inner paralyzing conflicts: the factors that produce the "intolerance of diversity" (e.g. Ken Eisold's hypotheses);
- conflicts between the belief that what is relevant for psychoanalysis consists in its training, practice and theoretical development and the notion that psychoanalytic presence in the real world and its joint work with other fields is equally relevant.

After that first inquiry, the Committee established that it had two target audiences: an internal one, namely the psychoanalytic community, and an external one, namely the other areas of the mental health field and the patients who seek help for their emotional suffering. Concerning the internal audience, the Committee acted through the IPA website, analytic meetings and congresses, the establishment of an international network of analysts interested and committed to a concern with the relevance of this kind of action for the future and the development of psychoanalysis, and through joint activities with other relevant IPA committees. Concerning the external one, we organized and encouraged the dialogue with relevant colleagues from other disciplines of the mental health field, actively inviting them to our meetings and attending theirs, organizing and stimulating a stronger analytic presence in journals and universities where our findings, research and clinical outcomes could be publicized.

About this book

This book has been conceived and edited in order to describe many of the concerns and possibilities that were identified and faced during the Committee's activity. The project was at first elaborated as a series of panels presented at the IPA Congress held in Boston (July 2015). Later on, it became an articulate editorial project that engaged the Committee for many months and became a three sections *work in progress*, aimed at illustrating the most promising facets of the very controversial (and sometimes frankly conflictive) boundaries between Psychoanalysis and Psychiatry.

The purpose of this book is not the pompous celebration of a new, great alliance between the disciplines that all together constitute the so called MHF, i.e. the *Mental Health Field* – a definition widely recognized as useful to designate the theoretical and practical changes that reshaped what once was simply named "psychiatry." Rather, the aim that these texts pursue is to prompt a better focused and, if necessary, clearer or even harsher collective discussion on the responsibilities, and possibilities, shared by the people working with that special sort of people who are the persons suffering of mental disorders and/or diseases.

If we look back to the histories of these disciplines, we have to recognize that there are at least three great families of etiological theories that have always alternated in taking the foreground (primacy, hegemony): the bio-genetic theories, the socio-genetic theories and the psycho-genetic theories (between these latter we count the psychoanalytic or psychodynamic theories). While the last two families have often been integrated to construct "psycho-social" approaches and conceptual models, the biological theories have for a long time found their allies in the field of the medical sciences and in the area of neurology. This latter family of theories studies the psychopathological phenomena with the model of "disease" as heuristic tool and has discovered the illnesses that are caused by infections, genetics and various deficiencies. The other families are much more uncertain about their taxonomic systems and now designate their objects as *Idealtypen*: "syndromes," "disorders," "relational patterns" or "states of mind."

Within the conceptual horizon opened by these hypotheses (yet too often assumed as they were already proven truths), the mental health professionals have imagined practical, and obviously intended as therapeutic, initiatives that have unfortunately been, frequently, idealized, becoming not methodologies whose efficacy had to be proven, but flags, shibboleths, magic symbols and logos of personal and professional identity. In the past of the MHF, the historical result was the abundance of crusades and religion wars: a tendency to the Balkanization of conflicts and a peculiar intolerance of different approaches to severe mental sufferance and the ensuing professional ailment.

It is possible that this summary is somewhat superficial and hopefully out of date.

So let's try to fix the novelties that have changed – we hope forever – the scenario. If we should clarify what makes possible the interdisciplinary dialogue that was so difficult in the past, the first words that come to our mind are the present *prudence* with which the techniques are now considered, and the much greater *respect* that characterizes the relationships between the different families of theories. In every discipline of the MHF a much deeper epistemological awareness has grown and the fundamental conceptual options, on which each theory is built, are more often clarified and challenged than taken for granted. The tight links that connected the etiological theories and the therapeutic approaches are now loosened and the biological, psycho-social and psychoanalytic families, that once behaved as conflicting tribes, seem more capable of a reasonable cohabitation. It's a double and intertwined movement: while growing on the one hand an always more accurate auto-critical attitude and the histories of the disciplines were slowly rewritten, on the other hand diminishing the interdisciplinary struggles and the amount of shared knowledge augmented.

In the psychoanalytic tradition, the pioneers of this methodological turn have been the authors (Winnicott, Bion, Bowlby, Kernberg, Ferro, Green . . .) who dared to rethink what were considered as established truths, and were able illuminate its inconsistencies both in theory and practice, and advance our knowledge in order to admit more clearly possibilities and limitations, and the need to work jointly with other authors or fields of ideas, both inside and outside the psychoanalytic realm.

In the psychiatric history, the caesura is represented by the anti-psychiatric movement, and other similar questioning (Basaglia, Foucault, Laing . . .) of the way traditional psychiatry treated patients and established networks of power and authoritarianism.

We don't want to give the reader the false impression that we are like Polyanna or Voltaire's Candide. The present world is far from being the better possible world for patients, families and professional alike, so the current situation challenges us, as members of the mental health field, to look for more rational ways of facing our similarities and differences in our ways of understanding mental suffering and its treatment.

So, the book is not intended as a collection of heterogeneous and separated/split contributions, but a *comprehensive review* of the positions that have proved to be most promising and helpful in order to rethink and ameliorate the cooperation between psychoanalysts and psychiatrists, and to offer materials that could be useful for thinking about the controversial areas, being informed about best practices.

Instead of denying the most controversial areas – see for instance the contributors to Part II: "Nosology, diagnosis and treatment" – the project was focused on a clear recognition of the intrinsic/inherent differences between the two disciplines and designed as an instrument that could help practitioners and leading figures to build new bridges of reciprocal understanding and joint cooperation.

After the forewords (IPA and WPA Presidents) and the introduction of the Editors, the book is divided in the following three parts/dimensions:

1. The Mental Health Field: global trends and local specificities

The first part is more traditional: essays that compare different regional perspectives (European, Latin American and North American) on the history and the present situation of a necessary but often conflicting relationship. The contributors to the chapter are psychoanalysts and leading figures in the field of psychiatry.

2. The clinical practice: nosology, diagnoses and treatments

The second part is a review of the methodologies that have been developed to deal with the clinical problems: how to understand the mental diseases and disorders and how to develop diagnostic procedures that keep together the aim of classifying something with the scope of building a relationship with someone. Instead of long and comprehensive essays, the Editors asked for short contributions that can help the readers to review and know the processes that made it possible to devise diagnostic tools such as the DSM-IV and the DSM-5, the OPD and, more recently, the PDM-2.

3. The formative dimension: teaching and continuous education

The third part is devoted to illustration/comment of examples of integration between psychiatry and psychoanalysis at the level of the teaching, training and continuous education of young psychoanalysts and residents in psychiatry. This part describes and briefly comments on examples of good and reproducible practices that may help the development of better relationships between the two disciplines.

Both psychoanalysis and psychiatry have changed a lot during the last two decades. Each of the two disciplines has developed its methods, studied the diagnostic categories that can benefit them and focused on the specific techniques and measures to be used in order to obtain clinical results. Having renounced the illusion of self sufficiency, psychoanalysis and psychiatry are perhaps ready for a new phase of cooperation and mutual recognition. The most advanced components of the two disciplines know that their future is one of further differentiation of their methods and better integration of different techniques and approaches.

This part is also focused on the too often neglected fact that these two disciplines deal with human contents (diseases, disorders and suffering human beings) by virtue of established human containers (institutions, organizations, staff, professionals and people). The focus here is also on the emotional burden of the *équipes* and teams that deliver treatments and care. These contributions describe and discuss new methods of understanding the recurrent crises of the institutional organizations and the intervention that can help the leaders and responsible figures to deal with the consequences of institutional instability. The theoretical idea behind these descriptions is the concept of "field" as a conceptual operator that can help the balanced appraisal (relativization) of different approaches and perspectives.

PART I

The Mental Health field
Global trends and local specificities

years, psychiatry has endorsed a new medical paradigm praising technology transference from clinical research and efficient management via a standardized decision process and service specialization grounded on population studies and randomized clinical trials. The main limitation of the experiment was a surprising disregard of the invaluable contribution of the quality of human relationship to efficient operating services. When managers came speaking the language of academic research and business schools, the capital of institutional commitment and psychotherapeutic culture gathered over a century of institutional psychotherapy was rapidly wasted. Together with the realm of a defective model of mental disorders, a way was opened to the return of those social biases, conventional mentalities and cultural prejudices threatening the empathy of every medical milieu confronting the mentally ill. No surprise, these drawbacks had devastating effects on quality of care becoming a serious obstacle to the valuable scientific intent of the entire project. Specialized treatment is indeed just an ultimate step of a service system machine requiring compassionate dedication to such a complex achievement. A third important factor calling for a closer relationship of psychoanalysis and psychiatry is the outstanding progress of both neuroscience and artificial intelligence leading to increased attention to the mind–brain frontier (Magistretti & Ansermet, 2004; Kandel, 2005; Edelman, 2006; Damasio, 2010). Together with the rapid move of the health system into an interdisciplinary framework, the enigma of the human prompts the revival of an integrative paradigm of medical illness and its treatment. It is of note that Freud showed extreme concern for this issue claiming in his late works that psychoanalysis endorses the Weltanschaung of science being threatened on one side by reduction to experimental psychology and on the other side by an elective drift into philosophical speculation and magic belief (Freud, 1932). It is of note, however, that while psychoanalysts are more aware of the several issues discussed above, yet psychoanalysis and psychiatry are increasingly being set apart, especially in the academic and institutional fields. Such an opposite move is even more alarming considering the simultaneous divorce of Subject and science in modernity culture (Touraine, 1992). To discuss this problem, this work will investigate the present irresistible rise of a new acute psychiatric patient. A prominent figure of the changing scene of contemporary psychiatry, the emotional crisis of these subjects has grown into an epidemic accounting for an overwhelming majority of psychiatric populations. The peak of the iceberg of a more widespread malaise, the vicissitudes of these patients highlight a new frontier of contemporary mental health and its clinical, institutional, cultural and epistemological relevance to the revived dialogue of psycho-analysis and psychiatry. This work is intended to study this intriguing issue using studies from others, data from clinical and service research conducted in Geneva and my own psychoanalytic works.

A new epidemic and its relevance to treatment innovation and better care delivery

Over the last several years, both the absolute number and the relative proportion of patients referred to acute psychiatric treatment has showed a tremendous rise. The trend started insidiously after World War II and became extremely widespread during the de-institutionalization era. Thereafter, this phenomenon led to relentless pressure on emergency rooms, psychiatric hospitals and outpatient centers. This epidemic was associated with a new diagnostic profile of the patient population almost consecutive with the surge of a new figure for acute psychiatric patients. Those schizophrenic, bipolar and mentally deficient subjects accounting, a few decades ago, for the overwhelming majority of hospital admissions were rapidly outnumbered by a newcomer exhibiting some combination of maladaptive reaction to adverse events and structured psychiatric ill-ness triggered by various social and medical problems. Impulsive and unstable, meeting diagnostic criteria for several diagnostic prototypes of the affective spectrum and personality pathology, abusing psychoactive substances, scoring high on suicidal risk scales, and often triggered by various social problems and somatic illness, these subjects are confronting both psychiatric services and private practice with dramatic clinical and ethical dilemmas. Their acute distress, severe risks and insidious long-term outcomes are indeed of serious concern since their problems do not respond well to the usual treatment. Too severe to be managed in an out-patient setting, not improving, or even worsening, where hospitalized, the new acute psychiatric patient accounts for an enormous consumption of useless, costly services with little benefit in a mental health system doing much but not taking care of his/her real needs.

Innovating acute treatment: a call for psychoanalytically inspired clinical research

The most intriguing issue among these patients is the valuable contain-ment of upsetting anxiety and chaotic mental functioning resulting in an exquisite mix of loss of emotional control, interpersonal conflicts, disordered behavior and helplessness. Together with personality disorder and a social profile facilitating rejection by close family, friends and caregivers (Andreoli et al., 1989), this factor accounts for a large proportion of the short-term and long-term outcome in these populations (ibidem). Equally important, psychotherapeutic intervention, and a system of service likely to provide it in adequate format, are the only treatment factors showing significant positive interaction with the outcome of these patients. Here we meet the clinical research problem calling for a closer relationship of psychoanalysis and psychiatry. The emotional crisis of the new acute psychiatric patient is strikingly similar to those storming episodes every psychoanalyst is used to going through with his/her patient in the psychoanalytic office. On both sides, an upsetting experience stems from a breach in the mentalization processes leading to a disorganized style of interaction and communication, maladaptive emotional reactions and cognitive distortions in a useless effort to gain some control (Bateman & Fonagy, 2004). Raising serious limitations to the psychoanalytic process and classic transference working through, this psychopathological enigma, and its relationship to compulsive repetition, have attracted enormous interest among psychoanalysts from pioneering works (Fenichel, 1945) to recent controversies (Green, 1997), plunging the psychoanalytic movement into an exciting debate (Foresti, 2013) and a number of endless inconclusive conflicts as well (Haynal, 1988). Considerable progress has come in the field from empirical investigations of impaired mentalization process and its root in attachment disorder as well as from empirical evidence of a significant association of attachment disorder, impaired mentalization and Borderline Personality Disorder (Fonagy et al., 2002; Mayes et al., 2007). Thriving on purely psychoanalytical material, A. Green (1997) has conceptualized the field as a "Clinique du reel" (see below)in contrast to a "repression related clinical field." The concept of "reel," derived from Lacan (1975), encompasses "what lies beyond the symbolic texture linking meaning, symptoms and repression," confronting the subject to the Freudian "Unerkannt," i.e. what cannot be told or written (for further discussion see: De Mijolla, 2002). The surge of the "Clinique du reel" would fall, according to Green, under sudden failure of the double barrier of watching the sensorial evidence of external reality and traumatic intrusion from the Es. The new acute psychiatric patient construct is primarily intended to extend the field to question the following issue: how much recent progress of psychoanalytic savoir and psychodynamic research is relevant to the real acute patient of general psychiatric services as well as to the clinical and institutional issues associated with its effective treatment? Classic psychoanalytic treatment, both on the coach and in a face to face setting, is feasible and useful among gifted, sensitive and socially privileged acute psychiatric patients with less impulsivity, paranoid reaction and a decreased load of additional axis I and/or axis II pathology. Yet, psychoanalytic treatment still requires among these subjects enormous flexibility, especially within acute emotional crises, and is hardly ever terminated. A larger subgroup of new acute psychiatric patients meets diagnostic criteria for Borderline Personality Disorder (APA, 2000), a prototype with special relevance to clinical research. A new generation of clinical trials (Bateman & Fonagy, 1999, 2008, 2009; Clarkin et al., 2007; Doering et al., 2010) has indicated that specialized psychodynamic psychotherapy based on various psychoanalytic models of disordered mental functioning is cost-effective among these patients. These works have provided a first demonstration that careful translation of psychoanalytic observations into testable research hypotheses is of significant medical and economic concern and may contribute to considerable advances in a field of enormous concern. Nevertheless, the Borderline Personality Disorder prototype accounts for a minority of new acute psychiatric patients and the practical impact of specialized psychotherapy in ordinary clinical environments is questionable. A very large majority of acute psychiatric patients belongs to a much wider and heterogeneous clinical field. Meeting more often severity than duration criteria for Borderline Personality Disorder, showing polymorphous co-morbidity and psychosocial profiles, these individuals are the enormous reservoir of a new psychotherapy need, both in terms of psychotherapeutic service culture and structured outpatient psychotherapy. Beyond impaired mentalization and traumatic anxiety, rupture, loss, separation and sudden discontinuity of human bonds are equally distinctive features of the syndrome. An issue widely investigated by previous psychodynamic studies (Horovitz et al., 1984), the pathological mourning process is at the forefront of the clinical evolution of these patients and a main therapeutic issue to which we have to respond to put an end to the emotional crisis accompanying psychiatric disorder among these persons. Simultaneously, their pain and despair tells psychiatrists and psychoanalysts about the insidious ability of disappointed love (Hill at al., 2011) to open the door of the "Clinique du reel," destabilizing the complex system of fantasies, identifications and inner object relationships inhabiting the underground of their Ideal.

Recent studies from our group (Burnand et al., 2002; Berrino et al., 2011; Andreoli et al., 2016) have shown the importance of paying more attention to this problem and its significant relevance to cost-effective crisis intervention at general hospital and outpatient psychotherapy. Various forms of specialized interventions focusing on disappointed love have shown thereafter superior efficacy and economic advantage compared to the usual good quality intensive treatment among unselected real patients with depression and/or severe personality disorders, a diagnostic subgroup accounting for a wide majority of the new acute psychiatric patient population (ibidem). Also important, psychoanalytically inspired acute treatment focusing on disappointed love has been found well adapted to provide a cost-effective intervention with equal impact either delivered from trained psychotherapists of from gifted caregivers with little psychotherapy training (ibidem).

Translating the legacy of institutional psychotherapy into contemporary service culture

Beyond medical and economic concern for individual treatment and specialized psychotherapy, the surge of such a new patient population calls for a renovated structure and enhanced operating efficiency of the mental health system as well as for a new service culture. Valuable provision of cost-effective acute care requires, indeed, an exquisite mix of empirical stand, compassionate dedication, inter-subjective skill and an aptitude for interdisciplinary work. Here is a second issue with special relevance to a closer relationship of psychoanalysis and psychiatry: the present call of the contemporary scene of mental health for an alliance of institutional psychotherapy and scientific medicine. While extreme mutual disregard has resulted, over the past years, in a war between evidence based medicine and institutional psychotherapy, the two respective paradigms call for some form of alliance. Nothing but an evidence-based medicine framework demonstrates that psychoanalysis easily becomes, especially in psychiatry, defensive against anxiety and purely speculative beliefs, facilitating avoidance, chaotic decision and final drift into the magic stance of popular medicine. Simultaneously nothing but an evidence-based service operating framework shows the permanent drift of doctors and caregivers who apparently endorse this model towards an erratic, unreliable decision process while confronted with a stressful encounter with an acute mental patient. Cutting across scientific medicine and dynamic psychiatry this trend highlights how both disciplines want to get rid of a companion they desperately need. Here we get to the important point of this paragraph. This is in keeping with paying simultaneous attention to service innovation, treatment research, training and supervision to develop a new psychiatric culture that enhances the dialogue of science and psychoanalytic savoir among caregivers. The first intent of this project should be reviving those political and humanistic values prompted by the institutional psychotherapy movement, inventing them in a new key more adapted to confronting the changing scene of contemporary psychiatry. Access and reaching out, structured assessment and a valuable decision process, service efficiency and staff cohesion go with a moral factor accounting for the quality of human relationships, careful recognition of the unique experience of a given patient and a curiosity with the virtual world of what goes on in the everyday interaction with his/her family and friends and the everyday walkabout of a psychiatric service. An important efficiency and effectiveness factor is, therefore, to resist the constant trend of simultaneously kicking out evidence-based guidelines and the human of the human of the acute disorder. The encounter with the "Clinic du reel" activates, among professionals, a compulsory reaction preventing them from adhering to the living inter-subjective reality of those relational events that are the best ally of the mentalization process and working alliance. A sustained interest for what is not yet accounted for by the objective reality of a given a-priori set of possibilities and attention to what opens wide, beyond the experience of discontinuity, the virtual field of a surprising experience, are the kingpins of psychoanalytic psychotherapy and psychoanalytic interpretation (Flournoy, 1987). This is even more important when the issue is to survive the enormous burden of impotence and helplessness arising from close involvement in the relationship with acute patients. To maintain resilience, and therefore a capacity of getting free of the grip of the "Clinique du reel," saves some capacity for playing with the reality of the present experience (Lane & Garfield, 2006). This is a natural gift psychoanalysts directly involved in operating services may teach with invaluable effect on efficient functioning of the mental health system. Globally speaking, I would define the moral factor we discussed above as an ability to maintain a friendship with the human whatever is going on in the room. Overall, this means surviving the upsetting world of mental illness without losing contact, on one side, with others as persons and citizens and, on the other side, with their very own capacity for caring for them. This is the spirit of institutional psychotherapy we should instill in contemporary psychiatry and its best legacy.

Treatment barriers: a new frontier of clinical supervision

An additional problem comes from the equally powerful attraction exerted, at the frontier of the "Clinique du reel," by a second force, the Imaginary (Lacan, 1975). This is in keeping with the continuous drift of the mentalization process into the powerful stream of illusion and wisdom where patients and professionals are involved in acute conflicts. Here the psychoanalyst easily recognizes the surge of the most profound unconscious voice of the Ideal watching on the border of the "Clinique du reel." A number of "treatment barriers" are simultaneously activated that are reflected by the various figures of sadistic institutional machine, perverse collusion, animistic feelings and dissociation among caregivers. Whatever its intensity, this phenomenon, widely encompassing Bion's basic assumptions (Bion, 1961), cannot be obviously worked through on the real scene of acute patient psychiatry. Much of the relentless tendency to adapt transference analysis and meta-psychological psychopathology to this world looks actually to me like a peculiar case of the above mentioned drift into the field of the Imaginary. Psychiatric science is not less vulnerable to such drift into illusion. Worthless oscillation of psychiatric paradigms reflects the epistemological impasse, making a fool of the Piagetian circle of sciences when psychiatry and its patient, this ultimate tomb of reason's illusions, becomes the point of the debate. In summary, the primary concern of the virtual agenda we can now set up is a system of services and a model of service management allowing professionals to be more aware of what is imported into the everyday treatment and care by continuous confrontation to the frontier of mental functioning uncovered by acute mental illness with unsparing sincerity. Second is service culture, reviving the potential for hospitality, which is an essential ingredient of service culture. Third is careful attention to treatment barriers both at the individual and institutional level. A typical case of the potential impact of this work is systematic ignorance and blaming, at the emergency room, of the otherwise obvious importance of disappointed romantic passion among patients referred with attempted suicide (Andreoli et al., 2016). A second case is in keeping with the shared belief, among borderline patients and caregivers, that treatment and care are just a comedy. Unfortunately this is sometimes true since patients, doctors and caregivers often do not really trust what they do. Let me also stress the importance of perverse complicity and sadistic attitude reflecting the loss of any maternal stance while the caregivers' group confronts depressive women suffering from their incapacity to hold a maternal position or adolescents hit by destructive vicissitudes of their sexual life. More than the transference issue, all this is a matter of the internal setting preventing a natural continuous shift, in the mental illness field, of medicine and psychoanalysis into healing wisdom, and sometimes into sorcery.

"Civilization and its discomfort" revisited

Crossing the gap between psychoanalysis and psychiatry is as much a clinical and institutional issue as a cultural and epistemological one. Psychoanalysis and medical psychiatry have contemporarily emerged from the confluence of neurology and humanistic concern for the mentally ill into the common project of discriminating the symptoms of mental disease and the various figures of human misery and social exclusion. Both psychoanalysis and psychiatry were rooted, therefore, in the spirit of modernity culture (Touraine, 1992) and the present crisis of the corresponding values (ibidem) may be a fundamental ingredient of their impaired dialogue. Here is another aspect of the significance of the new acute psychiatric patient to the purpose of this book. This epidemic reflects a more general subjective malaise echoing the "civilization discontent" Freud pointed to in one of his most fascinating works (1961[1930]) and provides an amazing confirmation of the topical importance of psychoanalysis to mental health. The "malaise of the modernity" is attracting tremendous attention since the triumph of the rationalistic philosophy of "Enlightenments" has unexpectedly led to increasing waste of those humanistic values this ideology was based on (Horkheimer & Adorno, 1997). A "totally administered society" (Adorno, 2000) is proving the claim that democracy will get in a sweet tyranny. Critical thinking is replaced by being politically correct, equal rights and fraternity have become standardization and disregard for difference and pluralism. Such an alienation of the political space is closing human minds to independence, participation and citizenship. A parallel "disenchantment of the world" (Wolfgang, 1989), has deprived the modern human being of those beliefs, myths and meta-narrative constructions (Lyotard, 1979), giving an affective meaning to his/her existence and interpersonal bonds. A parallel, irresistible rise of positivistic overestimation of facts and utilitarian mentality (Held, 1980) has led to an eclipse of meaningful objects filling our world with idols and advertisements (Baudrillard, 2004). Overall, the contemporary human being is losing that "feeling of existing" arising from the confluence of attachment to the autonomy of private life, concern for a common history and sense of universal truth. Increasing erosion of this lay version of the ancient metaphysical "ubi consistam" is exposing every human being to the tragic feeling of life that only well-educated philosophers were familiar with in the past (Touraine, 1992). Finally, modernity has gone with a "lure of heresy" (Gay, 2009), leading to relentless erosion of every established identity, tradition and form of expression, as well as to a seeking for novelty and authentic experience that turns too often into futility, egoism and the various figures of a new cult of addiction. Liberated and secured by extraordinary scientific, technological and political progress, the modern human being is ultimately threatened by tremendous alienation of its subjective experience, and lives thereafter in an era of emptiness and anomia while suddenly confronted with catastrophic change. Thereafter, a destabilized middle class crowds as much into the emergency rooms of the general hospital as into the waiting rooms of the psychotherapist. A tribute to civilization, the malaise of modernity has replaced, however, a previous worse alienation and helplessness with a more civilized form of narcissistic malaise. On the other hand, the acute distress of these patients is certainly triggered by a number of social and psychobiological factors but still rooted in the contradiction Freud's patients brought to the psychoanalytic couch, together with their unconscious rebellion against sexual and social repression and their quest for personal development and a new social identity. Yet, modernity is as easily given up to "the thing" of the event and consequent enormous need for psychological help. Notwithstanding, this is tremendous progress compared to the miserable hopeless human condition, sadistic social ties and magic healing their ancestors endured. Here is the price of "Clinique du reel" and the illusion that contemporary society has to pay for the hidden scene of its outstanding progress. Interestingly, enough philosophers, sociologists and psychiatrists do not pay attention to how much the malaise of sentimental life, and neurosis, are important in the mix.

Mourning the past and its inconclusive conflicts

The malaise of modernity culture has also great relevance to the present difficulty of developing a paradigm of mental illness that would escape the present mind–body, subjectivism–empiricism, reality–virtuality sterile opposition. To achieve this goal would be a pivotal step, putting an end to the inconclusive conflict which psychoanalysis and psychiatry are stuck in and their falling apart as well. Ultimately, we could resume the point as follows: the dialectic (so central to capturing the psychodynamic conception of conflict) is the main victim of the crisis of modernity values since opposition is hardly conceived today in terms other than antinomy, reconciliation or sum. Neurological psychiatry has endorsed from the beginning a monistic mechanistic perspective. On the psychoanalytic side, a symmetric belief has led to relentless attempts to transform psychoanalysis and psychiatry, psychoanalytic setting and institutional work, psychological psychopathology and mental illness into a coherent, homogenous and continuous field. This goes back to the difficult mourning of an illusion rooted in the first structural model, and its obstinate survival to Freud's abandonment of the project of a meta-psychological psychopathology. Freud was aware of how much this problem threatens the relationships of psychoanalysis and science (1932) and his late work has been of great concern among those authors who have studied the malaise of modernity (Habermas 1998; Adorno, 2000). According to Touraine (1992), modernity is rooted in a cult of rationality with potential evolution into an irremediable split of science and subject. Decreasing concern for subjective life in the political, scientific and economic worlds of rationality is actually responded to by the subjective world taking its revenge through a contemporary surge of aggressive irrationalism and intimistic withdrawal. This trend is reflected, as we have seen above, by psychoanalysts moving away from the scientific "Weltanschaung" and institutional commitment, and psychiatrists disregarding subjective experience, moral factors and humanistic concern. This drawback claims for equal respect of scientific knowledge and poetic truth, hermeneutical interpretation and empirical facts (Habermas, 1998). A typical case of this issue is provided from the share of borderline prototype among psychiatrists advocating for Bipolar Disorder or ADD and psychoanalysts attached to Borderline psychological structure, with on both sides strenuous refusal to accept the otherwise obvious evidence that this is just a syndrome, or a reaction, involving several distinct, heterogeneous ethiopathogenetic factors (Gunderson, 2001). Nothing but the illusion of defeating the Sphynx of being just human, and being thereafter rid of the radical alterity of the Subject and the body, has jailed human minds in the prison of the "crippled dialectic" of dualism and monism (Bateson, 1979; Searles, 2004) as well as in the alienating dialogue of helplessness and illusion (Freud, 1930). Overall, we can conclude that the frontier of psychoanalysis and psychiatry has been one of the victims of the many paradoxes associated with the postmodern crisis of western culture. To get out of this trouble we should rehabilitate the differences, practice both sides of their frontiers and praise the conflicts any honest dialogue involves. In other words, there is no other way to revive the relationship of psychoanalysis and psychiatry than being aware of scientific progress and more committed to institutional problems, while staying in touch with the subjective world of the psychoanalytic cure and the irreducible unique taste of its direct experience.

Conclusion

Before bringing this work to a close, we have to pay some attention to which ingredient is likely to give a genuine meta-psychological taste to such a complicated mix as an alliance of psychoanalytic expertise, institutional commitment and clinical research. The recipe is my very own of a given psychoanalytic and psychiatric history and it is therefore not exclusive of other advice. The natural conclusion of this work points to wise practicing of the lifelong vicissitudes of human love as being the factor giving to psychoanalytic skill a quite unique position and invaluable prize in the psychiatric world. Here is the stand my psychoanalyst can take to talk from to the subjective distress of his/her time pretending to have some citizenship in the medical world of mental illness. Hysterical and borderline patients have conveyed psychiatrists and psychoanalysts to a common goal, since their clinical vicissitudes and treatment shows so clearly this point. From the larger perspective of the malaise of modernity culture, the new acute psychiatric patient just reflects the new scene of the same basic contradiction of human sentimental life and its root in an evolutionary plan of the species, resulting in an irreducible conflict of social brain, instinctual animal machine and the human of the human. At the end of this brief travel on the frontiers of psychoanalysis and psychiatry we could therefore rephrase the Freudian "The Ego and the Id" (Freud, 1923) as follows: the ancient struggle of sexual drives and religious belief restarts today at an upper floor involving the ideal of modernity and adult love in a new conflict with an equally uncertain outcome. Together with extreme prematurity at birth (de Ajuriaguerra, 1980) and an animal instinctual machine destabilized by increased plasticity of an otherwise outstanding cortical equipment (Terrace, 2005), the predominant place taken in the human mental development by the inter-subjective relationship has introduced an irreducible contradiction in mammalian love. The

virtual sensual machine of this new love stems somewhere between failure of maternal instinct and the tickling reaction of the baby to maternal
touch (de Ajuriaguerra, 1980) and is simultaneously entangled in a sense
of belonging (Freud, 1914) that is a distinctive feature of what love was
when whom we loved was our world. Every psychoanalyst knows the
many ways this love was broken up and led first to traumatic helplessness, dramatic discrepancy of security and attachment need and sexual
excitement, as well as to the extreme burden of illusion, fault and awe
associated with the vicissitudes of its counter-investment process. Human
love is therefore inseparable from a virtual structure disorganizing the
adaptive machine of the pleasure/un-pleasure logic of the instinct. The
vicissitudes of acute mental patients show in turn how much the consequent need of illusion and idealization of human love is inseparable
from what becomes thereafter the worst enemy of security, comfort and
intimacy, making the human of the human even more prone to traumatic
separation, abandonment and loss. Not less important, we can observe
how much to be able to love is important in the most severe pathologies.
Everyone is simultaneously committed to turning around the traumatic
hole of their infancy and equally prone to suffering disappointed love,
adding to the "thing" of adverse event the demonic spin either facilitating
the arousal of the "Clinique du reel" or building a barrier to successful
achievement of traumatic mourning. A second aspect deserving final discussion leads us to the moral discomfort of mental illness and its institutions and to how psychoanalysts can contribute to responding to it. What
matters here is the quality of the counter-investment process transforming
the encounter with the radical discontinuity of the Subject, pointed to for
a long time by philosophers, either in a feeling of absence reloading the
momentum of desire or opening wide the sounding board of all our inse-
curities and becoming thereafter the source of a sense of defeat, helplessness and awe. Here lies the moral vulnerability and irrational momentum
continuously imported in medicine by acute mental disease. To be a psychoanalyst in the world of medical institutions is endorsing the complex
task of persuading other people that the constant effort of abolishing this
problem almost results in even worse trouble and failure. While this was
the main source of the discovery of transference phenomena, the job of the
psychoanalyst in psychiatry appears, however, less a matter of transference and interpretation than a capacity for watching what emerges from
the encounter with this limitation transforming treatment and institutional
care in a devastating machine. Equally important in this work is to sustain, without the support of the psychoanalytic setting, the Imago either

hit by the vicissitudes of the "Clinique du reel" or buried in the tomb of illusion and rationalization, perversion and depression. Considering this basic ingredient of mental health goes back to the mysterious power of the infant smile, maternal tenderness and paternal presence, here we are for the last time back to human love and to those figures that are the source of its eternal image. Watching some survival in psychiatry of this basic fuel of the psychoanalytic process, and every human life as well, psychoanalysts may add an invaluable factor to the alliance of psychiatry, institutional commitment and clinical research. Since the coach has so little place in such a far country, let us replace it by the motto: no science without affective truth.

Summary

The changing scene of contemporary mental health provides various opportunities to revive the controversial relationship of psychoanalysis and psychiatry. After psychodynamic psychotherapy gained better empirical grounding, new research has shown that specialized interventions inspired by psychoanalytic models of mental functioning show significant clinical and economic advantage compared to the usual psychiatric treatment. Simultaneously, extreme swing-back to a medical paradigm has stuck psychiatry in unforeseen difficulties calling for careful reconsideration of the potential contribution of institutional psychotherapy to enhance service efficiency. Additional attention to the closer relationship of psychoanalysis and psychiatry stems from neuroscience progress and from the move of health systems into an interdisciplinary framework leading, respectively, to growing interest for the mind–brain frontier and to increasing concern for a comprehensive model of medical illness. Little has been done, however, to raise this challenge and while a common effort would benefit both sides, yet psychoanalysis and psychiatry are falling apart, especially in the clinical, institutional and academic fields. To further investigate this problem, this work questions the present, irresistible surge of new acute psychiatric patients and the correspondent urgent need for innovative treatment and operating services. Using data from others and from studies conducted in Geneva, we discussed the main clinical aspects of this major mental health issue and its specific relevance to a closer relationship of psychoanalysis and psychiatry. The new epidemic of acute psychiatric patients is indeed the peak of the iceberg of a wider social, philosophical and moral malaise. Revisiting "Civilization and its discontent" in this new key, we have shown that both the clinical vicissitudes of the new acute patient and the new distress of modern society are entangled in a disappointing sentimental life and exquisite aptitude of contemporary human love to unmask a basic traumatic experience of discontinuity and the corresponding invincible drive of illusion, fault and awe on the human of the human. Here, is the new frontier of the relationship of psychoanalysis and psychiatry. Here, the psychoanalyst may find a fresh meta-psychological and epistemological stand to address the acute mental patient and their treatment. Mourning past relationships of psychoanalysis and psychiatry, he/she should establish a new alliance with institutional commitment and clinical research and talk from this unique position to contemporary mental distress pretending some citizenship in the medical world of mental illness.

Key words: psychoanalysis, psychiatry, acute psychiatric patient, mentalization, borderline patients, outcome research.

References

Adorno, T. W. (2000). *Introduction to sociology*. Cambridge: Polity.

American Psychiatric Association. (2000). *Diagnostic and statical manual of mental disorders* (4th ed., text rev.). Washington, DC: Author.

Andreoli, A., Gognalons, M. V., Abensur, J., Olivier, C., Mühlebach, A. L., Tricot, L., & Garonne, G. (1989). Suivi Clinique au long (2 ans) de 78 patients ayant fait l'objet d'une demande d'hospitalisation en situation de crise. *Archives Suisses de Neurologie et Psychiatre, 140*(5): 439–458.

Andreoli, A., Burnand, Y., Cochennec, M.-F., Ohlendorf, P., Frambati, L., Gaudry-Maire, D., & Frances, A. (2016). Disappointed love and suicide: a randomized controlled trial of "abandonment psychotherapy" among borderline patients. *Journal of Personality Disorder, 30*(2): 261–270.

Bateman, A., & Fonagy, P. (1999). Effectiveness of partial hospitalization in the treatment of Borderline Personality Disorder: A randomized clinical trial. *The American Journal of Psychiatry, 156*(3): 1563–1569.

Bateman, A., & Fonagy, P. (2004). *Psychotherapy for borderline personality disorder: Mentalization-based treatment*. Oxford, UK: Oxford University Press.

Bateman, A., & Fonagy, P. (2008). 8-year follow-up of patients treated for borderline personality disorder: Mentalization-based treatment versus treatment as usual. *American Journal of Psychiatry, 165*(5): 631–638.

Bateman, A., & Fonagy, P. (2009). Randomized controlled trial of outpatient mentalization-based treatment versus structured clinical management for borderline personality disorder. *The American Journal of Psychiatry, 166*: 1355–1364.

Bateson, G. (1979). *Mind and nature: A necessary unit*. New York: Hampton.

Baudrillard, J. (2004). *L'Intelligence du Mal ou le Pacte de Lucidité*. Paris: Galilée.

Berrino, A., Ohlendorf, P., Duriaux, S., Burnand, Y., Lorillard, S., & Andreoli, A. (2011). Crisis intervention at the general hospital: An appropriate treatment choice for acutely suicidal borderline patients. *Psychiatry Research, 186*: 287–292.

Binks, C. A., Fenton, M., McCarthy, L., Lee T., Adams, C. E., & Duggan, C. (2006). Psychological therapies for people with borderline personality disorder (Review). *Cochrane Database of Systematic Reviews*, (1). Art. No.: CD005652. DOI: 10.1002/14651858. CD005652.

Bion, W. (1961). *Experiences with groups*. London: Tavistock.

Burnand, Y., Andreoli, A., Kolatte, E., Venturini, A., & Rosset, N. (2002). Psychodynamic psychotherapy and clomipramine in the treatment of major depression. *Psychiatric Services, 53*: 585–590.

Condorcet, J.-A.-N. De Caritat, (2012). *Selected writings*. Oxford, UK: Oxford University Press.

Clarkin, J. F., Levy, K. N., Lenzenweger, M. F., & Kernberg, O. (2007). Evaluating three treatments for borderline personality disorder: A multiwave study. *American Journal of Psychiatry, 164*(6): 922–928.

Damasio, A. (2010). *Self comes to mind: Constructing the conscious brain*. New York: Pantheon.

Ajuriaguerra, J. de. (1980). *Manuel de Psychiatrie de l'Enfant*. Paris: Masson.

De Mijolla, A. (2002). *Dictionnaire international de la psychanalyse*. Paris: Calmann-Levy.

Doering, S., Hörz, S., Rentrop, M., Fischer-Kern, M., & Schuster, P. (2010). Transference-focused psychotherapy vs. treatment by community psychotherapists for borderline personality disorder: randomized controlled trial. *British Journal of Psychiatry, 196* (5): 389–395.

Edelmann, G. M. (2006). *Second nature: Brain science and human knowledge*. New Haven, CT: Yale University Press.

Fenichel, O. (1945). *The psychoanalytic theory of neurosi*. New York: W. W. Norton.

Ferruta, A., Foresti, G., & Vigorelli, M. (2012). *Le comunità terapeutiche*. Milan: Raffaello Cortina.

Flournoy, O. (1979). *Le temps d'une psychanalyse*. Paris: Belfond.

Fonagy, P., Gergely, G., Jurist, E. L., & Target, M. (2002). *Affect regulation, mentalization, and the development of the self*. New York: Other Press.

Fonagy, P., Roth, A., & Higgit, A. (2005). The outcome of psychodynamic psychotherapy for psychological disorders. *Clinical Neuroscience Research, 4*: 367–377.

Foresti, G. (2013). Freud's writings in the twenties: Theory construction and clinical research inhibitions, symptoms and anxiety. In S. Arbeiser & J. Shneider (Eds.) *On Freud's "Inhibitions, Symptoms and Anxiety"* (pp. 210–218). London: Karnac.

Freud, S. (1914). *On narcissism: An introduction*. Standard Edition, Volume XIV, pp. 73–102. London: Hogarth Press and the Institute of Psychoanalysis.

Freud, S. (1923). *The Ego and the Id*. Standard Edition, Volume XIX, pp. 12–59. London: Hogarth Press and the Institute of psychoanalysis.

Freud, S. (1930). *Civilization and its discontents*. 1961 Standard Edition, t. XXI, pp. 64–145 London: Hogarth Press and the Institute of psychoanalysis.

Freud, S. (1932). *The question of a Weltanschauung*. Standard Edition, Volume 22, pp. 158–184. London: Hogarth Press and the Institute of psychoanalysis.

Gay, P. (2009). *Modernism*. London: Vintage.

Green, A. (1997). *On private madness*. London: Karnac.

Gunderson, J. G. (2001). *Bordeline personality disorder: A clinical guide*. Washington, DC: American psychiatric publishing.

Habermas, J. (1998). *The philosophical discourse of modernity*. Cambridge, MA: The MIT Press.

Haynal, A. (1988). *The technique at issue: Controversies from Freud and Ferenczy to Michel Balint*. London: Karnac.

Held, D. (1980). *Introduction to critical theory: Horkheimer to Habermas*. London: Hutchinson.

Hill, J., Stepp, S. D., Wan, M. V., Hope, H., Morse J. Q., Steele, M., Steele, H., & Pilkonis, P. A. (2011). Attachment, borderline personality and romantic relationship dysfunction. *Journal Personality Disorders*, 25(6): 789–807.

Horkheimer, M., & Adorno, T. W. (1997). *Dialectic of enlightenments*. Santa Barbara, CA: Verso Books.

Horowitz, M., Marmar, C., Krupnick, J., Wilner, N., Kaltreider, N., & Wallerstein, R. (1984). *Personality styles and brief psychotherapy*. New York: Basic Books.

Kandel, E. K. (2005). *Psychiatry, psychoanalysis and the new biology of mind*. Washington, DC: American Psychiatric Publishing.

Lacan, J. (1975). *Les écrits techniques de Freud 1953–1954*. Paris: Editions du Seuil.

Lane, R. D., & Garfield, D. A. S. (2006). Becoming aware of feelings: Integration of cognitive-developmental, neuroscientific and psychoanalytic perspectives. *Neuro-Psychoanalyses*, 7(1): 5–39.

Leichsenring, F., & Leibing, E. (2007). Psychodynamic psychotherapy: A systematic review of techniques, indications and empirical evidence. *Psychology and Psychotherapy*, 80(2): 217–228.

Lyotard, J. F. (1979). *La condition postmoderne*. Paris: Les Editions de Minuit.

Magistretti, P., & Ansermet, F. (2004). *A chacun son cerveau*. Paris: Odile Jacob.

Mayes, L., Fonagy, P., & Target, M. (2007). *Developmental science and psychoanalysis: Integration and innovation*. London: Karnac.

Oury, J. (2003). *Psychiatrie et Psychothérapie Institutionnelle*. Nîmes: Les Editions du Champs Social.

Racamier, P. C., Bequart, P., Diatkine R., Paumelle, P. H., & Lebovici, S. (1970). *Le psychanalyste sans divan: la psychanalyse et les institutions de soins psychiatriques*. Paris: Payot.

Searles, J. R. (2004). *Mind: A brief introduction*. Oxford: Oxford University Press.

Stoffers, J. M., Völlm, B. A., Rücker, G., Timmer, A., Huband, N., & Lieb, K. (2012). Psychological therapies for people with borderline personality disorder. *Cochrane Database of Systematic Reviews*, 8, Art. no CD005652. 14651858. CD05. pub2.

Terrace, H. S. (2005). *The missing link in cognition*. Oxford: Oxford University Press.

Touraine, A. (1992). *Critique de la modernité*. Paris: Fayard.

Wolfgang, J. M. (1989). *The political and social theory of Max Weber: Collected essays*. Chicago, IL: University of Chicago.

CHAPTER TWO

Psychoanalysis and psychiatry in Latin America

Historical aspects and current challenges

Cláudio Laks Eizirik

Introduction

Forty years of constant contact with the fields of psychoanalysis, psychiatry and mental health, in their various forms and expressions, offered me the opportunity of observing different moments and movements of partnership and competition.

In this short period of time, historically speaking, I have witnessed and also participated in – sometimes adding impetus to – substantial changes in our field of activity: the exodus from the psychiatry macro-hospital and the advent of the general hospital; the idealization of psychoanalytical techniques and of the explanatory power of psychoanalytical theories; the introduction and growing use of drugs; community psychiatry and its difficulties; the appearance of shorter and more specific psychotherapies; the improvement in diagnosis through successive multicentric studies; the appearance and improvement of research into psychiatry and into correlated basic areas; the appearance of post-graduate courses and their continuous expansion; the increasing specificity of psychoanalysis and its therapeutic effectiveness in relation to patients whose access was considered limited; the establishment of programs for the treatment of specific psychiatric disorders and the consequent increase in their therapeutic effectiveness; the idealization of so-called biological psychiatry and of the explanatory power of the neurosciences; the growing presence and participation of the pharmaceutical industry in the daily life of psychiatrists and patients; the appearance of health-service provider companies and their interference in the privacy of the doctor–patient relationship; the changes in national health systems; the appearance of bioethics and their contribution to the study of the moral dilemmas in psychiatric, psychotherapeutic and psychoanalytical practice; the growing associative organization of Brazilian and international psychiatry; more open discussions of questions such as the patient's rights, the multiple forms of sexuality, psychiatric internment; the expansion of liaison services; the increase of the interface between psychiatry and medicine, neurology, neurosciences; the decrease of the interface between psychiatry and psychology, psychoanalysis and the humanistic areas; the current emphasis on evidence-based medicine and psychiatry and studies on efficacy and the effectiveness of different treatments (Eizirik, 2007).

Taking into account all these different moments and movements, I will now describe some of the main historical events that shaped the relation of psychoanalysis and psychiatry in Latin America, and then come back to the present and try to discuss some of the challenges for the future of this delicate but indispensable relationship.

Some historical highlights

Many years elapsed between the first time Freud and his method were named at an International Medicine Conference held in Buenos Aires in 1910 and the foundation of the Argentine Psychoanalytic Association in 1942. During those years, many philosophers, psychiatrists and intellectuals became familiar with Freud's work. Some of them exchanged letters with him, and one even sent an invitation to Freud for him to settle in Argentina.

Many pioneers were already meeting to study Freud's works and applying this newly acquired knowledge in treating patients at different hospitals. This was the case of Arnaldo Rascovsky, at Hospital de Niños (Pediatric Hospital), as well as Enrique Pichon Rivière and Arminda Aberastury at Hospicio de las Mercedes (the former Psychiatric Hospital). They lacked, however, personal analysis. This situation changed with Angel Garma's arrival from Spain and Celes Cárcamo's return from France in 1938. Both had been trained in Europe as psychoanalysts. Garma had been trained in Berlin and was a member of the German Psychoanalytic Society, and Cárcamo had finished his training at the French Psychoanalytic

Society. Shortly thereafter, Marie Langer, who had been trained in Vienna, joined the group.

In the group of interested and enthusiastic people starting analysis, different styles of training began to be transmitted according to the experience of the pioneers). This diversity in styles influenced the origin of one of the main traits of Argentine psychoanalytic thought: its pluralism and open-mindedness, which became the source not only of original creations but also of the potential of articulating different schools and authors. The situation radically changed in just four years. The Argentine Psychoanalytic Association was founded in 1942.

Argentine Psychoanalytic Association members usually held activities that helped to connect their society to Buenos Aires University, to other scientific societies, and to several hospitals. Both Garma and Rascovsky delivered lectures and gave classes at the Main Hall (Aula Magna) of the School of Medicine of Buenos Aires University. Their lectures are still remembered because of the large number of interested students who underwent analysis and later became outstanding analysts. The first time that Argentine Psychoanalytic Association members participated in a congress was at a neurology and psychiatry congress held in Buenos Aires.

This connection with hospitals and the university fluctuated depending on the country's political situation. There were times of expansion and others of contraction, especially during military dictatorships. It is worth highlighting, however, that the relationships with hospitals and universities were not carried out by the psychoanalytic institutions as such, but by their members, who either individually or in groups introduced psychoanalysis into psychopathology or psychiatry departments or to the chairs and deans at universities.

In the years following these developments, several psychoanalytically oriented institutions were founded. Among them, we may mention the Argentine School of Psychotherapy for Graduates, created by Argentine Psychoanalytic Association members, which has been transmitting psychoanalysis for 40 years; and the Child and Adolescent Psychiatry and Psychology Association, organized by Argentine Psychoanalytic Association members along with professors of the School of Psychology of Buenos Aires University. Another institution founded during this time was the Center for Research in Psychosomatic Medicine.

In the last years, the direct connection between psychoanalytic institutions and universities has increased as psychoanalytic societies search for official recognition. One may officially qualify as a psychiatrist or psychologist, but not as a psychoanalyst. This search for recognition is partly related to the fact that more recent generations perform their clinical practice mostly in relation to the new public health systems. Consequently, master's degree programs in some psychoanalytic specialties/specializations have been organized in cooperation with certain universities (Eizirik and Armesto, 2005).

In Brazil, psychoanalysis had its beginning in three main centers, São Paulo, Rio de Janeiro and Porto Alegre.

The main name in the beginning of psychoanalysis in São Paulo is that of psychiatrist and intellectual Durval Marcondes (1899–1981), who took the first initiative to organize a psychoanalytic movement in that city, beginning in 1924, when he graduated from medical school and took out a subscription to the *International Journal of Psycho-Analysis*; in 1926 he began corresponding with Freud, who encouraged him in successive letters.

In 1936, during the Marienbad Congress, Ernest Jones, then IPA president, heard that Dr. Adelheid Koch intended to emigrate from Germany because of the persecution against Jews, and was trying to get to Palestine, the United States, or Argentina. Jones suggested that Koch could move to Brazil.

After a few months to settle in, Dr. Koch went to see Durval Marcondes in July 1937 and immediately began her pioneering work of analyzing future analysts, teaching seminars and doing supervisions. For this purpose, a room at Dr. Durval Marcondes' office was used. She began with three physicians, one of them Marcondes himself, and a female sociologist. The inclusion of a sociologist made a lasting mark on the initial nucleus of São Paulo in that it accepted from the beginning non physicians as candidates. In the following years, Koch accepted new candidates, and her work, together with the work of those who finished their analyses and took up training functions, promoted the creation of the Psychoanalytic Group of São Paulo in 1944; it was officially recognized as a component society of the IPA in 1951.

The constitution of the Psychoanalytic Group of São Paulo was based on the synergy between Marcondes and Koch. Marcondes was the cultured, aristocratic psychiatrist from São Paulo, closely connected to art, a former teacher of literature who spoke and wrote very well, a friend of intellectuals, physicians and politicians, and a participant in the Modern Art Week in 1922. Adelheid Kock was the immigrant psychoanalyst who had trouble with the language and with the new, unknown culture and had to perform many different tasks, maintaining an analytic attitude amid such challenging circumstances, including a threat of being denounced for charlatanism for practicing psychoanalysis, which was considered an irregular and unacceptable method by some physicians.

As in São Paulo, the first decades of the twentieth century witnessed incipient expressions of interest in psychoanalysis in Rio de Janeiro, in the form of lectures and work performed by physicians and psychiatrists to disseminate Freudian ideas. Beginning in 1944, a group of young psychiatrists attempted to bring an IPA-trained psychoanalyst to Rio de Janeiro to begin analytic training. They invited Garma and Rascovsky to give lectures in Rio de Janeiro and counted on the help of both of them to invite Georg Gerö and, then, Daniel Lagache, who did not accept the invitation. Since the attempt was fruitless, the idea of establishing a psychoanalytic nucleus in Rio was put off, and in 1946 Alcyon Bahia, Danilo Perestrello, Marialzira Perestrello and Walderedo Oliveira traveled to Buenos Aires for analytic training.

Another group of psychiatrists who had remained in Rio contacted Ernest Jones, the president of the IPA, and once again requested that an analyst be suggested. Jones named Dr. Mark Burke, a member of the British Society. Burke arrived in Rio on February 2, 1948. A man with a great musical culture, and a violinist with a rare talent for languages, he would soon speak Portuguese correctly. Already in February, he began to analyze several candidates. Thus, the Brazilian Institute of Psychoanalysis was started, and, wishing to increase its training activities, the Institute requested another name from Jones, which led to the arrival of the German analyst Dr. Werner Kemper at the end of 1948. He immediately began to analyze another group of psychiatrists. Both Dr. Burke and Dr. Kemper started to teach seminars in 1949, and in Kemper's group, initially, Dr. Luiz Dahlheim (who later would become an important analyst) acted as interpreter and intermediary between the students and the teacher.

The early days of the institutionalization of psychoanalysis in Rio de Janeiro had the intense, dedicated participation of a growing number of young candidates who, on the one hand, learned from the pioneers despite the latter's limitations and, on the other, developed a great capacity to face complex situations and crises in associative life. Several members and candidates were very active at the university, both in the medical and psychology schools, as well as in the cultural life of the city.

The third main psychoanalytic center in Brazil is Porto Alegre, capital of the southernmost state of the country. Psychoanalytic ideas appeared there in the 1920s and developed in the following decades, through lectures and translations of Freud's books made by psychiatrists and professors of the medical school.

After his analytic training in Buenos Aires, where he was analyzed by Angel Garma, Mario Alvarez Martins went back to Porto Alegre in 1947, with his wife, Zaira Martins, a child analyst, beginning the analytic movement in that state. Mainly stimulated by their Argentinean colleagues, Mario Martins, Cyro Martins, José Lemmertz (these last two also trained in Buenos Aires) and Celestino Prunes (who trained in Rio) structured the Porto Alegre Psychoanalytic Society (SPPA), which was recognized by the IPA in 1963. Since its origin, the SPPA has been closely connected with psychiatry, Federal University of Rio Grande do Sul and the cultural milieu. Many of its members and candidates were and still are members of departments of psychiatry in the main medical schools of the city. At the same time, one of the pioneers, Cyro Martins, one of the best known writers of the state, was very active in the diffusion of psychoanalysis in the cultural milieu. The SPPA, in its development, shows a blend of the activities and personal trends of Mario and Cyro Martins (who were not relatives): the former turned inward, developing a continuous, persistent and patient work of training candidates, teaching and facing internal tensions; the latter performed his analytic function but, through his many books and lectures, also opened new channels and stimulated young people to join in and become interested in psychoanalysis.

These two trends must be stressed: the internal work aiming at a training with high standards, and the close links with psychiatry and a strong influence in the intellectual area. Possibly connected with the first trend, only in the late 1980s were psychologists accepted for training, which eventually corrected a distortion that had produced criticisms and the search for other training institutions. In the ensuing decades, members of the SPPA were also very active in developing group analytic psychotherapy, a trend that decreased in the 1990s. At the same time, members of the Society were extremely active in the development of psychoanalytic psychotherapy, and today analysts and candidates are teaching it at universities.

More recently, the influence of psychoanalysis in medicine and psychiatry has decreased, but there are several active university centers where research and doctoral studies in psychoanalysis attract many students. The delay, in some societies, to allow psychologists to train as analysts was an unfortunate policy that led many talented colleagues to look for their training elsewhere (Eizirik, 2002).

In Mexico, a group of psychiatrists began to meet in the 1940s (in Mexico City) to study Freud's works and then founded the Sigmund Freud

Study Group. Later, they trained in Buenos Aires at the Argentine Psychoanalytic Association, at Columbia University, in Paris, and at The Menninger Clinic. When they returned to Mexico, they were joined by others to constitute the Mexican Study Group of Psychoanalytic Association. In 1957, the IPA recognized the Mexican Psychoanalytic Association (APM) as a component organization (J. Vives & T. Lartigue, personal communication, 2004).

In its early days, the APM accepted only psychiatrists as candidates (with the exception of the biologist Luis Feder and the chemist Estela Remus), a situation that led many psychologists to create their own training institution. Later, the APM opened access to doctors in psychology and professionals with training in analytic psychotherapy. In the 1980s, the APM created a graduate center for training in analytic psychotherapy; today it has a doctoral program in psychotherapy and two master of science programs (one on analytic psychotherapy and the other on child and adolescent psychotherapy). Although in the first days members of the APM were very active in several universities, this presence decreased in the following decades.

The analytic movement in Venezuela began formally in 1965, when the first study group was constituted, with five members: Drs. Hernán Quijada (trained in Paris), Jaime Araújo and Antonio Garcia (both trained in Santiago de Chile), Guillermo Teruel (trained in London) and Manuel Kizer (trained in Buenos Aires). In 1971, with the inclusion of other colleagues, the Venezuelan Psychoanalytic Association (ASOVEP) was recognized by the IPA. Training of candidates began in 1969, and an intensive program of visits by distinguished analysts from the three IPA regions was developed. In 1975 a crisis emerged in the association that can be attributed to analytic intolerance among colleagues. This crisis led to an intervention by the IPA and required the help of members of the Colombian Society, who gave seminars and supervisions. There was a reconciliation in 1977.

The origins of psychoanalysis in Uruguay lie in the 1940s, while its development can be divided into two periods: the first runs from 1943 to 1961 and can be called the prehistory of the Uruguayan Psychoanalytic Association (APU), and the second extends to the present day. In the first period, Dr. Valentín Pérez Pastorini, a psychiatrist and professor at the medical school, had analysis with Angel Garma in Buenos Aires and influenced many young colleagues to study Freudian ideas. After his death, two of his patients, Drs. Rodolfo Agorio and Gilberto Koolhaas, took the lead, and a growing number of people interested in psycho-analysis tended to congregate around them. In 1954, Willy and Madeleine Baranger left Argentina, settled in Uruguay, and began their training activities. The act of foundation was signed in 1955 by 11 analysts. In 1957 the IPA, on the recommendation of the Argentine Psychoanalytic Institute, recognized the Uruguayan Study Group, and in 1961 the IPA recognized the Uruguayan Psychoanalytic Association as a component organization (Garbarino et al., 1995).

A major recent achievement was the recognition by the Uruguayan government of analytic training in the APU as a master's degree. As for the quality of its member's work, it can be illustrated by a study on con-troversies in psychoanalysis (Bernardi, 2002). Taking as an example the debates held in Buenos Aires and Montevideo during the 1970s, when the dominant Kleinian ideas came into contact with Lacanian thought, Bernardi, after a careful examination of different examples of argumenta-tive discourses, showed that the major difficulties encountered did not hinge on characteristics pertaining to psychoanalytic theories (i.e., the lack of commensurability between them), but on the defensive strategies aimed at keeping each theory's premises safe from the opposing party's arguments.

One of the first analysts with a complete training to arrive in Latin America, Allende Navarro was a pioneer of psychoanalysis in Chile; he began to analyze colleagues who would later become analysts. In 1934, Ignácio Matte Blanco returned to Santiago, after concluding his training at the British Society. The group of analysts that formed around these pioneers founded the Center of Psychoanalytic Studies, in 1946. In 1949, the IPA officially recognized the Chilean Psychoanalytic Association. Matte Blanco was a central figure in the development of psychoanalysis in Chile. He was a full professor in the Department of Psychiatry at the University of Chile Medical School, and master of a body of knowledge that integrated, at a high level, his abilities as an analyst, a psychiatrist, and a university professor. The greater part of the struggle to overcome the difficulties created by environmental influences fell on his shoulders; he was a stimulating leader of several generations of Chilean analysts, at the same time pursuing the objective of integrating psychoanalysis with psychiatry.

In Peru psychoanalysis was introduced in 1915, through the corre-spondence between Freud and Honorio Delgado, enabling the latter to be the first representative of psychoanalysis in Latin America (Engelbrecht & Rey de Castro, 1995). Delgado was a psychiatrist and the leading figure of the period between 1915 and the mid-1930s. Despite initial interest in psychoanalysis and several articles published in newspapers about it, Delgado eventually turned away from the field. In the 1930s, psychoanalysis attracted greater attention again, through the influence of the psychiatrist Carlos Alberto Seguin, who had undergone analysis in New York and, in spite of not concluding a full training program, had the main achievement of introducing a counter-model to traditional psychiatry as then represented by Delgado. The four founding members of the Peruvian Study Group and also some other of its future members were psychiatrists of the Seguin school before they turned to psychoanalysis.

In the late 1960s, the history of psychoanalysis in Peru entered its institutionalization phase. Saul Peña, Carlos Crisanto and Marx Hernández, all of whom had been trained in London, have worked in Lima since 1969, 1972 and 1974, respectively. Together with members of the second generation they founded the Peruvian Psychoanalytic Society, recognized by the IPA as a component society in 1987. From then on, contributions by Peruvian authors appeared at international congresses and national psychiatric and psychotherapeutic meetings, and in publications.

In Colombia, Freud's works were read by a select group of intellectuals soon after their appearance. Only after they were translated into Spanish by Luis Lopez-Ballesteros during the years 1922 and 1934 and published nearly simultaneously with the originals in German did they become more known in Colombia. One of the Colombian intellectuals influenced by Freud's ideas was the medical student José Francisco Socarrás, who would play a leading role in the future development of psychoanalysis in his country. In 1929 he introduced the teaching of analytic ideas in the School of Psychology; in 1930 he wrote his thesis on the fundamental principles of psychoanalysis. He then went to Paris where he trained and returned to Bogotá in 1950. Arturo Lizarazo did his training in Chile; he went back to Colombia in 1948 and became the first to start the practice of psychoanalysis in that country (Villarrel, 1995).

The two pioneers worked together and faced great resistance, even being attacked by some of the most well-known psychiatrists and by some priests as well. They were among the founding members of the Colombian Study Group, which was accepted as such by the IPA in 1957. Carlos Plata Mujica returned from his training in Buenos Aires in 1958 and has been a leading figure in Colombian psychoanalysis ever since. In 1961, the Colombian Psychoanalytic Society was recognized by the IPA as a component organization. In spite of the tensions, resignations and splits, which led to the formation of two other analytic groups linked to the IPA in Colombia, there is a continuous growth and several ties with psychiatry (Eizirik & Armesto, 2005).

Present challenges

It is possible to see, from this fragmentary historical account, how psychoanalysis, since its beginning in different countries of Latin America, kept a relation with psychiatry, and this relation presents nowadays challenges that will lead us in directions that tend to integrate or to disintegrate our field of knowledge and therapeutic action. I will describe and comment on some of these challenges.

Psychiatry and its basic sciences

Tension exists between the two main poles of thought in the mental health disciplines: the biological and the psychological. I do not include here the social pole because it does not seem to me that there is any major questioning of its relevance. The defenders of extreme biological view as well as the paladins of hardened psychological or psychoanalytic view admit that social factors play an important role, trying to attract it to their side. The real confrontation is between the explicative models, which are concentrated in psychoanalytical theories and those that derive from the neurosciences.

The pendulum, at this beginning of century, seems to swing powerfully toward the explicative power of the neurosciences, as in earlier decades it was psychoanalysis that was privileged. It is a difficult discussion because emotional aspects are at stake, and one should not disregard history, with all its traces of right and wrong, its exaggerations and possible arrogance of biological psychiatry today, something that was one of the trademarks of psychoanalysis in the previous decades. The present challenge, in my opinion, consists in recognizing the complexity and multi-determination of normal and pathological mental phenomena. Any form of reductionism, besides being arrogant, is essentially incorrect, due to the limited explicative extent of only one theory to understand manifestations that are as complex as those we study and treat.

The risk of a unidirectional view is its very tendency to allow the mechanisms of dissociation or fragmentation that are found in the postmodern world to also dominate the scientific sphere and to cause an impoverishment similar to the crisis in the models of identification that we witness in the virtual culture of our time.

Thus, I think we should recognize the existence of certain basic sciences, such as those mentioned and others of a psychological, biological and social nature and to find the ways in which it would be possible to integrate them, or to develop and maintain a dialogue respecting the specificities of each. Two interesting examples related to this have appeared in *Molecular Psychiatry* and in the *International Journal of Psychoanalysis*. In the first, Nemeroff (1999) summarizes and comments on the importance of studies that show that there is an increasingly impressive database concerning the long-term neurological consequences of untoward life events, e.g., child abuse and neglect, loss of parents. Such alterations appear to increase vulnerability in several major psychiatric disorders, including affective and anxieties disorders. A case control study by Agid et al. (1999) provides further evidence for such an association, thus confirming Freud's theories about early traumatic effects on mental health and disease. In the second, we find a series of papers in the main psychoanalytical journal exploring the development of the neurosciences and their possible repercussions on psychoanalysis.

Another stimulating interface is constituted by the various studies on the effectiveness of psychoanalysis and analytical psychotherapy, published as an open door review of outcome and process studies on psychoanalysis, and edited by Leuzinger-Bohleber and Kächele (2015).

Psychiatry as a medical specialty

The fact that psychiatry is a medical specialty is common knowledge. The challenge of the moment is the disturbing impression that it is becoming so medical that it can lose its specificity. We went to the general hospital, integrated ourselves into medical schools, we share the same space and the same worries. But our patients are different and, necessarily, the way we approach and treat them is different, too.

The doctor–patient relationship that we have tried to teach and valorize so much sometimes seems to be more learned and used by internists and pediatricians than by modern psychiatrists who are full of enthusiasm about technology and the therapeutic power of effective drugs, to the point of neglecting the person of the patient and of his or her family, with their internal worlds full of unconscious fantasies, expectations, fears and different anxieties (as Gabbard, 2017, discusses in this book).

Here, I want to characterize two common forms of reductionism that we need to avoid: either that of ignoring the necessity of combined treatments and adopting an exclusively psychotherapeutic or psychoanalytical practice, in cases where the indication for medication is evident, or that of becoming a prescription-writer, ignoring the emotional experiences and psychotherapeutic needs – at least as a support – present in all patients.

The doctor–patient relationship – in psychiatry and any form of relationship concerning a mental health professional – is specific, complex and involves, more than in other areas, the emotional response of the therapist or his/her countertransference. How this therapeutic instrument can be used has been known, since ancient times and more precisely in the last century, thanks to psychoanalysis. However, recent progress in the capacity of diagnosing and treating specific disorders in a purely manualized way may make us lose the ability family doctors had, and continue to have, of entering into emotional contact and, based on their own reaction, being able to identify what is happening with the patient.

In opposition to the current idealization of objectivity, and of a practice highly based on scales, I would like to recall another way of visualizing this concept:

> Objectivity is based on a kind of internal dissociation that enables the doctor to partially identify himself with the patient and to take himself (his own subjectivity or countertransference), partially, as object of his continuous observation. This position allows him to be relatively "objective" in relation to the patient.
>
> (Racker, 1957)

The understanding of the meanings and uses of countertransference, and, in a wider way, of the analytic field (Baranger & Baranger, 1961–2; Ferro & Basile, 2010, Eizirik et al., 2012), enhanced the therapeutic possibilities in mental health, regardless of the form of intervention adopted. And this issue leads us to the problem of the training of future psychiatrists.

Psychiatry and its practitioners

One of the most crucial and fascinating challenges of today refers to the kind of professional whom we think is best equipped for the next decades. If we consider complexity to be the trademark of our time, and that the natural trend points toward its intensification, the inference is that the present and future psychiatrist should be exposed to the widest possible range of learning experiences, kinds of patients and families, service "settings," theories and explicative models, and to be able to develop his/her critical thought and creativity.

Right from the start of training, access to research and participation in research groups should be stimulated. Experience has taught us that models of identification are the basis on which creative minds are built. This is a field in which the analytic training model reveals its usefulness very clearly, for it documents the possible ways in which to enable a professional to identify with a mental function whereby listening to the unconscious and searching for the meanings of normal and pathological mental manifestations become his central *modus operandi*.

Thus, the future professional needs the experience of personal, private and sufficiently long contact with several supervisors, who will allow him/her to observe how they think and develop their clinical thinking (Eizirik, 2014). Supervision, with its style of workmanship, teaching and contact, and its mutual learning experience, is at the core of establishing its multiplying potential. I think that there is a current risk of teaching excessively or exclusively in groups, be it of theoretical studies or of supervision of the activity with patients. Without an experience of contact with the present day representative of the craft-master, the notion of the indispensable human relationship, which is at the basis of any mental health service, will hardly be established in the mind of the student.

The professional of the future will have to face new situations, some that are arising and others that we have only heard of. Just as examples, the increasing presence of elderly people in the population and their specific problems, the questions of bioethical dilemmas, the multiple forms of sexuality and the presence of service provider companies are some of the challenges we will have to learn to face together with our young colleagues. Models and formulas useful in the past decades cannot continue to be practiced and taught without periodic critical reviews.

Finally, one paradoxical question relates to the psychiatrist's quality of life. This area is one of increasing study and relevance to multicentric studies, although the fact that professionals who dedicate themselves to mental health often have a poor or difficult quality of life. Some time ago, it was almost unthinkable that a person in this field would not look for his/her own analysis or psychotherapy in order to be personally and professionally better equipped. This is one of the questions in need of attention, especially in the light of a prevailing model in which the basic requisite is that of efficiency and outcomes, relegating quality of life and its relation to mental health practice to a less important place.

Some perspectives

If the present challenges I have tried to outline correspond approximately to the reality we are experiencing at the moment, the natural corollary is that some possible paths are offered to the mental health field.

The first of them would be that of progressive super-specialization and micro-specificities, in such a way that we would have several psychiatries, psychologies, etc., linked to different approaches, each developing its way of understanding and practicing the specialty, leading to the fact that the very notion of something called psychiatry, psychology, etc., without qualifiers, would lose its *raison d'être*. We would thus have total dissociation or fragmentation, with the constitution of theoretical and clinical feuds without bridges or attempts of any kind at communication. Such relatively independent parties would start to behave within the basic assumption of fight or flight described by Bion (1961).

The second possible scenario would be the definitive hegemony of biological psychiatry, which would be just another medical specialty, equal to the others, exclusively linked to its neuroscience basis, bringing neuropsychiatry back to life. Psychotherapists or psychoanalysts, or those who are connected to social approaches, would migrate to other, more agreeable and hospitable climates. For any kind of survival in a world so constituted, the submission to the New Order would be necessary, in a model that resembles the basic assumption of dependency described by Bion (1961).

A third scenario would consist in the maintenance of a large general specialty, mental health or psychiatry, psychology, nursing, etc. without qualifiers, like a large umbrella, able to shelter different trends and propitiate the development of specialties, while stimulating dialogue among several of them, and with those having other areas of knowledge.

Obviously I do not need a lot of imagination to figure out these three scenarios; they already exist, and we know exactly where they are. Maybe because I live in a state that borders other states and countries, maybe because I have spent so many years actively working, researching and teaching in the domains of psychiatry, mental health and psychoanalysis, maybe because I am a professor of a Department of Psychiatry where this really happens, for all these reasons. I think and hope that the third scenario is possible, because it seems to me to be the one that best serves our patients. Maintaining a space for thinking is the basic proposal of psychoanalysis, and I think that a model constituted like this, in the form of a work group (Bion, 1961), opens possibilities for stimulating integration, reducing dissociation and helping in the working out of mourning for past illusions through creative answers.

This may or may not happen. But I think our world and our horizons will be poorer, and our patients will have poorer care, if, somewhere in the future, we will no longer be able to continue and develop this integrative dialogue and practice.

References

Agid, O., Shapira, B., Zislin, J., Ritsner, M., Hanim, B., Murad, H. et al. (1999). Environment and vulnerability to major psychiatric illness: A case control study of early parental loss in major depression, bipolar disorder and schizophrenia. *Molecular Psychiatry, 4*: 163–172.

Baranger, W., & Baranger, M. (1961–2). La situación analítica como campo dinámico. *Revista Uruguaya de Psicoanálisis, IV*(1): 3–54.

Bernardi, R. (2002). The need for true controversies in psychoanalysis. *International Journal of Psychoanalysis, 83*: 851–873.

Bion, W. R. (1961). *Experiences in groups.* New York: Basic Books.

Cesio, F. (2000). *La gesta psicoanalítica en América Latina.* Buenos Aires: Editorial La Peste.

Eizirik, C. L. (2002). Emigration of European analysts to Brazil. Presentation at the *Plenary Session the Ninth International Meeting of the International Association for the History of Psychoanalysis, Barcelona, Spain, July 25.*

Eizirik, C. L. A. (2000). Psychoanalytic perspective on the future of mental health. In J. Guimón, & S. Zac de Filc (Eds.) *Challenges of Psychoanalysis in the 21st Century.* New York, Boston, Dordrecht, London, Moscow: Kluwer Academic/Plenum.

Eizirik, C. L., & Armesto, M. (2005). Psychoanalysis in Latin America. In E. Person, A. Cooper, & G. Gabbard (Eds.) *Textbook of psychoanalyis.* London: American Psychiatric Publishing.

Eizirik, C. L. A. (2007). Psiquiatria nos próximos 50 anos: a contribuição da psicanálise. *Revista de Psiquiatria do Rio Grande do Sul, 29*: 15–16.

Eizirik, C. L. (2012). História, histórias, passagens da psicanálise brasileira. *Revista Brasileira de Psicanálise, 46*: 77–81.

Eizirik, C. L. (2014). Discussion of the articles: Never ever stop learning more about supervision. *Psychoanalytic Inquiry, 36*: 642–643.

Engelbrechet, H., & Rey de Castro, A. (1995). Peru. In P. Kutter (Ed.) *Psychoanalysis international: A guide to psychoanalysis throughout the world*, Vol. 2: *America, Asia, Australia, further European countries* (pp. 160–173). Stuttgart-Bad, Cannstatt, Germany: Frommann-Holzboog.

Ferro, A., & Basile, R. (2010). *The analytic field: A clinical concept* (EFPP Series). London: Karnac.

Garbarino, M. F., Maggide Macedo, I., & Newe, J. C. (1995). Uruguay. In P. Kutter (Ed.) *Psychoanalysis international: A guide to psychoanalysis throughout the world*, Vol. 2: *America, Asia, Australia, further European countries* (pp. 174–185). Stuttgart-Bad, Cannstatt, Germany: Frommann-Holzboog.

Leuzinger-Bohleber, M., & Kachele, H. (2015). Open Door review of outcome and process studies in psychoanalysis. *IPA*. www.ipa.org.worldstolkinner

Nemeroff, C. B. (1999). The preeminent role of early untoward experience on vulnerability to major psychiatruc disorders: The nature–nurture controversy revisited and soon to be solved. *Molecular Psychiatry, 4*: 106–108.

Racker, H. (1957). The meaning and uses of countertransference. *Psychoanalytic Quarterly, 26*: 303–357, p. 348.

Stolkiner, A. (1988). Practicas en salud mental. *Investigacion y Educacion en Enfermeria, 6*(1): 31–61.

Victer, R. (1991). Elementos para uma compreensão da pré-história da SPRJ. *Revista de Psicanálise do Rio de Janeiro, 1*: 77–83.

Villarreal, I. (1995). Colombia. In P. Kutter (Ed.) *Psychoanalysis international: A guide to psychoanalysis throughout the world*, Vol. 2: *America, Asia, Australia, further European countries* (pp. 103–115). Stuttgart-Bad, Cannstatt, Germany, Frommann-Holzboog.

CHAPTER THREE

Psychoanalysis

Its glorious past, its troubled present, and its uncertain future

Allen Frances

Prologue: Acknowledging Darwin

Freud's biographer Ernest Jones called Freud "the Darwin of the mind." In fact, Darwin was the Darwin of the mind, with Freud as his great popularizer. Freud is the father of psychoanalysis and Darwin is its usually unacknowledged grandfather. Newton modestly described himself as a dwarf sitting on the shoulders of preceding giants. Freud was most certainly a genius, but he sat on the shoulders of psychology's greatest genius. Darwin had completely revolutionized the field with the stunning insight that human instincts and emotions have evolved from our primate ancestors, just as completely as had our bodily form. We are animals, a part of the grand tableau of creation, not its purpose. Human nature has evolved in just the same ways as have our bodily structures, via natural selection and sexual selection of reproductively successful chance variants – it was not preplanned or inspired by divine intervention. The best way to understand ourselves is to study the psychological steps in our evolution – as Darwin put it, we can learn more about human psychology by observing baboons than by reading great philosophers.

Darwin established that the mind and its consciousness are a product of brain functioning in a way not essentially different than digestion is a function of the gut. He understood that unconscious forces play a large role in influencing our behaviors, and much of our mental life is automatic and outside the control of reason or will. For Darwin, instincts are not completely fixed, but interact with experience to produce our feelings, thoughts, and behaviors – without us being much aware of their influence. Of note, he also pioneered in subjective introspection, including the self analysis of his own dreams.

For Darwin, the child is literally father to the man – we can learn much about the psychology of the individual and evolution of the species by carefully studying the maturation of behaviors in infants and children. Darwin's "A Biographical Sketch of an Infant" detailing his minute, naturalistic observations of the day to day emotional, intellectual, interpersonal, and moral development of his eldest son, created the field of child development.

Darwin demonstrated that psychology can be studied using the standard experimental and observational tools of science and he pioneered new methods of psychological research that have since become standards in the field. He used the recently discovered method of photography to study the universality of emotions and facial expressions. He conducted the first psychological surveys, creating a written instrument for gathering information from scientists and missionaries to show that human emotions are equivalent all around the world. Darwin proved that all people, despite differences in their current customs, are brothers and sisters within one human species, sharing the same basic emotions and intellectual endowment.

It is startling that Darwin made most of his major psychological discoveries before his thirtieth birthday and even before he realized that natural selection is the mechanism of evolution. He kept these findings buried in a drawer for 35 years before finally publishing them – partly because he was a meticulous collector of facts before presenting theories; partly because he realized that the world was not ready for his thoroughly materialistic view of man; and partly because he didn't like confrontation with critics.

Freud was only 26 when Darwin died and they never met, but almost all of his mentors were enthusiastic Darwinists. In Freud's day, psychologists and neuroscientists all spoke "Darwin" even if they didn't always realize it; just as today we all unconsciously speak some dialect of "Freud." Freud brilliantly and exhaustively fleshed out Darwin's skeletal psychological theories with rich and compelling examples drawn from his interpretation of psychiatric symptoms, dreams, the psychopathology of everyday life, myths, literature, and anthropological findings.

Lots of philosophers, scientists, and writers had explored the realm of the unconscious before and after Darwin. But Darwin was by far the most important because, by connecting the mind of man with our primate past, he was able to fill in so many of the blanks – explaining why we do what we do and feel what we feel.

Freud's fate

Freud was probably over-valued in his own lifetime and has been compensatorily undervalued since. He divided the contributions of psychoanalysis into three parts: psychoanalysis as a theory of human nature; psychoanalysis as a research tool; and psychoanalysis as a therapy. These three roles have fared differently in the crucible of history and will likely also face very different futures.

Psychoanalytic theory has been surprisingly robust at its center, but has turned out to be wrong and sometimes even silly at its margins. His descriptive observations about the power of unconscious thinking and conflict have largely been confirmed by the tools of modern neuroscience, cognitive science, and behavioral economics – usually without affording him the credit he deserves. Not surprisingly though, Freud was much less successful in his attempts to provide causal mechanisms connecting brain to behavior. His libido theory and metapsychology were creative and plausible attempts at explanation, given the primitive neuroscience tools available to him at the time, but seem quaintly dated now. No shame in that. All scientific theories are incomplete at best and in time all are superseded. We should not expect models based on the best of nineteenth century neuroscience to hold up very well in the face of powerful twenty-first century technology.

The problem is not Freud – he got the forest right and shouldn't be blamed if he couldn't always place the trees just where they belonged. But it is unfortunate, perhaps unforgivable, that subsequent psychoanalytic fundamentalists have religiously and literally worshipped Freud's written words and failed to do what Freud, himself a well trained neuroscientist, would surely have done – i.e., to forever modify psychoanalytic theory by incorporating into it the latest findings of neuro and cognitive science. Ever updating with new facts and ever shedding past fancies should become the ongoing task of future psychoanalytic theorizing.

Psychoanalysis as a research tool once had its uses, but always carried the heavy baggage of solipsistic observer bias and Hawthorne effect. Epistemology was not Freud's strong suit. He often developed his psychoanalytic theories first and then selectively sought their confirmation in his psychoanalytic practice. Memoirs of their treatments written by some of his patients describe a Freud who was anything but a neutral blank screen. It often seemed hard for patients to get a word in as Freud was so busy tying together their thoughts to confirm his own particular theories. Suggestible patients would also be all too eager to comply and agree.

Experience has shown that it is very easy to develop myriad opposing theories based on the same raw material of psychoanalysis and almost impossible to confirm or disconfirm any of them. The fiercely fought sectarian wars among the various schools of psychoanalysis reflect little more than the conflicting subjectivities of their founders, reified as universals by their all too loyal followers. Whatever value psychoanalysis had as a research tool played itself out very long ago. In this regard, it is a dead end.

Saving psychodynamic treatments

Which brings us to the aspect of psychoanalysis that interested Freud least – its value as therapy. Freud's early career was as dedicated neuroscientist, a pioneer in understanding neurons and their interconnections through synapses. Freud would have been content with life in the laboratory had his funding not run out, forcing him to make a living in the much less intellectually valued world of clinical practice. His attitude toward psychoanalytic work was more that of scientific researcher than therapeutic enthusiast or innovator.

Ferenczi, much more than Freud, was a complete clinician and the father of psychoanalysis as healing art and psychotherapy. He laid the groundwork for understanding the role of the interpersonal relationship, empathy, therapist activity, therapeutic alliance, the corrective emotional experience, and countertransference in both the process and outcome of therapy. He and Rank together developed brief psychodynamic therapy as an effective adaptation to real world constraints that often made impractical the demands of five times a week, regressive psychoanalysis.

Psychoanalysis eventually fathered most of the current day psychotherapies, but renounced its paternity and has suffered greatly from the loss of the rejuvenation its offspring could have provided. The analytic institutes and their associations have made the catastrophic mistake of betting the house on psychoanalysis in its original form. This restricted them to the very few patients and the very few clinicians willing and able to undergo its rigors. As a consequence, psychoanalytic institutes throughout the developed world are in a death spiral of irrelevance and decay. They find it increasingly difficult to recruit candidates and to find patients for them – not surprising since they are teaching an ossified and outmoded form of therapy that very few want to learn or to experience. With diminishing replacements in each new generation, the average age of analysts is approaching the geriatric. What was once the exciting new intellectual enterprise is now a dying cult, precariously maintained by its few remaining true believing acolytes.

Far more sensible would have been evolving psychoanalysis into a wide tent able to include all the various forms of short and long term psychodynamic therapy, family and group therapy, and especially the rapidly expanding cognitive/behavior therapy (developed by a psychoanalyst disaffected by the rigid exclusivity of analytic institutions and theorizing). Psychoanalysis could have retained its vitality and relevance had it seen itself as the progenitor, protector, and teacher of all forms of therapy, not just the fortress defender of its most extreme and exotic variant.

And psychotherapy badly needs defending and unification. It is in a David vs Goliath struggle against the pharmaceutical industry for the hearts, minds, and pocketbooks of potential patients. An accumulating literature confirms that brief psychotherapy is at least as effective and more enduring than medication for most people presenting with mild to moderately severe psychiatric symptoms. But most eligible patients wind up receiving meds, not therapy, because Big Pharma exerts great marketing muscle while psychotherapy is a mom and pop craft with no resources or skills in selling itself.

Needless and self-destructive sectarianism and civil wars within psychotherapy further weaken its credibility and its ability to present a united front. Sectarianism also results in an over-valuation of specific technique and undervaluation of the therapeutic relationship which the literature indicates is the major engine of change across all the various techniques. It is not too late for the psychoanalytic institutes to refashion themselves as psychotherapy institutes – teaching and researching all the various orientations and methods and championing them all. At the very least, the institutes should embrace all forms of psychodynamic therapy – as was originally suggested by Ferenczi and has also been proposed by many other innovators in the intervening century.

In much of the world, psychiatric training increasingly resembles training in internal medicine, with almost exclusive focus on drug indications and side effects. The trainees often crave opportunities to learn psychotherapy, but there are now few people within the academic centers able to teach it. In my view, the future of the psychoanalytic institutes as training centers depends on expanding their purview, breaking down walls, reducing unnecessarily onerous requirements, and responding flexibly to opportunity. Based on their past performance, analytic institutes are among the least adaptive and most hidebound of man's bureaucratic inventions. The smart money would not bet on their long term survival. But necessity is sometimes the mother of invention. Psychoanalysis began its existence as a creative, flexible, and exciting force. To survive, it must deossify and find a renewing fountain of youth. It would be a shame to let this important part of Freud's legacy die on the vine. Psychoanalysis is too important to be left to the psychoanalysts.

Acknowledgments

Much of this material was first presented as the 2013 Freud Memorial Lecture sponsored by The Freud Museum and King's College London and has also appeared in the Special Issue commemorating the 50th Anniversary of the Italian journal *Psicoterapia e Scienze Umane*, 2016, 50(3): 458–461. www.psicoterapiaescienzeumane.it/.

CHAPTER FOUR

Working together
Some institutional psychodynamics between psychoanalysts and psychiatrists

Robert D. Hinshelwood

The rift between psychiatry and psychoanalysis is at the organisational level. Here we investigate whether unconscious group psychodynamic relations interfere between disciplines who should be working together (but who can't).

Introduction

Psychoanalysis and psychiatry have lived alongside each other for more than a century, often under the same roof – marital partners whose divorce never quite happened. Early on Freud hopefully said, 'I cannot believe that psychiatry will long hold back from making use of this new pathway to knowledge' (Freud 1896, p. 221). But it did not turn out like that. In his biography, Ernest Jones mentions Freud's comment on the reception of this 1896 paper, 'According to Freud, the paper met with an icy reception. Krafft-Ebing [President of the Society of Psychiatry and Neurology in Vienna], who was in the chair, contented himself with saying: "It sounds like a scientific fairy-tale"' (Jones 1953, p. 28). And 20 years later Freud devoted one of his Introductory Lectures to the dire relations,

> Psychiatry does not employ the technical methods of psycho-analysis; it omits to make any inferences from the content of the delusion, and, in

pointing to heredity, it gives us a very general and remote aetiology instead of indicating first the more special and proximate causes. But is there a contradiction, an opposition in this? Is it not rather a case of one supplementing the other? Does the hereditary factor contradict the importance of experience? Do not the two things rather combine in the most effective manner? . . . Psychoanalysis is related to psychiatry approximately as histology is to anatomy: the one studies the external forms of the organs, the other studies their construction out of tissues and cells. It is not easy to imagine a contradiction between these two species of study, of which one is a continuation of the other.

(Freud 1917, pp. 254–255)

Instead of that happy continuation, the two branches of human understanding sadly avoid each other.

There has not been a lot of improvement in 100 years, although it has not always been bad. Adolph Meyer (1866–1950) in the US was very influential in pushing psychiatry towards a more integrated practice (Skull and Schulkin 2009). That movement of integration has lost ground again, so by 2000 a social scientist could say about psychiatric trainings in the US,

In the one domain, there is the scientist, the fearless investigator of truth. In the other there is the psychoanalyst, the wise wizard of insight. These two ideals embody different moral sensibilities, different fundamental commitments, different bottom lines.

(Luhrmann 2000, p. 158)

Psychiatry, Luhrmann conveyed, is an unhappy profession.

The consistent trend has been to develop psychiatric and psychoanalytic institutions with strict barriers confronting each other, evolving radically different aetiological concepts that keep each other at a distance through different terminologies and discourses. Regarding the conceptual differences, we have:

- Freud's initial distinction between hereditary, remote aetiology, versus the more special and proximate causes.

But newer discriminations have emerged

- one between treating symptoms and illnesses versus the treatment of persons and their experiences;

- and, another between objectivity with apparently scientific evidence using medical treatments versus a subjective approach understanding the power of relationships and narratives.

The institutional psychodynamics adhering to these polarities is the topic of this chapter.

Bio-psycho-social

The impenetrable quality of madness has led to many speculative views on its origins: biological and genetic; psychologically uncontained traumatic experiences; and socially constructed family scapegoating and stigmatising of roles. No one of the three contenders is clearly more convincing, although one has the commercial backing with the finance for a marketing advantage – I mean the drug companies advantage.

Advancing on all three fronts at the same time – biological, experiential and social – is a taxing demand, because each of the three appears to contend with the others. The empirical work of Spillius (1976 [1988] then working as Elizabeth Bott) in the mid-twentieth century is a model. She conducted an anthropological enquiry of a large mental hospital, and found that there were various unspoken discontents. There was an unconscious life to the attitudes and experiences that made up the job satisfaction (or dissatisfaction). Conflicting forces acting on the staff meant that whatever they did felt wrong from one or other point of view. They were caught in a triple pincer that demanded three things from them:

- They were asked to treat and *cure* their patients as taught in their own professional trainings;
- They were asked to *care* for people who were looking for a retreat, an asylum from the discontents of life itself;
- They were asked to control patients in a form of *custody*, those who society and family found too difficult to tolerate.

These three approaches represent the aspects of the bio-psycho-social model. Cure of mental illness is a bio-medical model of thinking and points us to symptoms and bodily or biological causes and treatments; care means engaging with the experience of patients who need respite and asylum (both mental and physical) from their own terrifying psychological experiences; and custody is the social and familiar response – out of sight and at a distance – that protects everyone in the wider society from the unpredictable threats and violence anticipated from the mad.

Cure, care and custody are conflicting tasks for the hospital to aim for, and they vied with each other within the organisation and among its staff. Each member of staff moved in this three dimensional matrix of attitudes and intentions. For instance, providing asylum for the unfortunately vulnerable patients, conflicts with another point of view – curing them so that they return to the situation in which they became disturbed. Spillius traced these incompatible aims to the contradictory needs of society at large, which also wants effective treatment for relatives and friends, humane care for them, and protection for themselves.

Complexity and conflict

These conflicting aims separate out and come to be reflected in separate groups within the hospital system. Staff are trained to treat and cure; patients want the sanctuary of an asylum; and relatives want their family members 'put away' in custody for the sake of the family. However, the tensions between these different tasks were not overtly expressed by the staff, and so not worked through. That meant individuals have to face three directions at once.

The hospital's solution was divisive to create schismatic groups. The functions were held by different people at different times and in different places. Instead of seeking some articulation between the separate attitudes, it seems the divisions were handled unconsciously, without full appreciation of how with three tasks, the individuals inevitably worked against themselves. In this way, an *internal* conflict became an external one. Individuals did not have to feel torn, and then to worry about their responsibility. Instead they held to a single aim and colleagues aimed at other tasks. At times, psychiatrists could represent custody when they sign a compulsory order, and nurses represent care; at other times, nurses are custodial, and doctors represent the treatment function; and so on.

Thus the three sets of attitudes could be conveniently held separate, by the individuals and the organisation, but at the cost that the organisation did not work as a whole, and the separate groups of people potentially grated on each other. Instead of an internal conflict to settle, there was a felt sense of working against someone else – an external conflict. So in the end, no one felt a proper job satisfaction; then morale falls (Hinshelwood 1979).

The conflicts remained unspoken and elusive, so the separation caused serious divisive results with schism, uncertainty and confusion for all. Nor are these conflicts overtly expressed in society, and in a way, the psychiatric organisations exist to take on these conflicts that society in general cannot handle. Spillius' organisational description illuminated divisions in the service that may apply to the psychiatrist–psychoanalyst one. Another example of the unconscious use of group relations, where individual conflict produced group dysfunction, is a piece of empirical work by Miller and Gwynne (1972), who study homes for physically handicapped people, and embodied a conflict between simple care, or 'warehousing', and a rehabilitative aim, called 'horticulture'. The conflict became a separation between different homes; some operated as if their inmates could do nothing and needed total care, and other homes operated as if their inmates could be restored to a full life. Both attitudes being unrealistic, need to be contained in an integrated way.

Moreover, innocent attempts at a conscious level to heal schisms of this kind between working groups will challenge the unconscious defensive system, and inadvertently threaten to provoke painful conflict. Therefore, such a reasonable approach based on sensible discussion will either fail or if successful release stress and conflict. In other words, there are strong and hidden forces to ensure failure that require a persisting schism between the apparently conflicting groups.

The question is whether the rift between psychiatry and psychoanalysis is a similar arrangement to cope with an unresolvable conflict, and with the unconscious benefit keeping the conflict in the form of an intergroup schism. Each group represents only one side of the conflict. People do not then have to worry about the conflict between custody and care for instance, or between medical and psychodynamic models. They can leave one or other attitude to others. These conflicts move their location from the identity conflicts inside people to the boundaries between institutionalised groups. This translocation turns the boundaries into barriers, away from mutual collaboration, and towards interdisciplinary conflict. The technical languages become foreign languages for each other. And worst of all differential value judgements grow up, identifying 'out'-groups as less worthy to co-operate with. The advantage is the self-evaluation that enhances confidence in comparison with other groupings. Freud knew this lack of respect,

> You will grant that there is nothing in the nature of psychiatric work which
> could be opposed to psycho-analytic research. What is opposed to psycho-
> analysis is not psychiatry but psychiatrists.
>
> (Freud 1917, p. 254)

However, psychiatrists might say something similar about psychoanalysts.

Freud looked from only one side, but elsewhere in a more neutral way Freud called it the narcissism of minor difference (Freud 1930, p. 114). Because of these advantage for each 'in'-group to devalue the 'other', there is a collaborative effort to establish these barrier-type boundaries' disciplines. However, that advantage is unconscious and the collaboration becomes maladaptive; it impedes inter-group co-operation and discussion, and being unconscious these group relations are frustratingly intractable. What then are the hidden conflicts and stresses that provoke these surface attitudes to each other? Let us return to this specific question after further consideration of the inter-group system.

Multidisciplinary team working

Despite these barrier effects, multidisciplinary team working had a place in the old institutionalised mental health hospitals. Roles and functions were prescribed by tradition, the psychiatrist with his team of nurses, psychologists, occupational therapists, etc. However, as care in the community has taken over from the old hospitals, that close, even rigid, integration has been steadily dismantled and the professions have separated themselves further from each other. Team working has therefore been increasingly emphasised, but, there is little evidence of specific training for professionals to work in a multidisciplinary way (Whyte & Brooker 2001). It seems to be generally assumed that people will work together in a collaborative way whenever given the chance, but there is little research evidence to corroborate that assumption. Where formal research has been done, it appears that the intuitive assumption is not necessarily the case (Atwal & Caldwell 2002; Burns & Lloyd 2004). For instance, a systematic study of music therapists showed a high rate of burn-out, for which the MDT did not apparently offer protection (Hills, Norman & Forster 2000). This may be a feature of the less powerful professions within the team. Verbal contribution to team discussion tends to vary according to discipline and the discipline's standing within the team; Sanson-Fisher, Poole and Harker (1979) showed that occupational therapists spoke less than nurses or doctors. This pecking order and interdisciplinary threat between OTs and nurses was confirmed by Jones (2006).

Jones found quite disturbing results in a study using participant observation and semi-structured interviews in a psychiatric team (in East London):

> To protect their role, clinicians attempted to protect role boundaries and function. This has also been described by Davies (2000) who found both medical and nursing staff intransigent in working towards collaborative ways of working.
>
> (Jones 2006, p. 25)

Intransigent is a strong word considering the self-evident benefits of working together. He continued: 'An intriguing finding is the readiness for some clinicians to establish for themselves a mandate to critique their colleagues' (p. 26). This is alarming because lack of support and institutionalised interdisciplinary criticism contribute to low morale (Maslach & Jackson 1982, Janssen, Jong & Bakker 1999). In the high stress work of mental health, observational methods have shown that workers do not always adhere to best practice.

Demonstration of one's superior understanding compared with other professionals becomes the more important task. Bowles and Jones (2005) summarise one of the themes of multidisciplinary working thus:

> [I]t appears that under certain circumstances, the whole system may work to shift responsibility in order to manage worker's anxiety more adroitly than, for example, working creatively to respond to people's needs.
>
> (Bowles & Jones 2005, p. 283)

A displacement of interest occurs; interest in treating the patient is overtaken by the alternative need to demonstrate the belief system of the professional group to which one belongs. Teamwork is a casualty in this system (see the symposium in *The Journal of Interprofessional Care* 15, in 2001, on team working in healthcare in general).

Working with patients

Not only do professionals of one discipline collaborate inexplicably poorly with other disciplines, but another group becomes caught up in this system of inter-group conflict, and devaluation. That further group consists of the patients. Professionals tend towards specific attitudes for somewhat similar reasons – that is unconscious reasons.

Take for instance the following occurrence:

> The patient was led into a quiet room for her relaxation therapy. She
> remained there with her nurse, who locked the door, and pressed a but-
> ton on a tape machine which played for 20 minutes. The nurse sat down
> and appeared bored from over-familiarity with the tape. At the end the
> nurse, wordlessly, switched off the machine, unlocked the door and led
> the patient out.

The role of care was interpreted as merely semi-custodial; keeping the
door locked, switching on the machine. Any personal quality to this
care functioning was pre-empted by the strictly mechanical interpretation, and exemplifying the quality Erikson (1956) called 'distantia-
tion'. In a remarkable book by Hardcastle et al. (2007), the interpersonal
distancing is revealed in conflicting unselfconscious accounts by both
users and carers:

> When I first arrived on the hospital ward two male staff took me to a
> side room. I desperately wanted to go to sleep. I hadn't slept well for two
> months . . . One was clearly more senior than the other and he wrote in the
> book whilst the other went through my belongings . . . After this job had
> been done, the junior one (who later told me he was a bank nurse, 'What's
> a bank nurse?') stayed in the side room with me. 'Why?' He started chat-
> ting about his personal difficulties. He may have thought this would be
> helpful . . .
>   I wanted to sleep
>   . . . He continued to talk. I was worried that if I told him to stop he
> wouldn't like me.
>
> (Hardcastle et al. 2007, pp. 23)

This painful form of contact, shallow and distancing, was also observed
by Donati (1989). She observed a touch-and-go form of relating in a long-
stay ward in a large mental hospital.

> Throughout the sessions while I was just sitting in an armchair, looking
> around, my contact with patients was largely restricted to exchange of smiles
> and looks. The patients very rarely spoke to others and this was not because
> of gross cognitive impairment as there were some who could play cards,
> chess, draughts, snooker extremely well, frequently beating the nurses!
>   Both patients and staff would break this isolation in two ways: (a) on
> their way in or out of the ward (is it time for OT?, how was the walk?, why
> don't you go out for a coffee?, how are you feeling today?); and (b) in brief

comments to the various passers-by who were captured momentarily with a challenging or appreciative or jokey comment from patients who were sitting in the armchairs as if waiting for something to happen. This touch and go behaviour involved everybody. This included the priest, whose two visits to the ward, while I was there, may now be mentioned.

(Donati 1989, p. 324)

The reason appeared to be a fear of engagement with mad patients. In settings intended to enhance the patients' social activity, staff constantly promoted a non-engagement that was visibly self-defeating. These kinds of phenomena could be explained on the basis that staff were wary and frightened of the patients' madness. The depersonalisation keeps an emotional distance from the disturbingly meaningless symptoms of psychotic patients (Donati 2000); and it resembled the findings of Menzies (1959) in her study of physical nursing.

It would appear that in physical nursing a large part of the anxiety that depersonalisation protects against is the nurses' feelings *for* their patients. In mental health, staff also feel for their unfortunate, suffering patients which, however, threatens to take over their own minds. However, in unconscious ways staff in mental health back away from the painful feeling – just because the sense of responsibility for dealing with that degree of pain has felt a back-breaking burden. The temptation for staff in mental health is to reconceptualise the nature of the problem, and to do so in such a way that their emotional distancing and depersonalisation is perfectly relevant. They *treat a disease* not a person. This shift of emphasis is unconsciously driven, and we could say, quite understandable. In the terms used above, there is an extra emphasis on cure, at the expense of care (Hinshelwood 1987, 1994, 2004).

The managerial intervention

Increasingly in recent decades a further 'discipline' has emerged as a player within this mosaic of groups. This is the growth of the management class within health care, as in all public service provision, stimulated by financial interests through insurance companies and pharmaceutical companies, and through political initiatives. In some ways, this is a group that intervenes within the whole system, and attracts attitudes, and relations, at the unconscious level as well as the conscious.

One result has been to support the emotional distancing noted above. The preferred form of management in the public services (most extreme perhaps in Britain) has been a realignment from a personal form of service provision to a 'commodified' form of service parcelled as products. Such an intervention has formed differential alliances with different disciplinary sub-groupings according to the conceptualisation typical of the discipline. For instance, supplying a pharmaceutical product is much closer to the managerial idea of service products, than say a service based on listening and thinking and exploring relational change.

However, this higher level support for the institutionalised depersonalisation of the clientele is not the only impact. Management, as a group, come to be seen as a group with responsibility; and indeed the group does adopt that position in part. Without the detailed skills of the professionals it does have a kind of overall responsibility, but is therefore wide open to be used as an agent for a total responsibility for everything, not just the task throughput, and the financial management, but also the unconscious system, with the intricate emotional attitudes and conflicts described above. In fact, the management training and practice is not well adapted to the unconscious level of inter-group relating. From my own experience of working within management, the conceptual model of a person used by an ordinary human resources department (known as HR, in Britain) is lacking in an understanding of the emotional relations with the work, the task and the clientele, and is at a loss usually even to consider an unconscious level to these emotions.

I have described how the relations between professional disciplines and patients have developed an emotional distancing (or institutionalisation) over many decades, perhaps centuries. The advent of HR has in some ways been an ally of the emotionally distancing set of attitudes that has been defensively adopted in psychiatry, with as Freud said that need to look to distant aetiologies, as opposed to proximal suffering.

The role of stress

Psychiatrists and psychoanalysts are humans too, and can be deleteriously influenced by stresses they feel daunted by. For the cultures of the two groups that makes them somewhat like patients, and risks shaming professionals who share such vulnerability. Nevertheless, the professionals in psychiatry do suffer stress in their work. The stress is of three kinds:

- the real risks of working with unpredictable people, a proportion of whom can be violent and dangerous;

- the lack of really good results (though some exist) and the consequent lack of appreciative feedback from people who have lost social skills;
- the confounding quality of the engagement with people who have lost the capacity to make meanings, to share the same reality, to express their experiences in comprehensible words, and indeed who have trouble capturing a sense of self or identity for themselves.

These stresses, which mental health professionals of all disciplines share, are rendered unconscious for much of the time, and therefore unshared. Instead they manifest themselves in various maladaptive institutional forms. There are a number of manifestations:

- One is the culture of depersonalisation mentioned already.
- At the same time there is a pervasive atmosphere of despair and help-lessnesss. This gets through into the staff, and they feel hopeless about helping.
- Psychotic patients use other, non-verbal routes to transmit affect, leaving the staff feeling a perplexity and aversion.
- There is often a connected culture of fear – something is going quickly out of control. This may be experienced as either madness or violence, a mind going out of control. This is frightening to us as mental health workers, no different from the public.
- There is another, less clear, fear. That is to do with a feeling that we will, ourselves, get madness inside us as well, and we will be contaminated, while there is no asepsis comparable to physical infections.
- The sense of *meaninglessness* in the patient's experience and anxiety creates a collective attitude that we are dealing with something that is without meaning, senseless; and this is connected to feeling overwhelmed by some*thing* out of control, leading to dismissal of the touch-and-go kind.
- The meaninglessness causes another reaction, the temptation for educated and trained professionals to jump in with their own meanings, with as explained an effect of cacophony as each discipline parades different meanings.
- Finally, we have unconscious expectations, and the suffering, stress and madness of the patients and clients provokes a particular impact on those of us doing the work. Indeed, we are often especially vulnerable as we were led into the work because of some ill or unhappy person in our own families. The urge to put them right is often very strong, and displaced onto the patients we work with. This motive

based on hardly appreciated unconscious and maybe phantasy motives, is common enough to encourage a common bond within a group of close colleagues.

The role of this plethora of cultural issues means that strong measures have to be instituted, and supported by the dynamics of the group. And the demands on leadership to contain these attitudes imply that the leading persons are the prime target for support – though often the most resistant to accepting it.

Treating versus suffering

I have singled out the conflict between cure versus care as a primary conflict in mental health work today. Treating symptoms is a very advantageous way of looking at the work. It has a clearly objective task, related to measurable (or quasi-measurable) symptoms, and there is a large and increasing pharmacopeia of medications; but in addition it is compatible with a set of attitudes that are emotionally distancing, and therefore protective of the professionals, who can be relieved of overwhelming stress. The situation is not as simple as Freud suggested; his recommendation of putting the distant aetiologies together with the proximal ones has to consider the obstacles of the inter-group dynamics. When Freud in 1917 considered this problem, he had not yet investigated the unconscious aspects of group dynamics sufficiently. He did so in 1921, and again in 1930, but did not come back to the problem with psychiatrists.

In fact, had Freud reconsidered things it might have been better to consider the psychiatrists' problems with psychoanalysts. To tell psychiatrists to attend to proximal causes is to tell them to come close to the suffering of their patients. Nevertheless, it is the advice of psychoanalysts. Freud's observations were put slightly differently more recently:

> We find it necessary to differentiate between the pain of a broken leg and the pain, say, of bereavement; sometimes we prefer not to, but exchange mental for physical pain and vice versa. Physician and psycho-analyst are alike in considering that the disease should be recognized by the physician; in psycho-analysis recognition must be by the sufferer too . . .
>
> The point that demonstrates the divergence most clearly is that the physician is dependent on realization of sensuous experience [feel, touch, smell, etc.] in contrast with the psycho-analyst whose dependence is on experience that is not sensuous. The physician can see and touch and

smell. The realizations with which a psycho-analyst deals cannot be seen or touched; anxiety has no shape or colour, smell or sound. For convenience, I propose to use the term 'intuit'.

(Bion 1970, pp. 6–7)

In other words, the psychoanalyst 'knows' the suffering by *feeling it with* the patient. That is not a recommendation that is likely to be welcomed!

I am here expanding the Spillius' 'oppositions', cure and care, and showing it is a conflict within psychiatry between distancing from the patient's suffering, and feeling it with him. It may be essential that a psychiatric service does both, but the patient suffers if the two aims are done in opposition. Yet the opposition seems inevitable. Unless . . . unless we could find a way of getting this message across as a completely understandable problem and conflict.

Conclusions

I have claimed that internal conflicts within individuals become conflicts between groups. Many years ago Elliott Jaques wrote,

> Individuals may put their internal conflicts into persons in the external world, unconsciously follow the course of the conflict by means of projective identification . . . and re-internalise the course and outcome of the externally perceived conflict by means of introjective identification.

(Jaques 1955, pp. 496–497)

This psychoanalytic model is appropriate for understanding the inexplicable antipathy between psychiatrists and psychoanalysts. Psychoanalysis is the science of unconscious experience. Although psychoanalysts often give explanations for consciously understood problems, it is the inexplicable where our expertise really lies.

References

Atwal, A., & Caldwell, K. (2002). Do multidisciplinary integrated care pathways improve interprofessional collaboration? *Scandinavian Journal of Caring Sciences*, 16: 360–367.

Bion, W. R. (1970). *Attention and interpretation*. London: Tavistock.

Bowles, N., & Jones, A. (2005). Whole systems working and acute inpatient psychiatry: An exploratory study. *Journal of Psychiatric and Mental Health Nursing*, 12: 283–289.

Burns, T., & Lloyd, H. (2004). Is a team approach based on staff meetings cost-effective in the delivery of mental health care? *Current Opinion in Psychiatry*, *17*: 311–314.

Davies, C. (2000). Getting health professionals to work together. *British Medical Journal*, *320* (7241): 1021–1022.

Donati, F. (1989). A psychodynamic observer in a chronic psychiatric ward. *British Journal of Psychotherapy*, *5*: 317–329. Republished in R. D. Hinshelwood and Wilhelm Skogstad (2000). *Observing organisations*. London: Routledge.

Erikson, E. H. (1956). The problem of ego identity. *Journal of the American Psychoanalytic Association*, *4*: 56–121.

Freud, S. (1896). The aetiology of hysteria. In *The standard edition of the complete psychological works of Sigmund Freud, volume III (1893–1899)* (pp. 187–221). London: Hogarth.

Freud, S. (1917). Chapter 16: Psychoanalysis and psychiatry. In *The introductory lecture. The standard edition of the complete psychological works of Sigmund Freud*, volume XVI (pp. 243–256). London: Hogarth.

Freud, S. (1930). *Civilization and its discontents. Standard edition of the complete psychological works of Sigmund Freud*, volume 21, (pp. 59–145). London: Hogarth.

Hardcastle, M., Kennard, D., Grandison, S., & Fagin, L. (2007). *Experiences of mental health in-patient care*. London: Routledge.

Hills, B., Norman, I., & Forster, L. (2000). A study of burnout and multidisciplinary team-working amongst professional music therapists. *British Journal of Music Therapy*, *14*: 32–40.

Hinshelwood, R. D. (1979). Demoralisation and the hospital community. *Group Analysis*, *12*: 84–93. Reprinted 2001 in R. D. Hinshelwood *Thinking about institutions*. London: Jessica Kingsley.

Hinshelwood, R. D. (1987). The psychotherapist's role in a large mental institution. *Psychoanalytic Psychotherapy*, *2*: 207–215.

Hinshelwood, R. D. (1994). The relevance of psychotherapy. *Psycho-Analytic Psychotherapy*, *8*: 283–294.

Hinshelwood, R. D. (2004). *Suffering insanity*. London: Routledge.

Janssen, P. M. P., Jonge, J. D., & Bakker, A. B. (1999). Specific determinants of intrinsic work motivation, burnout and turnover intentions: A study among nurses. *Journal of Advanced Nursing*, *29*: 1360–1369.

Jaques, E. (1955). Social systems as a defence against persecutory and depressive anxiety. In H. Klein, & R. Money-Kyrle (Eds.) *New directions in psychoanalysis* (pp. 478–498). London: Tavistock.

Jones, A. (2006). Multidisciplinary team working: Collaboration and conflict. *International Journal of Mental Health Nursing*, *15*: 19–28.

Jones, E. (1953). *The life and work of Sigmund Freud vol. 1*. London: Hogarth.

Luhrmann, T. M. (2000). *Of two minds*. New York: Alfred Knopf.

Maslach, C., & Jackson, S. E. (1982). Burnout in health professions: A social psychological analysis. In G. S. Sanders, & J. Suls (Eds.) *Social Psychology of Health and Illness*. Hillsdale: Erlbaum.

Menzies, I. (1959). The functioning of social systems as a defence against anxiety: A report on a study of the nursing service of a general hospital. *Human Relations, 13*: 95–121. Republished 1988 in Menzies *Containing Anxiety in Institutions*. London: Free Association Books; and in E. Trist and H. Murray (Eds.) 1990 *The Social Engagement of Social Science*. London: Free Association Books.

Miller, E., & Gwynne, G. (1972). *A life apart*. London: Tavistock.

Sanson-Fisher, R. W., Poole, A. D., & Harker, J. (1979). Behavioural analysis of ward rounds within a general hospital psychiatric unit. *Behavioural Research Therapy, 17*: 333–347.

Spillius, E. Bott (1976). Hospital and society. *British Journal of Medical Psychology, 49*: 97–140. Republished abridged as: Asylum and society. In E. Trist & H. Murray (Eds.) (1990) *The social engagement of social science, volume 1: The socio-psychological perspective*. London: Free Association Books.

Whyte, L., & Brooker, C. (2001). Working with a multidisciplinary team in secure psychiatric environments. *Journal of Psychosocial Nursing & Mental Health Services, 39*: 26–34.

CHAPTER FIVE

Psychoanalysis, psychiatry and medicine

Robert Michels

Psychoanalysis does not have an obvious relationship to psychiatry or medicine. It is not interested in psychiatric illnesses, but rather in how people adapt, how they cope with stress, including the stress of illness, rather than in the illnesses themselves. It is interested in the person's mind, not his body or even his brain. Psychoanalysis began outside of psychiatry, and Freud, himself a neurologist, never saw it as a part of psychiatry.

Freud's only visit to the United States, in 1909, was hosted by psychologists, not psychiatrists. Jung, a psychiatrist, was invited to the same conference, and was better known than Freud by American psychiatrists. Unlike Freud he had worked with Bleuler in Zurich, had conducted empirical research employing his word association methods on schizophrenic patients, and had published in English. Soon after the conference Freud and Jung had a falling out, and Freud became annoyed with two leading American psychiatrists who were enthusiastic about psychoanalysis—Smith Ely Jelliffe and William Alanson White—who maintained strong ties to Jung. Freud disliked America and Americans, and he returned to Vienna to develop his new science, viewing American psychoanalysis as an embarrassment. He had little contact with American psychiatry, then or afterward.

The middle of the twentieth century brought major changes. Several American psychiatrists went to Vienna to study with and be analyzed by Freud. More important, many prominent European psychoanalysts fled central Europe and settled in the United States. Freud himself wanted psychoanalysis to be independent from psychiatry and not restricted to physicians. He dreaded that it might, some day, become a chapter in a textbook of psychiatry. His view prevailed in much of the world. However American psychoanalysts both native and immigrant were attracted by the prestige of psychiatry and medicine, and opposed his anti-medical and anti-psychiatric stance. For more than half a century they succeeded in excluding non-psychiatrists from the American Psychoanalytic Association and tying themselves to psychiatry and to medicine. They constituted an elite group whose status in American psychiatry, medicine and society was enhanced by the exclusion of non-psychiatrist analysts, an exclusion that only came to an end with a lawsuit filed by a group of psychologists that was not settled until 1988.

The success of psychoanalysis in the world of psychiatry was remarkable. For several decades it dominated American psychiatry. As psychoanalysis arrived on the scene, psychiatry had become increasingly alienated from the rest of medicine, and surprising though it seems to a contemporary reader, psychoanalysis was hailed as promising closer ties to medicine and science. Through its prominence in psychosomatic medicine it meant a return from rural asylums for the insane to the teaching wards of academic medical centers. It offered an intellectually fascinating theory that promised a new understanding of mental life that seemed far more scientific than that provided by the humane and perhaps clinically helpful but theoretically unimaginative "nondynamic" psychiatry. It provided a counterpart to the somewhat disreputable physical treatments of convulsive therapies and lobotomies that were frightening to the public. Perhaps most importantly, it arrived with a reputation for clinical efficacy. Non-psychiatrist physicians who had received brief psychiatric training with a psychoanalytic orientation and then placed in the front lines of World War II returned home with stories of great therapeutic success in treating traumatized soldiers. They were enthusiastic about their clinical experiences and wanted to train as psychiatrists and psychoanalysts. The result was that psychiatry, and particularly psychoanalytic psychiatry was increasingly accepted by the public and by general medicine, and psychoanalysis was increasingly influential in psychiatry.

Psychiatry's enthusiasm for psychoanalysis faded over the next few decades. The theories of psychoanalysis were interesting, but they failed to generate a body of empirical research, were criticized for being unscientific, and came to be seen as historic relics rather than scientific theories.

Biologic psychiatry, beginning in the 1950s, developed successive waves of psychopharmacologic treatments that increasingly came to compete with the psychotherapies and psychoanalysis for the same population of patients. Perhaps most importantly, the psychodynamic psychotherapies that seemed so effective in treating the self-limited traumatic syndromes of the battlefield were much less effective when applied to the chronic mentally ill, while it became clear that their efficacy in treating acute trauma had little do to with their psychoanalytic theoretical foundation. Psychoanalysis had seemed to promise a strategy for developing a scientific psychiatry, but it failed to deliver on that promise and the sociocultural factors that supported its role faded away.

Before its decline, psychoanalysis came to dominate academic psychiatry as well as clinical psychiatry. Psychiatry was entering its golden age in academic medicine, and psychoanalysis was already at the peak of its golden age in psychiatry. However, they were not quite in phase with each other, and as academic psychiatry gained increasing status, its dominant theme shifted first to social psychiatry and then to biological psychiatry and neuroscience, while the influence of psychoanalysis waned.

Psychoanalysis seemed much more relevant to psychiatric practice and education than to psychiatric research. In the 1950s, American academic psychiatry was dominated by its educational mission. Beginning the 1960s, as academic psychiatry matured and moved closer to other fields of academic medicine, it became more like them as its research mission became increasingly prominent. Success was measured by research support and publications. Psychiatric research made immense strides, largely biologic research—first psychopharmacology, and later neuroscience, genetics and brain imaging. Psychological research, and particularly research in psychotherapy was much less prominent, and in psychoanalysis almost nonexistent. As academic psychiatry developed its scientific base its new leaders were more likely to be neuroscientists or biologic psychiatrists than psychoanalysts.

Psychoanalysis itself was changing simultaneously, independently of, and largely unrelated to the developments in psychiatry. Freud's death in 1939 ended an era in which there was a single accepted criterion for what was truly "psychoanalytic" and initiated a period of pluralism that continues to this day. Freud's early theories had been strongly biologic; they speculated about what was going on in the patient's mind and brain and emphasized constitutional determinants of behavior, innate drives that somehow led to mental events. His theories were also, of course, psychological, mentalist, but even these were formulated in ways that were comfortable to those familiar with the positivist scientific thinking of the day, and suggest the possibility of eventual neurobiologic reductionism. Freud believed that his method led to the discovery of previously existing although unconscious and therefore undetectable psychological phenomena, and that exposing them to the patient's consciousness would be curative. He had himself tried to construct neurobiological models of his psychology, but even though he eventually gave these up, this was not because he thought that they were inherently inappropriate, but rather because he thought that they were premature. The necessary neuroscientific knowledge base did not exist at the end of the nineteenth century. However, he had no doubt that mental life would someday be understood as the reflection of underlying neurobiologic processes. With today's neuroscience he would probably be an enthusiastic fan of "neuropsychoanalysis" and eager to make another attempt at his project for developing a scientific brain-based psychology. He did not want psychoanalysis to be a branch of psychiatry, but was quite comfortable seeing it as biological, and ultimately reducible to the functioning of the nervous system.

Why didn't American academic psychiatry, during its period of psychoanalytic leadership and its growing interest in research, develop a program of psychoanalytic research? Psychoanalysts were eager to be seen as scientific, and they cast their early theories in the language of science. However, they failed to develop a true scientific methodology and had little interest in testing their theories or in attempting to invalidate them. In fact, most of the theories that they embraced were not based on psychoanalytic data, but rather were borrowed from contiguous disciplines—initially neuroscience and cultural anthropology, later developmental psychology and linguistics. Psychoanalysts neither developed nor tested them, and in fact didn't treat them as scientific theories at all. Rather they used them as tools in the clinical process of searching for meanings, as sources of metaphor. The analytic process came to be seen more and more as an interpretive endeavor, developing new meanings, rather than searching for previously existing but unrecognized facts. The analyst and the patient co-constructed narratives, rather than uncovering forgotten memories. Psychoanalysis moved closer to the humanities rather than the sciences, and much as its practitioners admired science, borrowed its concepts, and aspired to be seen as scientists, their daily work and their intellectual interests moved them away from science, medicine and psychiatry, and toward hermeneutics. The goal was understanding, not explanation.

Freud wanted to develop an objective science of human subjectivity, and he viewed the psychoanalyst as a neutral observer of the patient's words and acts, data from which might be inferred the patient's inner experience. Contemporary psychoanalysts are not as confident in the analyst's neutrality or objectivity, and increasingly see the analyst's interpretations as reflecting the analyst's own inner subjectivity, while relying on the analyst's countertransference as an important contributor to the data. This shift, from the patient's words and acts to the analyst's experience and reactions, moves psychoanalysis even further from the rest of psychiatry, medicine and Popperian science.

I have mentioned the strong psychoanalytic interest in the theories and discoveries of adjacent sciences, if not in their methods. There has also been pressure within the psychoanalytic community for research on the treatment itself—its effectiveness, its indications, and so on. However, this pressure has largely come from those concerned with public health, health policy and economics. Clinical psychoanalysts have shown little interest in this kind of endeavor—the studies required would be long, expensive and difficult, and relate to the sciences of biostatistics and evaluation of treatment outcome, not to those of interest to psychoanalysis. Clinicians anticipated little from the results that would enrich their daily work. They had no doubt that their treatment worked, and had more confidence in the wisdom of their elders than in systematic empirical studies that explicated whether or how it worked. Studies of its effectiveness might be of interest to skeptics or to those concerned with public policy, but not to practicing psychoanalysts. Clinical psychoanalysts want to enrich their repertoire of potential interpretations, not to learn what percentage of their patients might be expected to improve by what percent on scales of psychopathology.

However, there is another reason that a research tradition in psychoanalysis has not developed, one that I believe is more important and has little to do with the potential value of empirical research but is embedded in the social structure of the profession. Most professional education occurs in university settings, and university cultures have a strong commitment to research. Faculty advancement depends on research productivity, and academic leaders are selected for their research, not their clinical or educational excellence. Psychoanalysis is different and virtually unique. Freud was suspicious of universities; he feared that they would attack and destroy his fragile creation, and psychoanalysis developed and largely continues outside of them. Psychoanalytic education is conducted in freestanding institutes, collections of practitioners with no full-time faculty, often meeting only at nights or on weekends, devoted to study and teaching, but with little interest, time or reward for research, and indeed often regard research activity with suspicion. Kernberg has compared these institutes to trade schools or seminaries. The result is that psychoanalytic research is almost, although not quite, an oxymoron.

Several aspects of the psychoanalytic paradigm are particularly critical for its relationship to medicine and psychiatry. First, its insistence on strict psychic determinism is in conflict with a major trend in contemporary psychiatry. Our growing understanding of neurobiology and of the genetic and biochemical correlates of psychiatric disorders have led to an increasing interest in understanding mental states as determined by brain states, rather than by preceding mental states. Of course, this interest is nothing new. Freud, discussing melancholic depression in 1917 wrote, "What is probably a somatic factor, and one which cannot be explained psychogenically, makes itself visible in the regular amelioration in the condition that takes place toward evening." Nevertheless, analysts try to understand meanings, while many modern psychiatrists are increasingly interested in understanding not only the form of mental life—such as diurnal variation in mood—but even the content—such as sexual, aggressive or suicidal wishes—as secondary to neural events. Clearly, these are not logically different positions as much as different perspectives and approaches, but different they are. However, this difference is far more fateful for the relationship of psychoanalysis to psychiatry than to medicine. For, while neurobiologic reductionism has been popular in understanding psychopathology and psychiatric disorders, it has had little impact on our view of nonpathologic adaptation or the clinical process. When we want to understand how a medical patient is coping with a myocardial infarct, or a surgical patient is anticipating a thoracotomy, or simply how someone is talking to a physician, what he is revealing and what he is concealing, we want to know his thoughts, feelings, wishes, and fears, not his serotonin receptor status or his threshold for kindling.

A second critical aspect of the paradigm, already suggested in the discussion of psychic determinism, is the psychoanalytic insistence on the continuity between normality and pathology. Freud's reconceptualization of hysteria did far more than enrich our understanding of a specific type of pathology; it provided a new paradigm for considering mental states, including both those that had been regarded as pathologic and others that had not, and thus it radically altered the conceptual relationship between the clinical pathologic syndromes of psychiatry and normality. Freud believed that hysterical patients were fundamentally normal and that the psychological mechanisms leading to their symptoms were normal mechanisms that could be recognized in anyone. The distinction between a hysterical patient and any other normal individual was of quantity, not quality, or at most was based on the social appraisal of a surface differentiation that overlay a hidden, deeper commonality. Anyone was capable of constructing a hysterical symptom, and such symptoms could be traced to universal themes and structures in mental life. Psychoanalysis was the tool for translating the apparently pathologic phenotype that seemed to be qualitatively different from the normal to deeper mental life that had created it. Furthermore, the deeper mental life that was first discovered in the treatment of neurotic patients was not only characteristic of the normal mind as well, but actually it became the key for unlocking the secrets of normal psychological development. In 1895, Freud wrote that he intended "to extract from psychopathology a yield for normal psychology. It is in fact impossible to form a satisfactory general view of neuro-psychotic disorders unless they can be linked to clear hypotheses upon normal psychical process." The focus of interest shifted from studying the various categories of pathology and the characteristics that differentiated each from the others to studying the universal mechanisms of all behavior, whether clinical syndrome or mundane experience, with the recognition that normality and pathology were expressions of the same fundamental processes, and the individuals were neither one nor the other, but rather both.

The fundamental distinction underlying nineteenth-century medicine, that between normal and pathologic, had been replaced by the fundamental distinction that defines the domain of psychoanalysis, between meaningful and meaningless. The same mechanisms that had first been discovered in such bold relief in the neurotic conditions formerly considered to be pathologic were studied in every area of behavior. Wishes, fears, defenses, conflicts were characteristic of what had been regarded as pathology, but more important, they were characteristic of the human condition. Freud repeatedly emphasized that "psychoanalytic research finds no fundamental, but only quantitative, distinctions between normal and neurotic life," that "there is no fundamental difference, but only one of degree, between the mental life of normal people, of neurotics, and of psychotics."

The corollary of these two aspects of psychoanalysis is that although it was developed as a treatment for mental disorders, unlike most other treatments in psychiatry, from its very beginning it was seen as relevant to normal psychology, and I would add particularly normal psychology under stress, conflict, or strong emotion. Indeed, the late Charles Brenner defined it as the study of the "mind in conflict." Further, while its relevance to the major disorders that concern contemporary psychiatry has been questioned, it's relevance to less severe aspects of personality disturbance or normal adaptation is largely unquestioned. Paradoxically, psychoanalysis today may be more relevant to medicine than to psychiatry, just as lifestyle and non-psychopathologic behavior patterns may explain more of the variance in the etiology of medical than of psychiatric disorders.

A third and final aspect of psychoanalysis critical for its relationship to medicine and psychiatry stems from its clinical method rather than its theory. Psychoanalysts are extraordinarily interested in the details of their patients' experiences. They spend hundreds of hours with a single patient, listening to every word and searching for nonverbal clues to feelings and hidden thoughts. As a result, they have become students of the clinical process, interviewing and communication. This procedure is an important basic science for all medical practice.

Today, psychoanalysis as a therapy is one treatment in psychiatry. It represents an important theme in psychiatric education, but for most students it provides a context for learning about human behavior and basic clinical skills, rather than a treatment that will be central to their future professional work. Patients with major psychiatric disorders are likely to seek help elsewhere, but psychoanalysis has had a steadily increasing role in the treatment of those individuals whose lives are limited by character pathology.

Psychoanalysis is a theory of mental functioning, one of mind and person, rather than brain and organism, or individual and culture. Its data consist of experiences observed introspectively or empathically and communicated largely verbally or symbolically. It is a theory about the experiential world of man, its origins, development, structure, and potential for change. In this regard, it relates to the most unique of man's biologic characteristics—his capacity for symbol use and symbol creation and for an organized experience of himself in the universe. Because psychoanalytic theory has been linked to a clinical treatment, it has largely emphasized those aspects of man's symbolic functioning that can interfere with his adaptation. Symbols can interfere with the most basic of biological processes. Other species kill in aggression, mate with lust, flee in terror, but man may kill for love, feel more anxiety than lust while mating, and flee from sexual pleasure. The symbolic structure of these behaviors, and the human interactions that may modify them, are the concerns of psychoanalysis. This concern has led to a special interest in early development, the origins of experiences concerning bodily needs, and the mental derivatives of these experiences in later adaptation.

As a result, psychoanalysis provides a framework for considering the experiences of patients, their response to stress and disease, and the alternate possibilities for integrating these factors into their lives. If there are diseases in which the patient's symbolic experience of himself in the world becomes part of his problem, and if a human interaction with a concerned other person could facilitate a change in that experience, then the psychoanalytic paradigm has a role in the understanding of that patient. It is particularly valuable in considering the sequelae of deviant developmental situations and, therefore, is of value in understanding adaptations to social and physical trauma, as well as primary psychopathology and its course.

References

Brenner, C. (1982). *The mind in conflict*. New York: International Universities Press.

Freud, S. (1895[1950]). *Project for a scientific psychology*. Standard Edition, vol. I. London: Hogarth.

Freud, S. (1913). *Totem and taboo*. Standard Edition, vol. XIII. London: Hogarth.

Freud, S. (1917). *Mourning and melancholia*. The Standard Edition of the Complete Psychological Works of Sigmund Freud, vol. XI. London: Hogarth.

Kernberg, O. (2000). A concerned critique of psychoanalytic education. *The International Journal of Psychoanalysis, 81*(1): 97–120.

CHAPTER SIX

Psychoanalysis and psychiatry
Between clinical culture and organizational culture

Mario Perini

P sychoanalysis and psychiatry, nowadays more than ever, rarely talk to each other, and when they do this they generally adopt attitudes of mutual mistrust and haughtiness, if not openly devaluating one another. Just as it happens to people, even cultures, the more they are in trouble or feel under attack, the more often they tend to fight and to become disrespectful to each other. And there cannot be many doubts that in recent years both disciplines in various ways and for different reasons have been going through a serious loss of credibility and growing socio-cultural marginalization.

For psychoanalysis this could appear as just the last of the recurring "down phases" that have occurred since its very foundation, and where its imminent death or celebrated funeral are announced, only to be soon followed by inevitable refutations and apparent evidence of good health. But here we should have no illusions: this crisis – whose symptom much more than the cause seems to be the growing popularity of cognitive and neurobiological approaches – is deep, systemic and doomed to worsen, unless psychoanalysis consents to undergo a brave review of its paradigms, methods and practices, and most of all to confront the external world's new challenges and turbulent transformations.

On the other hand, psychiatry does not seem to be faring much better. The mix of business orientation, political dilettantism, widespread corruption and wholesale cutbacks has come to reduce a complex and honored medical branch, that had been able to resurge from the asylum ruins by building bold bridges across the mind, the biology and the society, into a gasping, bureaucratic and sloppy system aimed at managing "wasted lives" (Bauman, 2004) and social peace, not to mention law and order issues. "Where can we place him/her?" and "What [medication] do we give him/her?" are actually the ritual questions within Mental Health services, while also revealing anxieties and discomforts that appear no longer dealt with by institutional containers and that have flooded by now a large part of the reflective space which should serve other and more sophisticated questions.

In a previous paper I wrote:

> The matching of psychoanalysis and psychiatry, in some ways natural and taken for granted, yet in other ways appears quite problematic. The term "psychoanalytic psychiatry," invented by A. A. Brill (1946), resumed by Paul Schilder (1951) and more recently reworded by Glen Gabbard (1990) and others as "psychodynamic psychiatry," did not generate after all an harmonious couple, while keeping a sort of taste of oxymoron and raising the suspicion of wanting to match the devil and the holy water; where each of the two "parts" would still seem rather inclined to demonize the other.
>
> (Perini, 2013a)[1]

As for the possibility of a cross fertilization between the two disciplines, I suggested on the one hand how psychiatry,

> ideally born to deal with human emotions, may sometimes come to prove so remote from them and so obtusely unable to manage emotions if not by displacing them into some building, classifying like insects or suffocating with some chemical substance;

and, on the other hand, how psychoanalysis, "originally conceived to explore the inner world from its psychopathological and behavioral derivatives, still may find so hard to contribute to clinical psychiatry and to face its dilemmas" (ibid.).

Evidence of such a failed encounter seemed to me the fact that most of the analysts working in the mental health services ended up by splitting their own psychoanalytic identity from their institutional roles, of clinicians, professors or managers, to recover it just in their private office.

At most, they would try "to insert into the body of the institution some psychoanalytically oriented curing practices or programs, such as long, short or focal psychotherapies, group therapies, or psychoanalytic supervisions" (ibid.), while generally giving up the idea of an effort to understand in psychodynamic terms the institution's response to those insertions.

The reasons for this "desertion" may be many, but the main one in my opinion is the lack of a profound reflection by the psychoanalytic community around some psycho-social objects such as group dynamics, issues of power and authority, money, work and organizational functioning; an absence that probably derives from a mix of mistrust, ignorance and conservatism, and that fostered among the analysts an explicit anti-institutional culture.

Another reason for such disengagement could arise from

a difficulty for the analyst to adapt to working within a setting which he/she does not own, could not establish, cannot manage, and which does not offer so many reflective spaces; and above all from the frustrating awareness of how little effectiveness show the traditional psychoanalytic tools, first of all interpretations, in giving rise to the desired changes inside the institution.

(ibid.)

Yet, the analysts showing a clear interest for social institutions and mental health services are not so rare, although at times in somewhat abstract and generic terms. An evidence of this is the 2012 National Congress of the Italian Psychoanalytic Society, which was held in Rome on unusual and unprecedented topics such as money, work, power and social rules; other indications come from recent online discussions on the IPS Mailing List about themes concerning the "outreach" or the "encounter between Psychoanalysis and Healthcare services."

With regard to the role of psychoanalysis in the practice of mental health services and in the exploration of the related institutional dynamics, I would refer the readers to my aforementioned paper (Perini, 2013a), the quoted debate on the IPS Mailing list (Campoli & Carnaroli, 2012) and the relevant however not so crowded literature on the subject (see particularly Racamier et al., 1970; De Martis et al., 1987; Correale, 1991, 2006; Hinshelwood & Skogstad, 2000; Bateman, 2004; Foresti & Rossi Monti, 2010; Plakun, 2012; Michels, 2015). Here I would instead address a basic question which could be usefully explored to understand an element of this sort of dialogue of the deaf that drives a wedge between psycho-analysis and psychiatry: the conflict opposing clinical cultures and organizational cultures.

Organizational cultures and healthcare systems: towards a "clinical theory of organizations"

The concept of organizational culture as an unconscious collective defense system, that Freud himself somehow sensed, was thoroughly explored by Bion, and further developed from different perspectives by Elliot Jaques and Isabel Menzies (Jaques, 1955; Menzies, 1959), the group analysis, the so-called "institutional psychotherapy," the various socio-analytic "schools," in the UK, USA, France and elsewhere. Nonetheless such concept is not a monopoly of psychoanalytic thinking. As early as in the 1970s, starting from a systemic paradigm and a "socio-technic" approach, Miller and Gwynne in their well-known Tavistock study entitled *A Life Apart* (Miller & Gwynne, 1972) discussed how institutions for chronic disabled people function, while differentiating two opposite cultural models: the *warehouse*, centered on the patient's dependence on care systems and substitutive assistance; and the *horticultural model*, centered on encouraging the patient's autonomy and on social stimulation. Their researches showed how each one of the two models also played a defensive role, the former through a disavowal of the patients' remaining resources and capacity for autonomy and development, the latter through a denial of their limits, difficulties and dependency needs; and both of them by trying to keep off the painful awareness that the institution's primary task was after all managing the inmates' "transition from social death to physical death" (ibid., p. 89).

On the other hand, even Franco Basaglia, whose thinking was mainly rooted in phenomenology, in his "anti-institutional" works explored the implicit function of the psychiatric hospital – marginalizing the insane and segregating insanity – in terms of a kind of protection at the same time social, political and psychological: a "safeguard of sane people from madness" and a defense against the anxiety for "having to recognize madness in its very origin, that is to say, from life" (Basaglia, 1968, 1984).

But the anti-institutional stance that Basaglia applied to the field of mental health and was nurtured by a radical social and anthropological pessimism towards the "inimical institution," in other areas of the philosophical and political thinking would become mitigated by elements of balanced pragmatism and the hope that organizations, while being inevitable, could anyway be created, managed and lived as "good enough" social objects. Thus, at the dawn of the building of the European Union Jean Monnet argued that "only institutions grow wiser" and reminded that if it is true that "nothing can be achieved without people," it is also evident that "nothing endures without institutions" (Monnet, 1976).

The effort that many have made – not everywhere and not always timely enough – to recover the meaning and the value of an institutional culture no longer among enemies to fight against, but rather among potential working instruments for the task of cure, has drawn an awareness from Basaglia's lesson: that just as for all clinical tools even this culture may fail, prove iatrogenic or counterproductive, be badly used or turn into abuse, stigmatization and perversity; after all the issue of power is inevitably intrinsic to it.

The concept of an *institutional clinic* has been proposed by DiMarco and Nosé in a book they edited in 2008 to review some of the seminal works of "sociotherapy" developed in the 1970s, from Tom Main to H. S. Klein, from Tosquelles to Racamier, from Fornari to Napolitani. This concept supports a "rehabilitated" view of the institution and its healing potential through the mutually complementary experiences of the modern therapeutic community, group analysis, and the socioanalytic research applied to the development of community mental health.

In their book's Foreword the editors point out how

> besides representing a possible way to facilitate the treatment of severe illnesses, institutional clinics may also become a response to ideological and technical excesses that have been so often denounced, in this way allowing that an appropriate balance may be maintained between technical devices, organisation, institution, and community.
>
> (Di Marco & Nosé, 2008)[2]

Such a bridge area connecting external reality with the internal world, and, at the same time, the individual with the organization has been also thoroughly explored by Edgar Schein, one of the most important scholars on organizational psychology, who, although not being a psychoanalyst, in his conception of organizational culture shows a wide concurrence and attunement of thought with psychodynamic approaches. Schein views organizational culture as

> A pattern of shared basic assumptions that the group learned as it solved its problems of external adaptation and internal integration, that has

worked well enough to be considered valid and, therefore, to be taught to new members as the correct way you perceive, think, and feel in relation to those problems.

(Schein, 1985, p. 12)

The originality of Schein is in the way he uses the *clinical method*, both for an analysis of organizational culture and for consulting to organizations (Schein, 1987). Regarding the consultancy work this method reveals its apparent roots in clinical psychology and in helping relationships of a therapeutic nature. When applied to organizational analysis "clinical method" means essentially

- being oriented to the relationship and the working alliance;
- putting an emphasis on wellbeing and the "health" of the system;
- showing sensibility to people's needs (the various stakeholders);
- paying attention to implicit, invisible elements (or, we might say, to "organizational unconscious");
- using emotions and feelings as an explorative instrument (in other words, using "countertransference");
- pursuing aims of organizational change by means of awareness and learning.

All these different approaches – the psychoanalytic thinking, the Tavistock socio-technical and systems psychodynamic model, Hinshelwood's organizational observation, Schein's dynamic perspective on organizational culture, the "institutional clinic" – have with time strongly inspired my way of exploring and working with mental health organizations. One might call such methodology *a clinical theory of organization*, as it relies upon a clinical conceptualization and an institutional practice that show an evident mutual inter-dependency, offering to organizational analysis a perspective more focused on both the complex system dynamics and the individual's emotional needs.

In particular, in the mental health field this methodology can work, so to say, in a "variable geometry" configuration, I mean, it can oscillate between two polarities according to different needs: on one side focusing on *the use of the organization* itself *as a clinical instrument*, namely for the aims of diagnosis, cure and rehabilitation of ill or suffering people (for example, the inmates of a therapeutic community), or, for other helping purposes; on the other side, trying to *employ clinical methods to explore how the organization is functioning*, as in the case of clinical/institutional consultancy offered to psychiatric teams to help them to cope with a change or a problem. These methods, which are mainly oriented at the "physiological" as well as the "pathological" processes inside organizational systems (Kets de Vries and Miller, 1984; Kets de Vries, 2000), are generally concerned with issues such as human relations, authority and leadership, communication, the socio-cultural environment, the emotional climate, myths and symbols, and the pursuit of awareness, job satisfaction and well-being.

From this point of view, a clinical theory of organization does not claim to be able to build universal interpretations to explain the life of institutions, but it merely inquires in depth their underground parts and shadow areas, exploring in particular the emotional and irrational aspects of individual and group behavior within an institution, and the way they influence the functioning of the institution itself: this implies how these factors impact on the institution's capacity to accomplish its primary task, the quality of relationships between members, between them and the organization, between the organization and the external environment, and in the last analysis the people's capacity of working creatively and managing themselves in their role, whether that of leader, follower or consultant.

Clinical and organizational cultures between co-operation and conflict

We must anyway admit that most of the organizational cultures nowadays operating within the business world and the public sector, even in healthcare institutions, are quite distant from clinical approaches developed by scholars such as Schein or the Tavistock researchers. Ostensibly afraid of getting closer to "the human factor" and perhaps vaguely aware of how difficult to recognize, understand and manage it may be, these cultures generally tend to repress it, to deny or minimize its importance through a massive use of splitting and projection. What results from such defensive activities is on the one hand the development of organizational dynamics dominated by mechanization and impersonality, on the other hand an increasing isolation that can disconnect structures from processes, practices and procedures from meanings, roles from persons, and institutional behaviors from underlying emotions.

Splitting and isolation, combined with the enduring myth of the rational nature of the organization, are among the main reasons that can explain why inside the healthcare system (and in general in social institutions) clinical and caring cultures coexist with administrative and managerial ones, usually ignoring each other or, worse still, fighting together, sometimes openly but more often in the shadow, with serious detriment for the quality of provided services and the involved people's wellbeing.

The growing business orientation in the welfare system – that in Italy has been carried out in a quite disharmonious and improvised manner under the pressure of the urgent need to control healthcare expenditure – is an eloquent example of the consequences following the failed integration of the two mentioned cultures. A triumphant managerial logic, essentially bureaucratic in its nature and based on procedures, and the prevailing reasons of accounts and expenditure control led on the one hand to a clinical practice systematically subdued to financial as well as political demands, while on the other hand this logic itself failed to realize a working alliance with clinicians aimed at a wise and responsible administration of resources that we can no longer see as limitless.

Even in mental health services the radical splitting between clinical and organizational cultures – which as said above usually do not talk or listen to each other, are reciprocally distrusting and destructively competing for resources, and sometimes do not even know of one another's existence – tends to reproduce within the different institutional applications giving rise to sets of cascades of splitting and fragmentation phenomena. The result is first a dissociation then an opposition or on the contrary a collusion involving areas, tasks, functions, roles, groups and processes that should instead coordinate themselves working together for a common primary task. This way decisions are made over the head of interested people, while nobody gives clear feedback about outcomes, crucial information is lacking because it gets lost or is jealously kept by someone, but on the other hand what is available is neglected; the center does not know anything about the periphery, and vice versa, who carries out control functions is denied any support, and who is oriented at giving support is careful not to bring about controls that might raise unpopularity and conflict; relevant envious movements spreading around divide administrative from technical staff, leaders from followers, doctors from nurses, hospitals from community services, front-line from back-office. And the whole system, already burdened with so many omnipotent expectations or consensus-hunting politics, becomes haunted by logics of emergency, procedural rigidity, risk avoidance and forced economies.

Such inconsistent and fragmented organizational cultures can only survive – and somehow go on functioning – at heavy emotional cost and provided that a constant split between thought and action is maintained.

The highly hierarchical structure of the healthcare system and a nearly complete lack of significant communication between the strategic top management and the operative first line are the most eloquent evidence of such splitting. Captains need to be left alone on the bridge while they plot their complicated routes, without being disturbed by the noises from the engine room or the stench from the hold, where crews' as well as passengers' anxieties, pain, rage, despair, odors and body fluids, blood, sweat and tears, are getting about. And, conversely, those dwelling in the belly of the ship probably do not want to know of reefs met during the navigation, escaped dangers, impending storms, namely everything that troubles the captain's sleep. But in this way who runs an organization ends up by losing the pulse of its members, their capacities, moods and loyalty; and those who obey "blindly" gradually come to lose their confidence in the leadership and the meaning of what they are doing.

Whenever action and thought do not feed back to each other (about processes and results, but also about the connected emotional experience) no learning cycle is enabled to start, shortcomings and errors fail to be detected and amended tending therefore to worsen or to recur, and in the last analysis a shared experience cannot emerge. The culture of splitting brings about at all levels of the organization waves of unthought and impulsive actions, driven by "basic assumptions," primitive emotions (Bion, 1961; Turquet, 1975; Lawrence, Bain & Gould, 1996), as well as stagnant areas filled with unproductive, inconclusive and self-referential thinking. And when the play gets rough or some accident occurs, then a cloud of projections comes to influence the organizational climate and behavior, so that inability to think, evacuation of guilt and rejection of responsibility are facilitated.

The organization thus loses contact with the reality and its mode of functioning becomes psychotic. The resulting institutional "sleep of the reason" then creates its typical monsters: paranoia (Jaques, 1976), mutual denigration, demoralization (Hinshelwood, 1979), witch hunting and scapegoating (Birchmore, 2000), bullying, mobbing, organizational malaise and burnout (Maslach and Leiter, 1997), perversion (Long, 2008).

During difficult times, containing anxiety and keeping the capacity to think may be felt as risky. And nowadays many organizational cultures, particularly in social and healthcare services, have turned to being risk averse (Sassolas, 2005): fearful, phobic and avoiding, they are afraid of any risk and whenever possible try to get rid of it; or, on the contrary, just as happens to counter-phobic adolescents, tend to deny risks and run to meet them by unawareness and defiance; or even, by avoiding examining their own abilities and responsibilities, convert risk into persecution and lay the blame on someone else.

Within contemporary cultures – from those pretending to rule the financial systems currently adrift to "defensive healthcare" with its procedural obsessions – what is probably occurring is a general flight away from the awareness of psychic life and the complexity of reality, both of which being sources of much anxiety and insecurity, that are already heavily pervading the world and none of the traditional social containers seems able to control any longer.

Mental health is also unavoidably implied in such a drift, and it is just on this "organizational" side that psychoanalysis might offer it a valuable contribution – obviously in co-operation with other disciplines and knowledges. Actually, it could explore what is going on "under the surface" pointing its lenses on a psychiatric institution as a dynamic system of relationships, a container of emotional processes, and a human multi-personal body, without forgetting anyway that it is also a socio-economic and cultural product.

Unfortunately this contribution is still a *work-in-progress*, confined to some diagnostic views and a series of working hypotheses, nothing that may look like an organic and steadily articulated strategy. However, following Hinshelwood's suggestions, it is possible to create, through a psychoanalytically oriented management of supervisions, meetings, leadership decisions, and even everyday life activities, what he simply calls "a reflective space" (Hinshelwood, 1995). In my opinion this is the essential element, although certainly not the only one, to install into the mental health system a solid, enlightened and safe enough "institutional container" that may be enabled to perform its basic transformative task, no matter whether you call it rêverie or alpha function (Bion, 1962), or toilet-breast (Meltzer, 1967): the task of dealing with toxic products of individual as well as organizational psychosis, turning them into added value in terms of awareness and wellbeing (Perini, 2013b).

Notes

1 Translated for this edition.
2 Translated for this edition.

References

Basaglia, F. (Ed.) (1968). *L'istituzione negata*. [The denied institution] Einaudi, Torino.

Basaglia, F. (1984). *Conferenze brasiliane.* [Brazilian lectures] Centro di Documentazione, Pistoia.

Bateman, W. A. (2004). Psychoanalysis and psychiatry: Is there a future? (Editorial), *Acta Psychiatrica Scandinavica, 109*: 161–163.

Bauman, Z. (2004). *Wasted lives: Modernity and its outcast.* Cambridge, UK: Polity Press.

Bion, W. R. (1961). *Experiences in groups.* London: Tavistock.

Bion, W. R. (1962). *Learning from Experience.* London: Heinemann.

Birchmore, T. (2000). Psychodynamics of scapegoating, persecution, bullying. Website, *Shame and Group Psychotherapy,* www.birchmore.org/Psychody namics_of_Scapegoating.pdf

Brill, A. A. (1946). *Lectures on psychoanalytic psychiatry.* New York: A.A. Knopf.

Campoli, G., & Carnaroli, F. (Eds.) (2012). Dibattito su: Psicoanalisi e servizi, quale incontro? [What happens when psychoanalysis and healthcare services meet? A debate at the Italian Psychoanalytic Society]. SPIWeb, www.spi web.it/index.php?option=com_content&view=article&id=2219:dibattito-su-psicoanalisi-e-servizi-psicoanalisi-e-servizi-quale-incontro&catid=256.

Correale, A. (1991). *Il campo istituzionale.* [The institutional field] Borla, Roma.

Correale, A. (2006). *Area traumatica e campo istituzionale.* [Traumatic area and Institutional field] Rome: Borla.

De Martis, D., Petrella, F., & Ambrosi, P. (1987). *Fare e pensare in psichiatria: Relazione e Istituzione.* [Doing and thinking in psychiatry. Relation and Institution]. Milan: R. Cortina.

Di Marco, G., & Nosé, F. (a cura di) (2008). *La clinica istituzionale: Origini, fondamenti, sviluppi* [Institutional clinic: Origin, grounding, developments]. Rovereto: Stella.

Foresti, G., & Rossi Monti, M. (2010). *Esercizi di visioning: Psicoanalisi, psichiatria, istituzioni.* [Visioning exercises: Psychoanalysis, psychiatry, institutions]. Rome: Borla.

Gabbard, G. O. (1990). *Psychodynamic psychiatry in clinical practice.* Washington, DC: American Psychiatric Press.

Hinshelwood, R. D. (1979). Demoralization in the hospital community. *Group Analysis, 11*: 84–93; and in *Thinking about institutions.* London: Jessica Kingsley, 2001.

Hinshelwood, R. D. (1995). Lo spazio riflessivo: Il gruppo come contenitore di psicosi [Reflective space: The group as a container for psychosis]. In A. Correale, C. Neri, & S. Contorni (Eds.) *Fattori terapeutici nei gruppi e nelle istituzioni.* [Therapeutic factors in groups and institutions] *Quaderni di Koinos,* n°2, pp. 29–37. Rome: Borla.

Hinshelwood, R. D., & Skogstad, W. (Eds.) (2000). *Observing organisations: Anxiety, defense, and culture in health care.* London: Routledge.

Jaques, E. (1955). Social systems as defense against persecutory and depressive anxiety. In M. Klein, P. Heimann, & R. Money-Kyrle (Eds.) *New directions in psychoanalysis*. London: Tavistock.

Jaques, E. (1976). *A general theory of bureaucracy*. New York: Halsted.

Kets De Vries, M. F. R. (2000). *Struggling with the demon: Essays on individual and organizational irrationality*. Garden City, NJ: Psychosocial Press.

Kets De Vries, M. F. R., & Miller, D. (1984). *The neurotic organization: Diagnosing and changing counterproductive styles of management*. San Francisco, CA: Jossey-Bass.

Lawrence, W. G., Bain, A., & Gould, L. (1996). The fifth basic assumption. *Free Associations*, 6/1(37): 28–55.

Long, S. D. (2008). *The perverse organisation and its deadly sins*. London: Karnac.

Maslach, C., & Leiter, M. P. (1997). *The truth about burnout: How organizations cause personal stress and what to do about it*. San Francisco, CA: Jossey-Bass.

Meltzer, D. (1967). *The psychoanalytic process*. London: Heinemann.

Menzies, I.E. P. (1959). The functioning of social system as a defence against anxiety: A report on a study of the nursing service of a general hospital. London: Tavistock; and in *Containing anxiety in institutions: Selected essays*. London: Free Association, 1988.

Michels, R. (2015). Psychoanalysis, psychiatry and medicine. Presentation at the IPA Congress, Boston 2015.

Miller, E. J., & Gwynne, G. V. (1972). *A life apart: a pilot study of residential institutions for the physically handicapped and the young chronic sick*. London: Tavistock.

Monnet, J. (1976). *Mémoires*. [Memoirs] Paris: Fayard.

Perini, M. (2013a). Un approccio psicoanalitico alle istituzioni della salute mentale [A psychoanalytic approach to mental health institutions]. *Psiche – Rivista di cultura psicoanalitica*, 1/2013, www.psiche-spi.it/Psiche/indice4.html.

Perini, M. (2013b). *Lavorare con l'ansia. Costi emotivi nelle moderne organizzazioni*. [Working with anxiety. Emotional costs in modern organisations]. Milan: Franco Angeli.

Plakun, E. (2012). Treatment resistance and psychodynamic psychiatry: Concepts psychiatry needs from psychoanalysis. *Psychodynamic Psychiatry*, 40: 183–209.

Racamier, P-C., Diatkine, R., Lebovici, S., & Paumelle, P. et al. (1970). *Le psychanalyste sans divan: La psychanalyse et les institutions de soins psychiatriques*. [The psychoanalyst without his/her couch: Psychoanalysis and mental health institutions]. Paris: Payot.

Sassolas, M. (Ed.) (2005). *L' Eloge du risque dans le soin psychiatrique*. [In praise of the risk in psychiatric care]. Toulouse: Ed. Erès.

Schein, E. H. (1985). *Organizational culture and leadership.* San Francisco, CA: Jossey-Bass.

Schein, E. H. (1987). *Process consultation, Vol. II: Lessons for managers and consultants.* Reading, MA: Addison-Wesley.

Schilder, P. (1951). *Introduction to a psychoanalytic psychiatry,* trans. by Bernard Glueck. New York: Inter. Universities Press.

Turquet, P. (1975). Threats to identity in the large groups. In L. Kreeger (Ed.) *The large group: Dynamics and therapy.* London: Constable.

PART II

The clinical practice
Nosology, diagnoses and treatments

CHAPTER SEVEN

What psychopathology can learn from neuropsychodynamic psychiatry?

A spatiotemporal approach

Heinz Boeker, Peter Hartwich and Georg Northoff

How can we link psychoanalysis, psychopathology and neuroscience? All three disciplines suppose different models. Psychoanalysis focuses on structure and form as well as on psychodynamic and mental mechanisms such as defense mechanisms. Psychiatry and psychopatology focus on symptoms as mental alterations which are most often associated with either cognitive, affective, social, or sensorimotor dysfunction. Finally, neuroscience searches fort the brain's neural activity during various cognitive, affective, social and sensorimotor tasks, e.g. task-evoked activity, and, more recently, investigates the brain's spontaneous or resting state activity. All three seem to employ different presuppositions and concepts that seem to be incompatible with each other.

How can we nevertheless link all three, psychoanalysis, psychopathology and neuroscience, to each other without amalgamating or reducing the former to the latter? For that, we argue, a common framework with commonly shared features is necessary. Based on our own investigations in psychoanalysis/neuroscience (Böker 1999, 2004; Boeker et al., 2000, 2013; Northoff et al., 2007; Northoff, 2011), psychopathology (Northoff, 2016a, 2016b), and neuroscience (Northoff, 2014), we suggest that such common framework consists in spatiotemporal features. By spatiotemporal features we do not mean the observable discrete point in time and space but rather structure, form and relation that as such are virtual and not observable rather than real and observable. We suppose that such spatiotemporal structure enables the description of psychodynamic mechanisms (such as defense mechanisms with introjection as paradigmatic example), psycho-pathology (such as depression as paradigmatic example), and neurosci-ence (such as the relationship between different neural networks within the brain's spontaneous activity as paradigmatic example). We therefore consider psychopathological symptoms in for instance depression as spa-tiotemporal symptoms of altered neuropsychodynamic mechanisms based on the spontaneous activity's spatiotemporal pattern.

Hence to link them we need to find a framework and features common to all three.

"Common currency" between experience and brain

How can we close the gap between experience and brain? Closing this gap is central for psychiatry since we need to understand the processes that transform abnormal neuronal into phenomenal states that psychiatric patients experience in first-person perspective. How can we apprehend these transformative processes, e.g., neuronal-phenomenal transforma-tion? For that we may want to search for a shared overlap or "common currency" between neuronal and phenomenal states that drives the trans-formation of the former into the latter.

The shared overlap or common currency between neuronal and phe-nomenal states, e.g., brain and experience, may consist in spatiotemporal features. On the side of the brain, it is the spontaneous activity (rather than its stimulus-induced or task-evoked activity that may be central in providing or constituting such spatiotemporal structure. The brain's spontaneous activity shows certain spatiotemporal features, a particular spatial and temporal structure in its neural activity that surfaces in and is transformed into phenomenal state, e.g., experience (see Northoff, 2014). One would consequently expect a common, similar or analogous spatio-temporal structure between the brain's spontaneous activity and the phe-nomenal features of experience.

Such common, similar, or analogous spatiotemporal structure between brain and experience amounts to what we describe as "spatiotemporal correspondence." The concept of spatiotemporal correspondence means that the brain's spontaneous activity and the phenomenal features of expe-rience show corresponding or analogous spatial and temporal features: the spatial and temporal configuration or structure of the neural activ-ity in the brain's spontaneous activity surface in the spatial and temporal features within which the contents of experience (such as specific objects or events including body, self and world) are integrated and thus structured and organized. For instance, a recent study of ours demonstrated that private self-consciousness is directly related to the temporal patterns of spontaneous or resting state activity across different frequency ranges (Huang et al., 2016). This suggests that mental features such as self may be rooted in spatiotemporal features of the brain's spontaneous activity. The self as mental feature may then be characterized in spatiotemporal terms, that is, by specific spatiotemporal schemata or structure rather than by cognition of particular contents (cf. Northoff, 2016).

Unlike Biological Psychiatry that focuses on the brain itself independent of its respective ecological context, Neuropsychodynamic Psychiatry emphasizes the integration of experience including the subject of experience within the ecological context of the world. There is continuity between experience and world, with such continuity often assumed to be mediated by the body, e.g., experience of the body as lived body (Northoff & Stanghellini, 2016). Such continuity between subject and world is deemed central for making experience including the first-person perspective itself first and foremost possible.

What exactly is the "common currency" that allows for continuity between experience and brain? The continuity between experience and brain may ultimately be traced to the continuity between world and brain. Let us give an empirical example. Duncan (Duncan et al., 2015) recently demonstrated that early childhood traumatic experience is manifest in adulthood in the spatiotemporal patterns of the brain's spontaneous activity (as indexed by entropy) which, in turn, impacts subsequent stimulus-induced activity in relation to aversive stimuli. The continuity between experience and brain can thus be traced to continuity between world and brain as it is manifest in the spatiotemporal pattern of the latter's spontaneous activity. One may consequently want to speak of "spatiotemporal continuity" between world and brain. The concept of "spatiotemporal continuity" refers to the fact that certain spatial and temporal features are continuous from world to brain as for instance when certain temporal differences in the environment (as between specific stimuli) resurface in the temporal difference of the brain's spontaneous activity. Psychopathological symptoms are conceived primarily in spatiotemporal terms rather than in cognitive (as in Cognitive Psychopathology), phenomenological (as in Phenomenological Psychopathology), affective (as in Affective Psychopathology), or neuronal terms (as in Biological Psychopathology) accordingly.

Three-dimensional neuropsychodynamic model

On the basis of a three-dimensional model encompassing the psychodynamic dimensions defense mechanisms, structure and conflict (cf. Mentzos,
2009), an analogous model was developed on the neuronal level. How can
this original, three-dimensional model of psychic illness be translated into
a neuro-psychodynamic context?

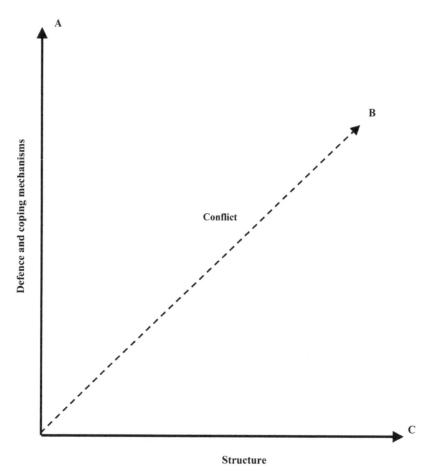

Figure 7.1 Three-dimensional neuro-psychodynamic model of mental illness

Note: A. Neuronal Processing in networks and regions and their interconnectivity; B.
Balance between extrinsic stimuli and intrinsic activity and their spatiotemporal structure;
C. Intrinsic activity and its spatiotemporal structure including the balance between self-
and object-specificity.

First dimension: Defense and compensation

The dimension of defense and compensation describes certain modes of intrinsically predisposed mechanisms for processing extrinsic life-events. In the context of the brain, the following question arises: what intrinsic predispositions does the brain use as mechanisms of defense and compensation?

The intrinsic activity of the brain may be characterized by different neuronal networks, for instance the default mode network, the executive network, the sensorimotor network, the attention network and the language network. These different networks are found in various regions. They are related to one another in a specific way: the default mode network (DMN) may be characterized particularly by the midline structures of the brain, whereas the executive network (EN) covers lateral pre-frontal and parietal regions. Functional imaging studies showed that both these networks are related to one another in a negative way, anti-correlating with one another. For instance, the activation of the DMN leads to a reduced activation of the EN and vice-versa. If the EN is strongly activated, for instance by cognitive processes, the activity in the DMN is reduced and the associated emotions or self-specific processes may be recruited in only a limited way. Because of the balance between different networks, there are predetermined mechanisms, by means of which extrinsic stimuli and tasks may be processed.

From a neuronal perspective, the different modes of defense and compensation of conflicts and/or traumata are analog to the resting state spatiotemporal structures' ability to modulate and adapt as well as to the resting state's self-specific organization.

Two different spatiotemporal axes are important: a longitudinal axis with a very long spatiotemporal scale, possibly reaching back into early childhood. Secondly, the mode of processing of the conflict or trauma depends on the interaction between a certain life-event at a specific time with the spatiotemporal structures of the involved conflicts or traumata. In the future, different mechanisms of neuronal processing that are analog to different mechanisms of defense in a neuropsychodynamic context may be investigated.

Second dimension: Conflict

How can the extrinsic–intrinsic interaction between the external reality and the internal psychic reality be translated into the neuronal context of the brain? The psychic conflict in a neuropsychodynamic perspective may be characterized as an interaction between the intrinsic resting state activity and the extrinsic stimuli, as resting state stimulus interaction or stimulus resting state interaction.

One limitation should be mentioned here: resting stimulus and stimulus resting state interaction describe specific mechanisms resulting from the interaction between intrinsic activity and an extrinsic stimulus. In contrast, conflict in a psychodynamic perspective is more a result than a mechanism. Focusing on the question of whether the resting state stimulus and stimulus resting state interaction and the interaction between intrinsic activity and an extrinsic stimulus result in different psychic conflicts will be highly significant for future neuropsychodynamic research on acute symptoms in psychiatric disorders.

Third dimension: Structure

The dimension of structure focuses on the organization of the personality and the psychic structure of the subject including her/his relationship to the object and to the self (Kernberg, 1975, 1976). Where can such a structure relating to the self and objects be found in the neuronal activity of the brain? The extrinsic activity of the brain focuses on the neuronal activity, which is triggered by certain extrinsic stimuli or tasks. This extrinsic activity should be differentiated from the brain's own activity which develops in the brain independently of extrinsic stimuli. This intrinsic activity is paradoxically called resting state activity – paradox because the brain is not continuously in the resting state. This can be seen for instance during sleep and dreams when the brain is still active despite a lack of certain stimuli or tasks.

The intrinsic activity has a specific spatiotemporal structure, but this should not be understood in a purely physical sense, but rather in a virtual sense or in a statistically based way (for instance like a computer program that remains invisible to a third party). This spatiotemporal structure is most probably constituted by the interaction between different networks and regions and the interaction between different fluctuations in different frequencies (0. 001–180 Hz). Recent studies showed that there is a continuous adaptation of a continuous variability, which is an essential characteristic of the intrinsic activity and its spatiotemporal organization. According to our own studies, it may be hypothesized that this spatiotemporal structure is essential for the transformation of purely neuronal processes into subjective experiences and phenomenal processes. Only if a certain extrinsic stimulus or task is integrated into this intrinsic activity, can something be consciously experienced.

A further analogy between the psychodynamic and the neuronal level concerns the self- and object-specificity. Intrinsic activity and its spatio-temporal structure show a strong overlap with the neuronal processes that underlie self-experience and are also at the same time greatly influenced by the outside world and its extrinsic stimuli. There is much evidence that particularly the midline regions show a strong overlap between intrinsic activity and activity by means of self-related stimuli (for instance by saying one's own name). This is only possible if specific self-related information is decoded by the intrinsic activity and its spatiotemporal structure. On the other hand, neuroimaging studies have shown that the intrinsic activity and its spatiotemporal structure may be strongly influenced by the outside world, especially by stressful life-events. Thus, intrinsic activity and its spatiotemporal structure would appear to fulfill the criteria for self- and object-specificity analogous to the structure in the psychodynamic context.

Neuropsychodynamic psychiatry may further contribute to the development of future diagnostic classification systems focusing on functional mechanisms in psychopathology and their subject-related application. Neuropsychodynamic psychiatry can thus contribute to a better understanding of irregular, turbulent and dynamic processes, which has long been standard practice in scientific models of complex systems.

Depression

Psychodynamics and psychopathology of the self in depression

In view of the development of the variety of psychoanalytic theories of depression (overview in Böker, 1999; Mentzos, 1995, 2009; Böker & Northoff, 2005; Gabbard, 2014), we will focus on the essential dimensions of depression, which are related to Freud's outstanding contribution "Mourning and Melancholia" (Freud, 1917). According to this, the reactivation of earlier experiences of loss in childhood, the introjection of the lost objects in childhood, which are connected with negative emotions, and the current loss of object relations which are connected to the loss of the self, may be described as psychodynamic essentials of depression. The early loss of objects in childhood is part of the bio-psycho-social vulnerability of persons likely to develop a depressive disorder in later life. The fixation on the mental representation of the lost objects involves great psycho-energetic exertion, which Freud compared to an "open wound" taking psychic energy from the self and object representations. This regressive process leads to both the outer world and the self being completely depleted of representations.

Depressed persons develop an increased inner focus and are no longer able to focus on the outer world. This self-focused attention is the focus of perception of interpersonal relationships. This information is derived from sensory perceptions that react to changes in somatic activity (Ingram, 1990). The attention shifts from the exteroceptive sensory system to the interoceptive sensory system, which processes somatic stimuli.

Attribution of negative emotions to one's own self

The self in depression is attributed to negative emotions (failure, guilt, hypochondric fear of illness and death, in some cases connected with depressive delusion). Positive emotions are no longer connected with one's own self. These scrupulous tendencies correlate with the number of former suicide attempts and are risk factors for suicidal behavior.

The cognitive processing of the own self (rumination) increases the depressive mood and develops into an increasingly dysfunctional mechanism of compensation that is connected with the self-focused attention and a repetitive focus of one's own negative emotions (Ingram, 1990; Treynor et al., 2003; Rimes & Watkins, 2005). This increasingly so-called "analytical self-focus" contrasts with the reduced experience-based self-focus ("experiental self-focus").

It may be hypothesized that the increased inward focus in depression corresponds with psychodynamic processes, especially introjections and identification of the self with a lost object. Finally, the significance of the actual loss of objects corresponds with the increased cognitive processing of the self because the cognitive processing no longer focuses on the actual loss, but on the loss of objects with which the self is identified ("decreased environmental focus").

The decoupling of the self in depression

The development of neuropsychodynamic hypotheses of the altered self-reference in depression is based on the investigation of the emotional–cognitive interaction in depressed patients, which focused on the neurophysiological correlates of depressive inhibition and the neurophysiological substrates of negative cognitive schemes and the neuropsychological deficits (overview in Northoff et al., 2002, 2005, 2007; Böker & Northoff, 2005, 2010; Grimm et al., 2008, 2009; Walter et al., 2009; Boeker et al., 2012). To sum up, depression may be characterized by reduced neuronal activity in the left dorsolateral prefrontal cortex and increased activity in the right dorsolateral prefrontal cortex. The neuronal activity in the left dorsolateral prefrontal cortex cannot be modified by emotional valence. The severity of depression correlates with the activity in the right dorsolateral prefrontal cortex. Connected with the reduced deactivation in the pregenual ACC (default mode network), depressed persons cannot shift their attention from themselves to the outside world (Grimm et al., 2008). The degree of helplessness and the severity of depressive symptoms correlate with the reduced deactivation in the PACC and PCC. The signal intensities in different subcortical and cortical midline regions (DMPFC, SACC, precuneus, ventral striatum, DMT) were reduced significantly. On the basis of these empirical results, it may be concluded that the increased negative self-attributions – as typical characteristics of an increased self-focus in depression – may result from altered neuronal activity in subcortical–cortical midline structures in the brain (especially from hyperactivity in the cortical–subcortical midline regions and hypoactivity in the lateral regions).

On the basis of neuropsychological, neurophysiological and neurochemical findings and, as we mentioned, psychodynamic dimensions of depression, neuropsychodynamic hypotheses on the disturbed self-reference in depression were developed and related to psychodynamic and specific neuronal mechanisms of depression.

Increased resting state activity and reactivation of early object loss

The resting state activity in the brain represents the intrinsic activity of the brain and should be differentiated from the brain's activity induced by somatic stimuli or outside stimuli. It may be hypothesized that the empirically validated induced resting state activity in depression is a predisposition for reactivation of early object loss experiences in the subject.

PET-studies in major depression underline the decreased resting state activity especially in the lateral anterior cortical midline regions (PACC, VMPFC, compare Mayberg, 2002, 2003a, b; Phillips et al., 2003). Alterations in neural activity were shown in ventral regions of the so-called default mode network (DML) in depressed patients (reduced deactivation, that is negative BOLD-reactions, compare Greicius et al., 2007; Grimm et al., 2009; Sheline et al., 2009). Furthermore, a translational meta-analysis of resting state studies in depressed patients and in animal models confirm resting state hyperactivity in ventral, cortical midline regions (PACC, VMPFC, Fitzgerald et al., 2007; Drevets et al., 2008; Alcaro et al., 2010; Price & Drevets, 2010).

In contrast to the anterior midline regions, posterior midline regions (PCC, precuneus/cuneus) and the superior temporal gyrus (STG) show hypoactivity in the resting state (Heinzel et al., 2009; Alcaro et al., 2010). The hyperactivity in the anterior midline regions and the hypoactivity in the posterior midline regions result from a disturbed balance between anterior and posterior midline regions in acute depression and a disturbance in the default mode network in depression (Raichle et al., 2001; Buckner et al., 2008).

How can these results be related to psychodynamic mechanisms, especially the reactivation of early loss in childhood? Early traumatization causes alterations in developing processes that may contribute to the development of early immature defense mechanisms (Feinberg, 2011). Traumatization in early childhood was found in a large subgroup of depressed patients (experiences of loss, divorce of parents, physical or sexual abuse, compare Böker, 2000; Nemeroff et al., 2003; Gabbard, 2005). Traumatic life-events may cause biological alterations on the genetic, hormonal or anatomic-structural level (Feder et al. 2009). It may be hypothesized that traumatic life experiences interfere with the development of the VMPC and especially the ventral anterior subcortical–cortical midline regions as an essential part of the default mode network (DMN). Anterior midline regions are especially involved in the processing of the degree of self-reference of different stimuli, whereas the posterior regions are likely to be involved in the processing of social and non-self-related stimuli (Qin & Northoff, 2011).

Furthermore, it may be assumed that early traumatic experience of object loss is associated with the desperate attempt to relate the self to the lost object in order to develop a self-object relationship and to experience the lost object as a self-object. In connection with this, possible hyperactivation, especially in the anterior midline regions, may be induced, which finally contributes to a disbalance in the posterior midline regions.

The retrieval of early traumatic experiences in the context of current experiences of object loss triggers a reactivation of the same neuronal patterns used in the early development of a relationship to the object. In view of the early object loss, depressed patients develop a psychological predisposition to attribute a high degree of self-reference to lost or disappointing objects. Therefore, a neuronal predisposition for the development of hyperactivity in the resting state in anterior midline regions when object loss is experienced in adulthood is induced.

Reduced resting state-stimulus-interaction and introjection in correlation with negative emotions

Resting state–stimulus interaction includes the interaction between two different modes of neural activity: the intrinsic activity of the brain and the stimulus-induced activity (induced by stimuli from the outside world and/or the own body). It may be hypothesized that resting state–stimulus interaction in depression is reduced because of increased resting state activity and that the resting state–stimulus interaction is associated with introjective processes in the interaction between self and the object world connected with negative emotions. Functional activation paradigms (emotional, cognitive) showed dysfunctional activation patterns, especially hyperactivity, in the ventral cortical midline regions in patients with major depression during resting state and emotional stimulation (Elliot et al., 1998, 2002; Mayberg et al., 1999, 2000; Davidson et al., 2003; Canli et al., 2004; Fu et al., 2004). In other brain regions, especially in the reward system (VS/N. accumbens, right and left amygdala), dysfunctional activation patterns were found during positive and/or negative emotional stimulation in MDD (Kumari et al., 2003; Canli et al., 2004; Lawrence et al., 2004; Surguladze et al., 2004). These dysfunctional activation patterns may be interpreted as the neurophysiological basis of the "negative affective bias," that is the focusing of negative emotions that is related to the inability to process positive emotions (Phillips et al., 2003; Mayberg, 2003a, 2003b; Heller et al., 2009; Heinzel et al., 2009; Grimm et al., 2009). The reduced deactivation in cortical–subcortical regions was correlated with the severity of depression and the degree of hopelessness. A direct association between reduced resting state–stimulus interaction and the severity of depression may be assumed (Grimm et al., 2009).

Further studies focused on the biochemical basis of the reduced resting state stimulus interaction. It could be shown that increased resting state activity in the PACC is associated with the concentration of the neurotransmitter glutamate (Northoff et al., 2007; Walter et al., 2009; Alcaro et al., 2010; Sanacora, 2010). A disbalance between neuronal inhibition and excitation in the anterior midline regions in depressed patients may be assumed. The induced resting state activity in the brain inhibits the neuronal processing of stimuli from the outside world. Stimuli from the outside world cannot be related to one's own self or connected with emotional valence. Nevertheless, these psychological mechanisms are still active and are mediated by the induced resting state activity. From a psycho-energetic perspective, the energy that is usually used for the development of self-relatedness and the connection with emotions (emotional valence) is related to early stimuli that are related to early object loss and the induced resting state activity.

The change from current to early stimuli may contribute to an increase of introjective processes in a neuropsychodynamic perspective. The reactivated stimuli from the past are related to the self and negative emotional valence. Stimuli that are connected with early object loss are introjected and related with negative emotions. It may be assumed that this process corresponds with an introjective type of depression (Blatt, 1998) that is characterized by an increased interpersonal relatedness.

Reduced stimulus–resting state interaction and the loss of current object relations

It may be hypothesized that the modulation of the resting state activity by means of stimulus-induced activity and the stimulus–resting state interaction in depression is reduced because of the increased resting state activity. Reduced stimulus–resting state interaction probably leads to dysfunctional development of the neuronal structure and organization that is associated with dysfunctional processing of current experiences of loss. The reduced stimulus–resting state interaction can be seen in three different patterns: first, interoceptive stimuli no longer modify the resting state or baseline activity of the brain (Wiebking et al., 2010); second, exteroceptive stimuli are no longer associated with value and reward (Kumar et al., 2008; Dichter et al., 2009; Pizzagalli et al., 2009; Smoski et al., 2009), and third, exteroceptive stimuli no longer induce or constitute cognitive processing (Goel & Dolan, 2003a, 2003b; Northoff et al., 2004; Grimm et al., 2006).

On the basis of these empirical results, Phillips et al. (2003) and Mayberg (2003a, 2003b) developed a model of the altered reciprocal functional interaction between ventromedial and dorsolateral prefrontal cortex in MDD (model of ventro-dorsal dissociation) where reciprocal modulation of neural activity in depression is reduced because of reduced deactivation in the medial regions and reduced activation of the DLPFC (Grimm et al., 2008; Carhart-Harris et al., 2008). The disturbed modulation of the lateral prefrontal cortical resting state most probably contributes to a reduced stimulus-induced activity triggered by cognitive stimuli. From a neuropsychodynamic perspective, the reduced stimulus resting state activity and the reduced exteroceptive neuronal interaction contributes to a reduced constitution of objects which also results from the reduced emotional valence and reward. Current object relationship experiences lose their emotional significance.

Reduced reciprocal modulation – as the third part of the reduced stimulus resting state interaction – contributes to a reduced activation of cognitive processes by exteroceptive stimuli. In this way, the "object cathexis" is reduced (Carhart-Harris et al., 2008). Furthermore, it may be assumed that the disturbed reciprocal modulation may be an adaptive mechanism by which the depressive self is finally disconnected from the significance of current object relationship experiences. From a psycho-energetic perspective, the result is a further reduction of object cathexis. The depressed patient attempts to constitute and cathect compensational objects from his inner world. The inner world encompasses interoceptive stimuli of the body and cognitive stimuli instead of external objects.

A neuropsychodynamic approach to depression may be summarized as follows: The self and the changes in self-experience are core dimensions in depression and of psychoanalytical theories of depression. The experience of self-related depression can be characterized as the experience of the loss of the self. A mechanism-based approach was developed, focusing on the psychodynamic, psychological and neuronal mechanisms in healthy and depressed persons. On the basis of empirical results concerning emotional–cognitive interaction in depression, neuropsychodynamic hypotheses of the self in depression were developed. First, it may be assumed that the empirically validated increased resting state activity in depression is a pre-disposition for the reactivation of experiences of early loss. The term "experiences of object loss" not only focuses on traumatic relationship experiences, but also encompasses the loss of the self in a significant relationship structure.

Second, it may be hypothesized that the resting state–stimulus interaction in depression is reduced because of the increased resting state activity and that it corresponds with introjective processes of the self in the relationship with objects (correlated with negative emotions).

Third, it may be hypothesized that the modulation of the resting state activity by means of stimulus-induced activity and the stimulus–resting state interaction in depression is reduced because of the increased resting state activity. Dysfunctional development of the neuronal structure and organization results from the reduced stimulus–resting state interaction, as displayed in the processing of current experiences of loss.

The increased resting state activity in depression is especially associated with an increased resting state activity in the default mode network (DMN). By means of this, changes in the complete spatial temporal structure of the intrinsic activity of the brain and the dysbalance between default mode network and executive network (EN) are induced. The reciprocal or negative interaction between DMN and EN is shifted in the direction of the DMN. This disbalance causes an abnormal increase in the internal mental contents, whereas externally oriented actions are decreased. The increased inward focus (with strong ruminations) and a reduced outward focus (with a reduced relationship to the outside world) are core symptoms in depression. The depressed patient is no longer able to differentiate between external stimuli and his/her own self (caused by the increased resting state activity in the DMN which cannot be modified by external stimuli).

The question of why adaptive mechanisms are activated in the disturbed context of the increased resting state activity may be answered by mentioning the central aim of these neuropsychodynamic mechanisms: to maintain at all costs the subjective existence of the self in view of the experienced threat of loss of the self. It is neither lesions nor disturbances of adaptive neuronal mechanisms that generate depressive symptoms, but rather increasingly dysfunctional mechanisms of compensation on the basis of the increased resting state activity.

Some limitations of this neuropsychodynamic approach to depression concern the problem of investigating psychodynamic dimensions of depression by means of operationalized studies (compare Böker & Northoff, 2010; Boeker et al., 2013). Further studies are necessary to validate the increased resting state activity in depression. Possible therapeutic consequences of the neuropsychodynamic approach to depression involve the necessary emotional attunement in psychoanalytic psychotherapy of depressed patients and the adequate timing of therapeutic interventions (confer Stern, 1985; Böker, 2003). The hypotheses that have been developed in the context of the neuropsychodynamic model of depression may be used for more specific psychotherapeutic interventions, aiming at specific mechanisms of compensation and defense, which are related to the increased resting state activity and the disturbed resting state–stimulus interaction. Moreover, in a future "brain-based psychoanalytical psychotherapy" of depression, the enabled processes of development and separation will be based on new experiences in the context of the therapeutic relationship.

Schizophrenia

Today we see the etiopathogenesis of the heterogeneous illness commonly called schizophrenia as a complex interaction between somatic-genetic factors, the psychological environment and the individual personality structure. From the viewpoint of descriptive symptomatology, patients can be differentiated into groups: e.g. a paranoid-hallucinatory group with positive symptoms, such as hallucinations, catatonia and delusions; a non-paranoid group with symptoms such as attention deficit, restricted affect, anhedonia and social withdrawal; a coenesthetic schizophrenia group with aberrant symptoms of the experienced body (Leiberleben), and more groups as well.

The psychopathological symptoms are understandable in a psychological way and also from a somatic perspective. Therefore any treatment should consider both aspects, e.g. psychotherapeutic methods and antipsychotic medication.

In the past, classical psychoanalytical understanding and treatment of the illness by Freud's followers was not successful enough, especially not in severe psychotic inpatients. Our focus is to explain that many results of neuroimaging studies can be seen in relation to psychopathological symptoms and can even lead to new aspects of a neuropsychodynamic/neuropsychoanalytic approach that we call neuropsychodynamic psychotherapy.

From the multitude of studies showing aberrant neuronal functions, only some of the most important ones will be mentioned here. Whitfield-Gabrieli et al. (2009) showed hyperactivity and hyperconnnectivity of the DMN (default mode network) in schizophrenic persons and also in their first-degree relatives. Holt et al. (2011) showed that abnormal anterior-to-posterior midline connectivity is related to self-specificity processing in patients with schizophrenia. An abnormal resting state activity and imbalance between anterior and posterior midline regions (hyperconnectivity) were also observed in many other studies. The resting state spatiotemporal structure does not operate properly in schizophrenics; therefore they are not able to modulate and adapt the pathologically increased hyperconnectivity. The result is that we see a precondition of a possibility of what is to be observed on the phenomenal level: the change or even deterioration of the consciousness of the self. The idea behind this is that the neuronal (= prephenomenal) virtual spatialtemporal structure does not correspond properly with the phenomenal spatial-temporal structure of the self-experience, so that psychoanalytically speaking, schizophrenics suffer from self-fragmentation (Kohut, 1973; Kernberg, 1976 which may be seen as a trans-phenomenal concept. The "trans-phenomenal level targets the implicit yet operative matrix that underlies these anomalous subjective experiences" (Northoff & Duncan, 2016). Our emphasis is to find treatment methods that are able to connect fragments with each other, or in other words that strengthen or even restore the spatiotemporal structure of the self. The bottom-up version would be to influence the spatiotemporal neuronal prerequisite of the possibility of the self experience e.g. with antipsychotic medication, while the top-down version would be to use psychodynamic methods, including e.g. creative therapies and self-mirroring, which may have an additional influence on neuronal activity in CMS (cortical midline structures).

The anticorrelation between DMN and CEN (central executive network, lateral regions of the prefrontal and parietal cortex) in healthy persons is mentioned above. The crucial point in schizophrenics is that the balance of the connectivity between DMN and CEN changes, depending on the amount of the abnormally high resting state activity and hyper-connnectivity in the CMS (Northoff et al., 2004; Vanhaudenhuyse et al., 2011; Wiebking et al., 2014a, b; Northoff, 2015). The result is that external mental content is now no longer reduced when internal mental content is strong and schizophrenics lose the clear distinction between internal and external mental content. Northoff describes this confusion as "self-environment blurring." Psychodynamically speaking, loss of ego-boundary cathexis takes place (Federn, 1958) and the barrier between what is inside and what is outside cannot be distinguished. Also the idea of the schizophrenic "dilemma" between self-relation and object-relation, as referred to by Mentzos (2011), could also apply here.

Depending on whether the accentuation of a disorder is more in the direction of DMN or CEN, we suppose psychopathological symptoms change from attentional dysfunctions (Hartwich, 1980) to delusion and to a strange sense of agency. The connectivity between other regions of the brain, however, should also be taken into account, e.g. orbito-frontal dysfunction and catatonia (Northoff and Boeker, 2003). Some studies demonstrated abnormally high resting state activity in the auditory cortex during auditory hallucinations. This may be related to the DMN and CEN and their relation with the auditory cortex. In the resting state, the

DMN seems to be less connected to the auditory cortex, which, in contrast, is rather strongly connected to CEN. Such disengagement of DMN functional connectivity from auditory cortex and the latter's association with CEN may account for the assignment of an external origin to hallucinated voices, rather than relating them back to an internal origin (Northoff and Qin, 2011).

Robinson et al. (2015) referred to the sense of agency (SoA), which means the self as the subjective experience that oneself is the agent of perception, action, cognition and emotion. German psychopathology called this "Meinhaftigkeit" (Schneider, 1962) and ego-activity (Scharfetter, 1986) which means functioning as a self-directing unity that appears to be disrupted in individuals with schizophrenia. It is hypothesized that, when on the neuronal level the abnormal resting state hyperactivity in medial prefrontal regions as part of the DMN is given, while there is resting state hypoactivity in lateral prefrontal regions as part of the CEN, patients may misattribute the source that generates a stimulus on the phenomenal level. In psychopathology, the corresponding result is the loss of the self-reference of the sense of agency, together with thought insertion, meaning the psychopathological experience that ideas, voices, orders and other influences are forced into the patient's head by some powerful authority from the outside.

Why does the schizophrenic create such symptoms?

When there is a state of losing the ego-boundary and symptoms such as delusion, signs of catatonia or perceptions of coenesthesia etc. are formed, we can ask the question, why do patients create such symptoms?

Ideler (1847, p. 11) was one of the first to attempt psychodynamic interpretations of schizophrenic symptoms: "Psychoses show the stressful effort of consciousness to reorganize the self." He understood delusions as a defense against unbearable situations. Freud, who may have known Ideler's writings, mentioned Schreber's case: "The delusional formation, which we take to be the pathological product, is in reality an attempt at recovery, a process of reconstruction. Such a reconstruction after the catastrophe is successful to a greater or lesser extent" (Freud, 1911, p. 74). Bleuler (1911), Benedetti (1987), Scharfetter (1986), Mentzos (2011) and others followed this line of thought and also regarded psychotic symptoms as compensatory attempts to restructure and reorganize the constitution and construction of self and objects, including self-object differentiation. In a neuropsychodynamic context, these compensatory mechanisms cannot be regarded as defense mechanisms in the proper sense of the term.

Due to the lack of psychological structure and organization, the rather amorphous compensatory mechanisms in psychosis do not reach the level of defense mechanisms in a proper or a narrow sense, and may thus be conceptualized as either "paraconstructions" or defense mechanisms in a wider sense (Hartwich, 2006). In connection with the view of neuronal mechanisms and their different abnormality in various psychiatric diseases, we call many of the symptoms "neuropsychodynamic paraconstructions," which means that their pathogenesis is biological *and* psychodynamic. Therefore the conception of defense mechanisms from only a psychodynamic point of view should be changed because of the direct link between psychodynamic and neuronal mechanisms. Symptoms used to make a diagnosis are seen from this perspective and help create a nosology which is biological and psychodynamic.

We suppose that not only the psyche but also the brain have counter-regulations against the danger of breakdown of the spatiotemporal structure of the self. We see these counter-regulations as very basic and see an analogy with the somatic area. For example, if the body is injured and bleeds, blood immediately coagulates to protect the body. Another example is forming antibodies. We suppose that there are also comparable protection mechanisms in our psyche. This may also be true for our brain on hormonal and neuronal levels. Schizophrenics may use this kind of protection against the danger of the deterioration of the self. Because they are not able to build real reconstructions, they create instead neuropsychodynamic paraconstructions as delusions, catatonic, coenesthetic symptoms etc.

The concept of *neuro-paraconstruction* can be explained using the example of delusion (delusion of persecution, delusion of pregnancy, delusion of jealousy etc.). Our hypothesis is that the disturbed balance between DMN and CEN may be the neuronal precondition that corresponds with the beginning of the confusion between inside and outside experiences. This causes a dangerous insecurity for the consciousness of the self. Depending on the strength of the personality structure, psychic and neuronal systems try to protect the self by creating e.g. delusional ideas that are subsequently followed by an individual delusional system. Such a paraconstruction of delusion is able to strengthen the self in such a way that the patient is not able to question or even give up the new system of his view of the world, because he needs this kind of protection, otherwise the spatiotemporal construction of the self would disintegrate rapidly. This means that therapists should *respect* the neuropsychodynamic paraconstructions as a counter-regulation, which is essential for the patient's stability to survive. This explains the patient's firm hold on the symptoms. Our therapeutic aim is to go beyond the paraconstructions, that means to use methods that, as mentioned above, have conclusive effects and can stabilize the spatiotemporal construction of the self, e.g. "glue" together the self-fragments.

How can we combine neuronal aspects with psychodynamic therapy?

One possible strategy: compensation

Compensation would mean enhancing and increasing neuronal mechanisms that may be able to compensate aberrant connectivity, e.g. with creative therapeutic methods (Arieti, 1976; Hartwich & Fryrear, 2002). When a person is in a state of creativity, enhanced neuronal activity in the temporal and parietal regions can be found, sometimes with a sudden increase of high frequency (summarized by Kandel, 2012). Therapists may be able to strengthen these neuronal activities using therapeutic methods that stimulate and unfold creativity with the help of expressive media such as painting, sculpture, music, movement and poetry. We postulate that such creative therapies could modify the hyperconnnectivity in a positive way. In the future, more specific nuances in creative therapies could be investigated on the basis of neuronal compensation, which refers to the interaction and relation between the phenomenal and neuronal level.

Another compensatory mechanism could involve self-related processing (Northoff, 2011, 2014; Northoff et al., 2009). Neuroimaging studies have demonstrated that words and pictures that are highly related to the individual's self are considered to be more emotional than those that show a rather low degree of self-relatedness. On the neuronal level, a meta-analysis (Northoff et al., 2006) underlines that there is a concentration of neuronal activation in the cortical midline structures, the premotoric and bilateral parietal cortex. Huang et al. (2016) showed that the MPFC region (medial prefrontal cortex) is closely linked to self-related processing.

In psychopathology the mirror phenomenon is well known as "signe du miroir." This was first described by the French psychiatrists Delmas (1929) and Abély (1930). Some schizophrenic patients look in the mirror for hours in order to "find themselves"; this can be interpreted as an "autotherapeutic habit" (Scharfetter, 1986) to stabilize themselves when there is a danger of deterioration. On the phenomenal level and even

on the neuronal level, they may unconsciously use the activation arising from self-related processing. This corresponds with empirical studies about video-mirroring in schizophrenics which showed an increase of
ego-strength in experimental investigations (Hartwich, Lehmkuhl, 1979).
The neuronal activation coming from the self-related processing could
be enhanced using audiovisual mirroring systematically. There may be a
positive influence on the abnormal resting state activity and its imbalance
in interaction by improving the spatiotemporal structure of the self also on
the phenomenal level.

Neuronal aspects of countertransference

Countertransference, especially in the treatment of psychotic patients,
should be given a broader definition.

> This definition serves to attenuate the pejorative connotation of counter-
> transference – unresolved problems in the treater that require treatment –
> and to replace it with a conceptualization that views countertransference
> as a major diagnostic and therapeutic tool that tells the treater a good deal
> about the patient's internal world.
>
> (Gabbard, 2014)

For the therapist working with schizophrenics, the common countertransference is impatience, fear, anger and feelings of distance. Often there is
a countertransference obstacle, because the therapist has to bear the psychotic disintegration of his patient. In this case, he should learn what we
call "chaos-aptitude" (Hartwich, 2007). It may be considered normal that
the therapist wants to protect himself from his own self-fragmentation,
which is why he builds countertransference-resistance. When he becomes
aware of this in his psychodynamic setting, he is more likely to realize the
patient's danger of self-fragmentation at an early stage.

Neuropsychodynamic therapists can benefit by bearing in mind the
imagination of abnormal neuronal events in the brains of their psychotic patients, e.g. hyperconnnectivity and DMN–CEN imbalance. The
danger of their own self-fragmentation will then be reduced. By considering not only the phenomenal, but also the neuronal perspective,
the therapist's paradigm can be changed, resulting in a reduction of his
countertransference-resistance. This being the case, more therapists could
attempt to treat psychotic patients neuropsychodynamically.

Conclusion

Neuropsychodynamic psychiatry bridges the gap between psychoanalysis, psychiatry and neuroscience (cf. Boeker, Hartwich & Northoff, 2017). Neuropsychodynamic psychiatry encompasses a novel approach to psychopathology and its psychodynamic dimensions, namely to perceive psychopathological symptoms in terms of their underlying spatiotemporal features. Spatiotemporal psychopathology assumes correspondence and continuity between the spatial and temporal features of the brain's spontaneous activity on the one hand, and the spatial and temporal structure underlying psychopathological symptoms on the other hand. Such spatiotemporal correspondence has been exemplified by ruminations and the experience of loss of the self in depression.

Further, neuropsychodynamic psychiatry assumes continuity between the spatial and temporal features of the world and those of the brain entailing spatiotemporal continuity. Such spatiotemporal continuity is disrupted, for instance, in schizophrenia, which may be central in constituting hallucinations and delusions.

Neuropsychodynamic psychiatry aims to complement and extend phenomenological psychopathology beyond the phenomenal boundaries of experience and thus towards the brain. Specifically, spatial and temporal features shared by both experience and the brain should correspond with each other; the changes in the spatiotemporal structure of the brain's spontaneous activity are assumed to surface and translate into abnormal spatiotemporal structuring on the phenomenal level of experience, resulting in the various kinds of psychopathological symptoms.

Methodologically, this requires twofold access: the neuropsychodynamic psychiatrist and psychoanalyst needs access to subjects' experience while, at the same time, he requires access to the brain's spontaneous activity, just as the spatiotemporal neuroscientist. This will ultimately enable neuropsychodynamic psychiatry to bridge the gap by providing time and space as a "common currency" between experience and the brain, e.g., by their shared spatiotemporal features.

References

Abély, P. (1930). Le signe du miroir dans les psychoses et plus spécialement dans la démence précoce. *Annales Médico-psychologiques*, *88*: 28–36.

Alcaro, A., Panksepp, J., Witczak, J., Hayes, D. J., & Northoff, G. (2010). Is subcortical-cortical midline activity in depression mediated by glutamate and GABA? A cross-species translational approach. *Neuroscience and Biobehavioral Reviews, 34*: 592–605.

Arieti, S. (1976). *Creativity*. New York: Basic Books.

Benedetti, G. (1987). Psychotherapeutische Behandlungsmethoden. In K. P. Kisker, H. Lauter, J. E. Meier, C. Müller, & E. Strömgen (Eds.), *Psychiatrie der Gegenwart, Bd 4*. Berlin, Heidelberg, New York: Springer.

Blatt, S. J. (1998). Contributions of psychoanalysis to the understanding and treatment of depression. *American Journal of the Psychoanalytic Association, 46*: 723–752.

Bleuler, E. (1911). *Dementia praecox oder Gruppe der Schizophrenien*. Leipzig: Deuticke.

Böker, H. (1999). *Selbstbild und Objektbeziehungen bei Depressionen: Untersuchungen mit der Repertory Grid-Technik und dem Giessen-Test an 139 PatientInnen mit depressiven Erkrankungen*. (Monographien aus dem Gesamtgebiete der Psychiatrie). 329 pp. Darmstadt: Steinkopf-Springer.

Böker, H. (Ed.) (2000). Depression, Manie und schizoaffektive Psychosen: Psychodynamische Theorien, einzelfallorientierte Forschung und Psychotherapie. 433 pp. Giessen: Psychosozial-Verlag. (3rd ed.) 2001.

Boker, H. (2003). Sind Depressionem psychosomatische Erkrankungen? Vierteljahresschr. *Naturforschende Ges. Zür, 148*: 1–16.

Böker, H. (2004). Persons with depression, mania and schizoaffective psychosis: Investigations of cognitive complexity, self-esteem, social perception and object relations by means of the repertory-grid-technique. In B. F. Klapp, J. Jordan, & O. B. Walter (Eds.), *Role repertory grid and body grid: Construct psychological approaches in psychosomatic research* (pp. 119–146). Frankfurt/M: VAS – Verlag für Akademische Schriften. Reihe Klinische Psycholinguistik.

Böker, H., & Northoff, G. (2005). Desymbolisierung in der schweren Depression und das Problem der Hemmung: Ein neuropsychoanalytisches Modell der Störung des emotionalen Selbstbezuges Depressiver. *Psyche Zeitschrift für Psychoanalyse und ihre Anwendungen, 59*: 964–989.

Böker, H., & Northoff, G. (2010). Die Entkopplung des Selbst in der Depression: Empirische Befunde und neuropsychodynamische Hypothesen. *Psyche Zeitschrift für Psychoanalyse und ihre Anwendungen, 64*: 934–976.

Boeker, H., Hell, D., Budischewski, K., Eppel, A., Härtling, F., Rinnert, H., von Schmeling, C., Will, H., Schoeneich, F., & Northoff, G. (2000). Personality and object relations in patients with affective disorders: Idiographic research by means of the repertory grid technique. *Journal of Affective Disorders, 60*(1): 53–59.

Boeker, H., Schulze, J., Richter, A., Nikisch, G., Schuepbach, D., & Grimm S. (2012). Sustained cognitive impairments after clinical recovery of severe depression. *Journal of Nervous and Mental Disease, 200*: 773–776.

Boeker, H., Richter, A., Himmighoffen, H., Ernst, J., Bohleber, L., Hofmann, E., Vetter, J., & Northoff, G. (2013). Essentials of psychoanalytic process and change: How can we investigate the neural effects of psychodynamic psychotherapy in individualised neuro-imaging? *Frontiers in Human Neuroscience, 7*: Article 355.

Boeker, H., Hartwich, P., & Northoff, G. (2018). *Neuropsychodynamic Psychiatry*. New York: Springer.

Buckner, R. L., Andrews-Hanna, J. R., & Schacter, D. L. (2008). The brain's default network: Anatomy, function, and relevance to disease. *Annals of the New York Academy of Science, 1124*: 1–38.

Canli, T., Sivers, H., Thomason, M. E., Whitfield-Gabrieli, S., Gabrieli, J. D., & Gotlib, I. H. (2004). Brain activation to emotional words in depressed vs healthy subjects. *Neuroreport, 15*: 2585–2588.

Carhart-Harris, R. L., Mayberg, H. S., Malizia, A. L., & Nutt, D. (2008). Mourning and melancholia revisited: Correspondences between principles of Freudian metapsychology and empirical findings in neuropsychiatry. *Annals of General Psychiatry, 24*: 7–9.

Davidson, R. J., Irwin, W., Anderle, M. J., & Kalin, N. H. (2003). The neural substrates of affective processing in depressed patients treated with Venlafaxine. *American Journal of Psychiatry, 160*: 64–75.

Delmas, F.A. (1929). Le signe du miroir dans la démence précoce. *Annales Médico-psychologiques, 87*: 227–233.

Dichter, G. S., Felder, J. N., Petty, C., Bizzell, J., Ernst, M., & Smoski, M. J. (2009). The effects of psychotherapy on neural responses to rewards in major depression. *Biological Psychiatry, 66*: 886–897.

Drevets, W. C., Price, J. L., & Furey, M. L. (2008). Brain structural and functional abnormalities in mood disorders: implications for neurocircuitry models of depression. *Brain Structure and Function, 213*: 93–118.

Duncan, N., Hayes, D., & Northhoff, G. (2015). Negative childhood experiences alter a prefrontal-insular-motor cortical network in healthy adults: A preliminary multimodal rsfMRI-fMRI-MRS-dMRI study. *Human Brain Mapping, 36*(11): 4622–4637.

Elliot, R., Sahakian, B. J., Michael, A., Paykel, E. S., & Dolan, R. J. (1998). Abnormal neural response to feedback on planning and guessing tasks in patients with unipolar depression. *Psychological Medicine, 28*: 559–571.

Elliot, R., Rubinsztein, J. S., Sahakian, B. J., & Dolan, R. J. (2002). The neural basis of mood-congruent processing biases in depression. *Archives of General Psychiatry, 59*: 597–604.

Feder, A., Nestler, E., & Charney, D. (2009) Psychobiology and molecular genetics of resilience. *Nature Reviews Neuroscience, 10*: 446–457.

Federn, P. (1958). *Ichpsychologie und die Psychosen*. Frankfurt am Main: Suhrkamp.

Feinberg, T. E. (2011). Neuropathologies of the self: Clinical and anatomical features. *Consciousness and Cognition, 20*: 75–81.

Fitzgerald, P. B., Sritharan, A., Daskalakis, Z. J., de Castella, A. R., Kulkarni, J., & Egan, G. (2007). A functional magnetic resonance imaging study of the effects of low frequency right prefrontal transcranial magnetic stimulation in depression. *Journal of Clinical Psychopharmacology, 27*: 488–492.

Freud, S. (1911). *Psychoanalytic notes on an autobiographical account of a case of paranoia. Standard edition, vol. 12.* London: Hogarth Press.

Freud, S. (1917). *Trauer und Melancholie.* GW X (pp. 427–446). Standard Edition.

Fu, C. H. Y., Williams, S. C. R., Cleare, A. J., Brammer, M. J., Walsh, N. D., Kim, J., Andrew, C. M., Pich, E. M., Williams, P. M., Reed, L. J., Mitterschiffhaler, M. T., Suckling, J., & Bullmore, E. T. (2004). Attenuation of the neural response to sad faces in major depression by antidepressant treatment: A prospective, event-related functional magnetic resonance imaging study. *Archives of General Psychiatry, 61*: 877–889.

Gabbard, G. (2005). *Psychodynamic psychiatry in clinical practice.* Arlington, VA: American Psychiatric Press.

Gabbard, G. O. (2014). *Psychodynamic psychiatry in clinical practice* (5th ed.). Washington DC: American Psychiatric Publishing.

Goel, V., & Dolan, R. J. (2003a). Explaining modulation of reasoning by belief. *Cognition, 87*: 11–22.

Goel, V., & Dolan, R. J. (2003b). Reciprocal neural response within lateral and ventral medial prefrontal cortex during hot and cold reasoning. *Neuroimage, 20*: 2314–2321.

Greicius, M. D, Flores, B. H., Menon, V., Glover, G. H., Solvason H. B., Kenna, H., Reiss, A. L., & Schatzberg, A. F. (2007) Resting-state functional connectivity in major depression: Abnormally increased contributions from subgenual cingulate cortex and thalamus. *Biological Psychiatry, 62*: 429–437.

Grimm, S., Schmidt, C. F., Bermpohl, F., Heinzel, A., Dahlem, Y., Wyss, M., Hell, D., Boesiger, P., Boeker, H., & Northoff, G. (2006). Segregated neural representation of distinct emotion dimensions in the prefrontal cortex: An fMRI study. *NeuroImage, 30*: 325–340.

Grimm, S., Beck, J., Schüpbach, D., Hell, D., Boesiger, P., Bermphol, F., Niehaus, L., Boeker, H., & Northoff, G. (2008). Imbalance between left and right dorsolateral prefrontal cortex in major depression is linked to negative emotional judgment: An fMRI study in severe major depressive disorder. *Biological Psychiatry, 63*: 369–376.

Grimm, S., Ernst, J., Boesiger, P., Schuepbach, D., Hell, D., Boeker, H., & Northoff, G. (2009). Increased self-focus in major depressive disorder is related to neural abnormalities in subcortical midline structures. *Human Brain Mapping, 30*: 2617–2627.

Hartwich, P. (1980). *Schizophrenie und Aufmerksamkeitsstörungen.* Berlin, Heidelberg, New York: Springer.

Hartwich, P. (2006). Schizophrenie. Zur Defekt- und Konfliktinteraktion. In H. Boeker (Ed.) *Psychoanalyse und Psychiatrie* (pp. 159–179). Heidelberg: Springer.

Hartwich, P. (2007). Psychodynamisch orientierte Therapieverfahren bei Schizophrenien. In P. Hartwich, & A. Barocka (Eds.) *Schizophrene Erkrankungen* (pp. 33–98). Sternenfels: Wissenschaft & Praxis.

Hartwich, P., & Lehmkuhl, G. (1979). Audiovisual self-confrontation in schizophrenia. *Archiv für Psychiatrie und Nervenkrankheiten, 227*: 341–351.

Hartwich, P., & Fryrear, J. L. (2002). *Creativity, the third therapeutic principle in psychiatry.* Sternenfels: Wissenschaft & Praxis.

Heller, A. S., Johnstone, T., Shackman, A. J., Light, S. N., Peterson, M. J., Kolden, G. G., Kalin, N. H., & Davidson, R. J. (2009). Reduced capacity to sustain positive emotion in major depression reflects diminished maintenance of fronto-striatal brain activation. *Proceedings of the National Academy of Sciences of the United States of America, 106*: 22445–22450.

Heinzel, A., Grimm, S., Beck, J., Schuepbach, D., Hell, D., Boesiger, P., Boeker, H., & Northoff, G. (2009). Segregated neural representation of psychological and somatic-vegetative symptoms in severe major depression. *Neuroscience Letters, 456*: 49–53.

Holt, D. J., Cassidy, B. S., Andrews-Hanna, J. R., Lee, S. M., Coombs, G., Goff, D. C., Gabrieli, J. D., & Moran, J. M. (2011). An anterior-to-posterior shift in midline cortical activity in schizophrenia during self-reflection. *Biological Psychiatry, 69*: 415–423.

Huang, Z., Obara, N., Davis, H., Pokorny, J., & Northoff, G. (2016). The temporal structure of resting-state brain activity in the medial prefrontal cortex predicts self-consciousness. *Neuropsychologia, 82*: 161–170.

Ideler, K. W. (1847). *Der religiöse Wahnsinn.* Halle: Schwetschke.

Ingram, R. E. (1990). Self-focused attention in clinical disorders: Review and a conceptual model. *Psychological Bulletin, 107*(2): 156–176.

Kandel, E. (2012). *Das Zeitalter der Erkenntnis. Die Erforschung des Unbewussten in der Kunst, Geist und Gehirn von der Wiener Moderne bis heute.* München: Siedler.

Kernberg, O. F. (1975). *Borderline conditions and pathological narcicissm.* New York: Jason Aronson.

Kernberg, O. F. (1976). *Object relations theory and clinical psychoanalysis.* New York: Jason Aronson.

Kohut, H. (1973). *Narzißmus.* Frankfurt am Main: Suhrkamp.

Kumar, P., Waiter, G., Ahearn, T., Milders, M., Reid, I., & Steele, J.D. (2008). Abnormal temporal difference reward-learning signals in major depression. *Brain, 131*: 2084–2093.

Kumari, V., Mitterschiffthaler, M. T., Teasdale, J. D., Malhi, G. S., Brown, R. G., Giampietro, V., Brammer, M. J., Poon, L., Simmons, A., Williams, S. C. R., Checkley, S. A., & Sharma, T. (2003). Neural abnormalities during cognitive generation of affect in Treatment-Resistant depression. *Biological Psychiatry, 54*: 777–791.

Lawrence, N. S., Williams, A. M., Surguladze, S., Giampietro, V., Brammer, M. J., Andrew, C., Frangou, S., Ecker, C., & Phillips, M. J. (2004). Subcortical and ventral prefrontal cortical neural responses to facial expressions distinguish patients with bipolar disorder and major depression. *Biological Psychiatry, 55*: 578–587.

Mayberg, H. (2002). Depression, II: Localization of pathophysiology. *American Journal of Psychiatry, 159*: 1979.

Mayberg, H. S. (2003a). Modulating dysfunctional limbic-cortical circuits in depression: Towards development of brain-based algorithms for diagnosis and optimised treatment. *British Medical Bulletin, 65*: 193–207.

Mayberg H. S. (2003b). Positron emission tomography imaging in depression: A neural systems perspective. *Neuroimaging Clinics of North America, 13*: 805–815.

Mayberg, H. S., Liotti, M., Brannan, S. K., McGinnis, S., Mahurin, R. K., Jerabek, P. A., Silva, J. A., Jekell, J. L., Martin, C. C., Lancaster, J. L., & Fox, P.T. (1999). Reciprocal Limbic-Cortical Function and Negative Mood: Converging PET Findings in Depression and Normal Sadness. *American Journal of Psychiatry, 156*: 675–682.

Mayberg, H. S., Brannan, S. K., Tekell, J. L, Silva, J. A., Mahurin, R. K., McGinnis, S., & Jarabek, P. A. (2000). The metabolic effects of fluoxetine in major depression: Serial changes and relationship to clinical response. *Biological Psychiatry, 48*(8): 830–843.

Mentzos, S. (1995). *Depression und Manie: Psychodynamik und Psychotherapie affektiver Störungen*. Göttingen, Zürich: Vandenhoeck & Ruprecht.

Mentzos, S. (2009). *Lehrbuch der Psychodynamik* (5th ed.). Göttingen: Vandenhoeck & Ruprecht, 1911.

Mentzos, S. (2011). *Lehrbuch der Psychodynamik. Die Variationem der funktionsbezogenen Dynamik Psychotischer Störungen*. Göttingen: Vandenhoek & Ruprecht (7. überarbeitete Auflage, 2015).

Nemeroff, C. B., Heim, C. M., Thase, M. E., Klein, D. N., Rush, A. J., Schatzberg, A. F., Ninan, P. T., McCullough, J. P., Weiss, P. M., Dunner, D. L., Rothbaum, B. O., Kornstein, S., Keitner, G., & Keller, M. B. (2003). Differential responses to psychotherapy versus pharmacotherapy in patients with chronic forms of major depression and childhood trauma. *Proceedings of the National Academy of Sciences of the United States of America, 100*: 14293–14296.

Northoff, G. (2011). *Neuropsychoanalysis in practice*. New York: Oxford University Press.

Northoff, G. (2014). *Unlocking the Brain. Volume II. Consciousness*. New York: Oxford University Press.

Northoff, G. (2015). Is schizophrenia a spatiotemporal disorder of the brain's resting state? *World Psychiatry, 14*(1), 34–35.

Northhof, G. (2016a). Neuroscience and Whitehead I: Neuro-ecological model of brain. *Axiomathes, 26*: 219–252.

Northhoff, G. (2016b). Is the self a higher-order or fundamental function of the brain? The "basis model of self-specificity" and its encoding by brain's spontaneous activity. *Cognitive Neuroscience, 7*(1–4): 203–222.

Northoff, G., & Boeker, H. (2003). Orbitofrontal cortical dysfunction and "sensomotor regression," a combined study of fMRI and personal constructs in catatonia. *Neuropsychoanalysis, 5*: 149–175.

Northoff, G., & Duncan, N. W. (2016). How do abnormalities in the brain's spontaneous activity translate into symptoms in schizophernia? *Progress in Neurobiology*, PMID 27531135 DOI: 10.1016/j.pneurobiol.2016.08.001.

Northoff, G., & Qin, P. (2011). How can the brain's resting state activity generate hallucinations? A "resting state hypothesis" of auditory verbal hallucinations. *Schizophrenia Research, 127*: 202–214.

Northoff, G., & Stanghellini, G. (2016). How to link brain and experience? Spatiotemporal psychopathology of the lived body. *Frontiers in Human Neuroscience, 10*: 172.

Northoff, G., Bogerts, B., Baumgart, F., Leschinger, M. D., von Schmeling, C., Lenz, C., Heinzel, A., Scheich, H., & Boeker, H. (2002). Orbitofrontal cortical dysfunction and "sensori-motor regression": A combined study of fMRI and personal constructs in catatonia. *Neuro-Psychoanalysis, 4*: 149–175.

Northoff, G., Heinzel, A., Bermpohl, F., Niese, R., Pfenning, A., Pascual-Leone, A., & Schlaug, G. (2004). Reciprocal modulation and attenuation in the prefrontal cortex: An fMRI study on emotional-cognitive interaction. *Human Brain Mapping, 21*: 202–212.

Northoff, G., Richter, A., Bermpohl, F., Grimm, S., Martin, E., Marcar, V. L., Wahl, C., Hell, D., & Boeker, H. (2005). NMDA Hypofunction in the posterior cingulate as a model for schizophrenia: An exploratory Ketamine administration study in fMRI. *Schizophrenia Research, 72*(2–3): 235–248.

Northoff, G., Heinzel, A., de Greck, M., Bermpohl, F., Dobrowolny, H., & Panksepp, J. (2006). Self-referential processing in our brain: A meta-analysis of imaging studies on the self. *Neuroimage, 31*: 440–457.

Northoff, G., Walter, M., Schulte, R. F., Beck, J., Dydak, U., Henning, A., Boeker, H., Grimm, S., & Boesiger, P. (2007). Gaba concentrations in the human anterior cingulate cortex predict negative BOLD responses in fMRI. *Nature Neuroscience, 10*: 1515–1517.

Northoff, G., Schneider, F., Rotte, M., Matthiae, C., Tempelmann, C., Wiebking, C., Bermpohl, F., Heinzel, A., Danos, P., Heinze, H.J., Bogerts, B., Walter, M., & Panksepp, J. (2009). Differential parametric modulation of self-relatedness and emotions in different brain regions. *Human Brain Mapping, 30*: 369–382.

Phillips, M. L., Drevets, W. C., Rauch, S. L., & Lane, R. (2003). Neurobiology of emotion perception II: Implications for major psychiatric disorders. *Biological Psychiatry, 54*: 515–528.

Pizzagalli, D. A., Holmes, A. J., Dillon, D. G., Goetz, E. L., Birk, J. L., Bogdan, R., Dougherty, D. D., Iosifescu, D. V., Rauch, S. L., & Fava, M. (2009). Reduced caudate and nucleus accumbens response to rewards in unmedicated individuals with major depressive disorder. *American Journal of Psychiatry, 166*: 702–710.

Price, J. L., & Drevets, W. C. (2010). Neurocircuitry of mood disorders. *Neuropsychopharmacology, 35*: 192–216.

Qin, P., & Northoff, G. (2011). How is our self related to midline regions and the default-mode network? *NeuroImage, 57*: 1221–1233.

Raichle, M. E., MacLeod, A. M., Snyder, A. Z., Powers, W. J., Gusnard, D. A., & Shulman, G. L. (2001). A default mode of brain function. *Proceedings of the National Academy of Sciences of the United States of America, 98*: 676–682.

Rimes, K. A., & Watkins, E. (2005). The effects of self-focused rumination on global negative self-judgments in depression. *Behavior Research and Therapy, 43*: 1673–1681.

Robinson, J. J. D., Wagner, N. F., & Northoff, G. (2015). Is the sense of agency in schizophrenia influenced by resting-state variation in self-referential regions of the brain? *Schizophrenia Bulletin, 42*: 270–276.

Sanacora, G. (2010). Cortical inhibition, gamma-aminobutyric acid, and major depression: There is plenty of smoke but is there fire? *Biological Psychiatry, 67*: 397–398.

Scharfetter, C. (1986). *Schizophrene Menschen* (2nd ed.). Münich: Urban & Schwarzenberg.

Schneider, K. (1962). *Klinische Psychopathologie* (6th ed.). Stuttgart: Thieme.

Sheline, Y. I., Barch, D. M., Price, J. L., Rundle, M. M., Vaishnavi, S. N., Snyder, A. Z., Mintun, M. A., Wang, S., Coalson, R. S., & Raichle, M. E. (2009). The default mode network and self-referential processes in depression. *Proceedings of the National Academy of Sciences of the United States of America, 106*: 1942–1947.

Smoski, M. J., Felder, J., Bizzell, J., Green, S. R., Ernst, M., Lynch, T.R., & Dichter, G. S. (2009). fMRI of alterations in reward selection, anticipation, and feedback in major depressive disorder. *Journal of Affective Disorders,* *118*: 69–78.

Stern, D. N. (1985). *The interpersonal world of the infant.* New York: Basic Books.

Surguladze, S. A., Young, A. W., Senior, C., Brébion, G., Travis, M., & Phillips, M. J. (2004). Recognition accuracy and response bias to happy and sad facial expressions in patients with major depression. *Neuropsychology, 18*: 212–218.

Treynor, W., Gonzalez, R., & Nolen-Hoeksema, S. (2003). Rumination reconsidered: A psychometric analysis. *Cognitive Therapy and Research, 27*: 247–259.

Vanhaudenhuyse, A., Demertzi, A., Schabus, M., Noirhomme, Q., Bredart, S., Boly, M., Phillips, C., Soddu, A., Luxen, A., Moonen, G., & Laureys, S. (2011). Two distinct neuronal networks mediate the awareness of environment and of self. *Journal of Cognitive Neuroscience, 23*: 570–578.

Walter, M., Henning, A., Grimm, S., Schulte, R. F., Beck, J., Dydak, U., Schnepf, B., Boeker, H., Boesiger, P., & Northoff, G. (2009). The relationship between aberrant neuronal activation in the pregenual anterior cingulate, altered glutamatergic metabolism and anhedonia in major depression. *Archives of General Psychiatry, 66*: 478–486.

Whitfield-Gabrieli, S., Thermenos, H. W., Milanovic, S., Tsuang, M. T., Faraone, S. V., McCarley, R. W., Shenton, M. E., Green, A. I., Nieto-Castanon, A., LaViolette, P., Wojcik, J., Gabrieli, J. D., & Seidman, L. J. (2009). Hyperactivity and hyperconnectivity of the default network in schizophrenia and in first-degree relatives of persons with schizophrenia. *National Academy of Sciences, 106*: 1279–1284.

Wiebking, C., Bauer, A., de Greck, M., Duncan, N. W., Tempelmann, C., & Northoff, G. (2010). Abnormal body perception and neural activity in the insula in depression: an fMRI study of the depressed "material me." *World Journal of Biological Psychiatry, 11*: 538–549.

Wiebking, C., Duncan, N. W., Tiret, B., Hayes, D. J., Marjańska, M., Doyon, J., Bajbouj, M., & Northoff, G. (2014a). GABA in the insula: A predictor of the neural response to interoceptive awareness. *Neuroimage, 86*: 10–18.

Wiebking, C., Duncan, N. W., Qin, P., Hayes, D. J., Lyttelton, O., Gravel, P., Verhaeghe, J., Kostikov, A. P., Schirrmacher, R., Reader, A. J., Bajbouj, M., & Northoff, G. (2014b). External awareness and GABA: A multimodal imaging study combining fMRI and [18F]-flumazenil-PET. *Human Brain Mapping, 35*: 173–184.

CHAPTER EIGHT

Reflections on psychoanalytic supervision changes in psychiatry

Stefano Bolognini

L ike several other colleagues, I belong to that category of analysts who began and had been primarily educated as psychiatrists (in my case, in several institutional structures: Psychiatric Hospital, Day Hospital, Territorial Equipes); for more than 30 years now, I have maintained a constant connection with that professional area, working as a supervisor of psychiatric *équipes*: a task shared by a large number of psychoanalysts all over the world.

I recognize – again, like many of us – that I would have become a very different psychoanalyst had I not gained this experience in the Mental Health Service; had I not learned so much from other psychiatrists, from psychologists and from the nursing staff working there; and, above all, had I not clinically got in touch with those wasted states of Self and with those seriously regressive and dissociated levels of mental life which only in Psychiatry can be closely and deeply experienced, studied and treated, together with other competent colleagues.

So, I am officially acknowledging here the educational debt I owe to the psychiatric school and its related environment.

I think I can also say that psychiatry, in turn, would not be what it is today, had it not encountered psychoanalytic thinking and especially the psychoanalysts' way of being and working institutionally: even in the harshest and most ideologically opposed environments, as well as in services that are more structured in an integralistically pharmacological sense, an inevitable cultural osmosis has nonetheless occurred over the past decades.

It seems to me that, in any case, much of what is inherently "post-analytic" is passed from psychoanalysis to psychiatry, with the effect of contributing towards humanizing professional practices and vision, even if this is not always officially recognized, and at times can even be imitative and disregardful.

For many decades now in psychiatry, the specific contribution most commonly requested from psychoanalysts is supervision of psychiatric *équipes*.

A number of experienced psychoanalysts are asked for supervisions in the Mental Health Service sectors in many countries today, even if this often happens in an unofficial and institutionally conflictual way.

It should be clear that the work of the supervisors there is not aimed at planning the classical psychoanalytic treatment of patients, but mainly at working through and improving the emotional environment of the psychiatric *équipes*, which are generally affected by the overwhelming and confusing resonance of pathological impacts and influences generated in the institutional field.

The mental health field is subject to substantial tensions and problems, such as: a disinclination within the social context, and sometimes on the part of the operators themselves, to recognize, tolerate and process the psychic pain underlying the pathology; to respect with humanity the relational incapacity of individuals and families; to take responsibility for long-term treatments and patient–therapist interdependencies that are very often heavy to bear over time, on both sides.

This work involves using the psychoanalytic view of the human mind, of the specific person, of the group he/she belongs to and of the therapeutic relationship, in order to help the operators to work in a very different way from the psychic "non-working" by which many individuals and groups tend to unconsciously defend themselves from anxiety (mainly to avoid coming into contact with their own feelings, and/or those of others).

On the whole, it is a challenging and ambitious task in a difficult field.

Nevertheless, for decades, analysts in many countries have been collaborating with psychiatric *équipes* by intensively exploring and sharing their direct experiences and contacts with their patients and with their serious, dramatic, sometimes mysterious or bizarre pathologies, as well as with the context that hosts their consultations, hospitalizations and treatments.

The main overarching goal of this work is to "*give sense to what may seem senseless*" in the daily interaction with their patients, when possible, and to improve the "*liveability*" of the interpsychic institutional environment.

The extent to which supervisions have contributed, throughout all these years, towards making the psychiatric environments more liveable, towards keeping the operators psychically alive and sensitive, towards reopening perspectives and lowering the levels of tension and impenetrability of so many patients, is clear to all those who for years have sat down together in a room to talk constructively about clinical work, periodically and patiently, resonating together in the face of more or less sustainable or disorganized stories and thoughts shared within the work groups.

A problematic landscape

It is almost impossible to describe in uniform terms the history of the psychoanalytic practice of supervision in the Mental Health Services all over the world: each country has its own history, related to the diffusion of psychoanalysis in its territory, and to the specific relationship between local psychoanalysts and the psychiatric community.

Generally speaking, one could say that in the majority of countries the interaction between the two areas has been based more on personal links between individuals than on inter-institutional agreements: rarely have psychoanalytic institutes or societies been officially consulted for an institutional supervision.

The previous personal analytic treatment of some (or many) psychiatrists was the real starting point of several interdisciplinary collaborations, while the university, as the third pole of an ideal institutional triangle (Mental Health Services, Psychoanalytic Institutes and University) rarely promoted such initiatives, unless, of course, a psychoanalyst also happened to be an academic professor.

As everyone knows, there was a very different history in North America after the Second World War, when the psychoanalytic influence on Psychiatry flourished, with a number of famous analysts appointed as Clinic and Faculty Chiefs in the US.

This trend is in dramatic decline today.

Also in Argentina the psychoanalytic presence and influence in public institutions was very strong, thanks to the capillary analytic activity and the cultural trend in that country before and after the dictatorial régime. Now, there is a more encouraging trend there, thanks to the immense cultural popularity of psychoanalysis which is a peculiarity of that country.

In Europe the general situation was more complex, even if the enormous prestige of the British psychoanalytic school deeply influenced the feasibility of a psychoanalytic approach in the hospitals and therapeutic communities; one can cite, as a macroscopic consequence, how the general custom of separating mothers and children in the hospitals progressively changed, mainly after remarks by psychoanalysts, with further resonance and consequences across the whole of Europe. There was a relevant connection of psychoanalytic institutions such as the Tavistock Clinic or the Hampstead with the medical world, supported by the communication skills of professionals such as Balint, Winnicott, Bowlby, Bion and others.

In other areas, such as Italy, France, Switzerland, Germany and Scandinavia, the personal prestige of individual psychoanalysts facilitated their call-up by hospitals and services for team supervisions.

However, the aim of this paper is not to illustrate the history and geography of the general influence of Psychoanalysis on Medicine and on Psychiatry.

My specific interest lies, instead, in describing how psychoanalytic supervision has changed over the years, from its beginnings as the intervention of a super-expert in an under-cultured professional *équipe*, reaching a whole new level of collaboration today between two different professional competences, combining supervision and inter-vision processes with a group dynamics perspective.

The need and the consequent request for help

The request for psychoanalytically oriented intervention and help in the Mental Health Service is usually expressed by one or more members of a professional team who experience some degree of discomfort with their conditions at work. Sometimes the request comes from the chief of the team, sometimes from the other members.

The analysis of the initial request is extremely important, since the reasons for calling on a psychoanalyst to collaborate can vary enormously and can imply very different underlying processes.

The most appropriate motivation is an honestly expressed need of the team to be helped in the perception, representation, containment, mentalization and metabolization processes which psychiatric work, with its frequently unbearable rhythms and traumatic intensity, imposes on the staff in an overly limited or condensed way.

In such cases, the supervision becomes the only time and place where "normal enough" steps can be taken in the exploration and revisitation of unelaborated individual and group experiences.

The staff members can evoke, describe, share and analyse more in depth institutional occurrences and processes that had previously been bypassed and that remained to occupy the team in a disturbing way, without any real elaboration.

In other cases, however, the secret source of the request for an intervention of a psychoanalyst is much less benign in its deep motivation: i.e., when a part of the team deeply and implicitly asks for the engagement of a "counter-chief", of an antagonist of a contested official leader of the Service, and a conflictual, divisive development will probably take place, if the psychoanalyst doesn't realize this kind of unconscious plan is underway.

On the other hand, a similar motivation could derive from a Service chief's need to present a strong new ally (a respected "friend or brother-like" psychoanalyst) to put a stop to a possible rebellion against him by part of the staff; I am deliberately mentioning here these unpleasant and de-idealizing cases in order to facilitate a realistic evaluation of the different situations where a supervision can be requested.

Another problematic situation may arise if the *équipe* includes professional competitors of the analyst, who could, consciously or unconsciously, attack and boycott his role and work. Idealization of the analyst's status, rivalry and envy, oedipal and pre-oedipal fantasies can create serious transferential obstacles to collaboration inside the team.

On the other hand, the supervisor has to constantly monitor his/her countertransference and his/her illusions and ambition.

After 30 years of supervision practice in the public services, I can say that the narcissistic illusion of the psychoanalyst, who may initially delude him/herself to be a sort of "deus ex machina", has to be substantially reduced: the call from a team for supervision is a potentially powerful narcissistic temptation for any analyst, whose grandiosity and need for valorization could be subtly excited by the role (= *one* individual *for many* dependent people . . .) and by the supposed, gratifying recognition of his/her competence, whereas the initial motivations for such a request could be, frankly, far less romantic.

Understanding the real source and motivation behind a supervision request can be the first, fundamental step for initiating a fruitful collaboration.

Who is the official customer? And who is the real one?

This is a fundamental question, since in many countries supervisions are administratively registered and officially paid for by the National Health Systems, while in other countries they frequently appear to be unofficial and sometimes almost secret, more or less as if the team that requested the supervisions should behave like a private patient, needing some confidentiality.

The effects of the institutional supervision

I have no hesitation in confirming that this profound, continuous and extensive (albeit unacclaimed) work within the *équipes*, carried forward for decades with such dedication by analysts and psychiatrists in joint collaboration, has contributed to bringing about considerable changes in psychiatry.

There have been internal changes among doctors, psychologists, social workers, and especially the nursing staff, who are now able in many cases to think, to feel, to communicate and to interact with each other and with their patients by elaborating fantasies and emotional states that were previously unthinkable (or at least unmentionable), in a process of gradual humanization and familiarization with the inner world and its most perturbing paths.

On the whole, the mental activity of an *équipe* bears many similarities to the functioning of the individual mind.

By this I mean that, like individuals, working groups also encounter natural and foreseeable difficulties in maintaining a functioning activity of thought when that thought has to confront internal and external realities that produce distress or pain.

Just as an individual defends him/herself from contact with distress and pain by not thinking, in the same way psychiatric *équipes* defend themselves – classically – by not creating circumstances in which an activity of thought is likely to develop.

For this basic reason the *équipe* meeting and the supervision are activities desired by all from a cultural point of view, but are in fact very difficult to maintain on a regular basis and to render physiological in institutional life.

It is well known that many experiences of supervision start out at full speed with a following wind, only to falter in hopeless patches of dead calm before finally petering out in a relatively short time under some administrative pretext.

I therefore consider it a sign of the *équipe*'s mental health if they are able to work under supervision with good continuity: just as it is a positive sign, in an individual psychotherapeutic treatment, when the patient is sufficiently able to keep to the rhythm of the sessions, that is, the contact not only with the therapist, but above all with her/himself.

Being there, working together, thinking together, listening and associating are not obvious activities: the fact that an *équipe* manages – albeit conflictually – to maintain a good continuity in this group work, is an elementary but essential indicator of its functional state.

The "group mind" can falter from time to time or take breaks for a diversionary digression, but it is important that it is able, for a sufficient time, to *"take care of the object"*, that is, the patient and the therapeutic relationship.

This characterizes a working group; this basic parameter is fundamental and should be monitored as a functional indicator.

The moments of (albeit necessary) narcissistic withdrawal from the object and the interruptions to the supervision session due to official causes (typical of every psychiatric facility: administrative reasons, service calls, more or less compelling emergencies) are also substantial indicators.

When the group mind "is there" and works, the group agrees to explore the experience, to face the contact with what is painful, with what seems to make absolutely no sense and what did not go as hoped, with what not everyone agrees on and what some would prefer not to think about.

It is there that you see the quality, expertise and experience of a specialist *équipe*.

This work can have a direct impact on the management of the pharmacological aspects of treatment, but also and above all on the relational strategies to be adopted with the patient, and on the experience of the operators, whose attitude towards the patient is usually different, once the less comprehensible elements of the relationship have been worked through.

Technical notes

In essence, the contribution of psychoanalysis to groups working in the institutional environment today has neither a Super-Ego style (= *"this is the way it should – or shouldn't – be done!"*), nor a narcissistic oracle style (= *"the analyst-guru"*): instead its contribution is creative and sometimes reparative, cultured and patient, based on a shared construction of the sense and discovery of the experience, the fruitful germination of thought under initially arduous conditions, and the transformation of the unthinkable into the *"at least partially thinkable and communicable"*.

Above all, I would say that we have moved progressively *from "supervision" to "inter-vision"*.

This corresponds to the contemporary evolution in analytic technique towards a search for inter-psychic levels facilitating exchanges (between two minds, in analysis) and internal processes (inside and among the different levels of the same individual mind; in this case, a group mind).

The supervisor acts (at least *also*) as a proactive factor in the mental flow of associations, emotions, representations, memories, fantasies and elaborative thoughts produced by the group.

Exactly like in an individual treatment, the direct interpretive activity of the supervisor on the presented clinical material is neither the only nor the main work: the main object to focus on is the way the group feels, works, maintains its capacity to think or not think, and allows its members to cohabit and to cooperate.

This "work in progress" is another step forward in the fight against the alienation of thought and feeling in institutions; and our expectation is that these shared experiences can help young people working in the Mental Health field to understand that there is a psychiatry that espouses psychoanalysis without imitating it, but also without fearing it; and vice versa.

How supervision has changed

More specifically, supervision has changed exactly as psychoanalysis changed during these decades.

At the beginning, the analyst was mainly a *"sujet supposée savoir"*: knowing the psychoanalytic theory and clinic, he was expected to bring to the psychiatric team an interpretive key for disclosing the unconscious meaning of the patient's mind and behaviour, accordingly with the current main streams of the psychoanalytic trend.

The very initial stages of the psychoanalytic supervision, as I had the opportunity to reconstruct from memories of older colleagues, were based, frankly, on partial equivalents of "lessons": the analyst received a clinical presentation (usually from one of the youngest colleagues), and after some further investigation the supervisor framed the case into a conceptual interpretative area, aimed at clarifying an official "psychoana-lytic vision" on the presented issues.

This procedure – quite infantilizing, initially reassuring but then usu-ally boring, near to the saturation point and conclusive in itself – declined rapidly, because of its undeniable infertility.

The further evolution in supervision technique recalls the famous proverb usually attributed to Confucius: "Give a man a fish, and you feed him for a day. Teach a man to fish, and you feed him for a lifetime."

The academic lesson-like explanatory supervision was equivalent to "giving a fish for one day"; the *équipes* in difficulty needed something else.

Year by year, the supervision technique became increasingly dynamic and based on interlocution between the expert and the working team, even if the spotlight still focused on the psychoanalyst, who honestly brought his personal theoretical "credo" inside the Service group mind.

So, for years, in the Freudian perspective the many libidinal phases, their fixations and styles, the castration anxieties and Oedipal conflicts could be highlighted in the institutional context, both regarding the patient and their caregivers.

In a Kleinian milieu, the split parts which projectively affected the clinical scene and the groupal functioning had been systematically inves-tigated, reducing their fragmentation and projection, and possibly re-introjected and integrated.

In a more Winnicottian atmosphere, the capacity of the team for hold-ing function and the utilization of intermediate spaces between Self and Not-Self could more specifically have been co-experienced and explored by the supervising analyst.

In a Bionian view, the enrichment of the possibly poor and traumatic elements presented, via a reverie function in an actively creative mental container (the analyst's mind) was supposed to be a main transforma-tional factor.

However, what I want to underline here is that, even after the natural decadence of the "lesson-like" supervisions, for a long time the protago-nism of the psychoanalyst still remained central and crucial, both in the expectations of the team and in the personal style of the supervising ana-lyst her/himself.

Basically, the success of a psychoanalytic supervision in a public Ser-vice seemed to depend primarily on the more or less impacting capacity and talent of the supervisor in suggesting new points of view and new interpretations.

I remember with pleasure some unforgettable, absolutely brilliant contributions by highly respected analysts (from Italy and also from other countries) on clinical materials during supervisions at my Service, and I can say their words remain engraved in my memory.

Nevertheless, today I can also say that their performances sounded more like personal VIRTUOSITIES than part of an evolutionary process of the working team.

Benefits of institutional supervision

I have no doubt, based on my experience and that of many colleagues, that such a substantial commitment of resources and financing can be useful and meaningful for the fate of patients and can also constitute a form of worthwhile investment for the community.

This is true in general, but it is even more so in the case of young patients: besides the obvious and primary aspect of individual suffering, their pathology, at such a "pivotal" age, can be the prelude to a progressive psychiatrization.

In many cases, supervision does not at all revolutionize the basic structural difficulties of the patients treated by the *équipe*, but very often it changes the level of intensity, relative comprehensibility and subsequent containability of the pathological aspects.

The management of inpatient or outpatient care, and subsequently that in the family context or in other facilities, can be configured with improved understanding and with the hope of passing through the further turbulences in more liveable conditions.

Those who work in this field can be helped to develop, through supervision/inter-vision, a very realistic sense of the importance of small measures of progress and the ability to pass through moments of crisis, advancements and setbacks, ruptures and recompositions, like steps in a process that does not lead to any miraculous events; yet, the small daily transformations are the real testing ground for the work being done, and take on a very special significance, since they can powerfully influence whether an individual takes one path rather than another in life, in their affects and in the positive or negative developments of their underlying pathology.

The équipe as a clinical theatre

Another aspect of the high level of specificity involved in institutional supervision work is the gradual realization, on the part of the operators, of the roles they play (sometimes voluntarily and knowingly, sometimes not) in the shared scene of daily cohabitation with patients.

Factors such as the regularity of the meetings, the continuity of the *setting* and the intensity of the cohabitation in residential, semi-residential or brief hospitalization, while offering an opportunity for dialogue, especially with nurses, also facilitate and accentuate the onset of multiple transference.

Soon enough the patients determine the true characteristics of the operators, including those that may be less obvious at first, and they add their projections, instinctively recreating internal and external scenarios that implicate the care providers beyond their preconstituted intentions and their theoretical notions.

Supervision can progressively highlight some typical forms of transference, enabling them to be recognized and possibly used in a somewhat conscious way.

For example, the primary nature of the atmosphere surrounding a form of intimacy attuned to sounds and rhythms, in which the generally maternal characteristics of the therapeutic environment were quickly invested and used with high levels of regression; the natural inclination of some young and dynamic operators to represent a sort of "expert and competent older brother", vitalizing compared to faint or inconsistent internal objects, and at the same time capable of counterposing a valid limiting barrier to the demands of omnipotence and aggressive drives that certain subject patients fear are uncontainable; the potential parental roles of health professionals who are in charge of regulating the pace, duration and mode of hospitalization, as well as assigning some management roles, while faced with parental figures who are sometimes insufficient and incapable of modulating basic relational functions.

In a supervision some of these transference currents can take on substance, colour and comprehensibility, in a more appropriate and productive way for the *équipe* members, by identifying the deep meaning of some of their phantasmatic investments, or by simply making them more aware of "what was brewing" in a certain period.

What is certain is that an *équipe* that is articulated and varied in its composition (both in terms of professional skills and, if you will, the "characters" that make it up) offers a potentially very wide range of transference options, of which the patient's subjective scenario can take advantage; and that the importance of the *casting*, in this complex type of care, is by no means negligible, indeed it constitutes a technical factor in itself.

On many occasions I have had the chance to appreciate the flexible, intelligent, serene (and sometimes even witty) way in which some operators have been able to recognize certain transference and countertransference configurations underway, without shrugging them off prematurely and, instead, preparing with patience and mutual support to "play" them with the patient: in this way, they did not shy away from these relational opportunities that often revealed themselves to be the most important factor in effecting significant changes in the field.

CHAPTER NINE

The person with the diagnosis

Glen O. Gabbard

When departments of psychiatry in academic settings were chaired by psychoanalysts, the concept of psychiatric diagnosis involved an understanding of who the patient was. In our contemporary era, when psychoanalysts are rarely found in academic leadership positions, psychiatric diagnosis in some cases may be relegated to a 15 minute interview and a symptom check list. In some centers the interview is enhanced by genomic data, brain scanning, and laboratory tests that will determine what medications are likely to be most effective based on the patients' genetic characteristics. One of the unfortunate casualties of this approach to psychiatric diagnosis is that the *person* with the illness is not considered as a central feature of diagnostic investigation. Hippocrates is reported to have said centuries ago, "It's more important to know what sort of person has a disease than to know what sort of disease a person has." Indeed, as the quotation implies, the personhood of the patient is seen as essential to medicine in general, not only to psychiatry.

It is ironic that the phrase *personalized medicine* now is often associated with genomic characteristics rather than an understanding of the person. To be sure, a backlash has occurred in response to this reductive approach to medical and psychiatric diagnosis. Horowitz et al. (2013) point out that even in nonpsychiatric illnesses, such as cardiovascular disease, such factors as diet, behavior, stress, and culture may be far more relevant than genetic features in determining risk. They have argued for a shift of emphasis from genomics to personal attributes of the patients and their environments. Hence, they view the term "personalized medicine" as a misnomer. After all, genomic expression is highly influenced by environment. Experience leads to the laying down of neural networks that become the basis of self-image and expectations of how others will behave (Gabbard 2014). Representations of people, objects, and situations are stored in the brain in the matrix of connections, i.e., the synapses. They serve as ghostly figures of self and other that haunt individuals throughout their lives. As bioethicist Alex Mauron (2001) has pointed out, personal identity is not necessarily overlapping with genomic identity. Monozygotic twins with identical genomes may be highly distinct individuals.

Hence an essential perspective that psychoanalytic thinking brings to the training of psychiatrists, one that must never be lost, is that we are diagnosing persons, not simply illnesses. While the official diagnostic nomenclature of psychiatry has a role to play and consists of many valid diagnoses, that construct alone is insufficient to understand the person and inform the treatment that follows from the diagnosis.

The search for the "person"

In the interest of simplifying complexity, we are prone to think of the *person* as a synonym with the *self*. However, as we shall see, the reduction of the notion of person to the concept of self is facile but not accurate. As philosophers such as Strawson (2009) have pointed out, the term "self" is embedded in a context that involves philosophical, religious, psychological, and psychiatric perspectives that are heavily theory-driven and extremely diverse. In psychoanalytic thinking, for example, the notion of self has been used to indicate an intrapsychic representation as well as a structure that includes subjective experience or personal agency (Guntrip 1968, Kernberg 1982, Sutherland 1980). One of the central challenges in using the concept of self is that it is both subject and object. In the following sentence, "I think of myself," there is the self as the phenomenal "I" of philosophy and self as representation. These two concepts of self are combined in one sentence that illustrates both the subject and the object roles of the self. We can certainly not limit the notion of the self to conscious contents of the mind since we are all masters of self-deception and split off shameful aspects of ourselves while repressing unacceptable feelings. Memory certainly plays a significant role in the development of the self because much of the self representation that we use to think about ourselves is the aggregate of personal memories and the social personas associated with them.

These considerations lead us into the problem that the self is both conscious and unconscious. Much of the choices, impulses, fleeting thoughts, and reactive feelings reflect disavowed parts of the self that are largely unconscious. The philosopher Thomas Nagel (1986) made the point that we can use the term "I" to describe oneself even though our actual self-knowledge of who we are is quite limited and confused. So in considering the role that the self construct plays in understanding the person we must recognize its limitations. There is a mismatch between the way that we think, feel and act, on the one hand, and the narrative we have internalized from childhood that bears the weight of our moral value system and our conscience.

Moreover, we must avoid the naïve view that the self-concept is monolithic. In psychoanalytic discourse, it has become widely accepted that while we might wish to maintain an illusion of a continuous self, the reality is that we are all composed of multiple discontinuous selves that are constantly being shaped and defined by real and fantasized relationships with others. Schafer (1989) understood this phenomenon as a set of narrative selves or storylines that we develop to provide a coherent account of our lives. Mitchell (1991) noted that a paradox of psychoanalytic work is that as patients learn to tolerate multiple facets of themselves, they begin to experience themselves as more durable and more coherent. What we know as the self is context dependent. Different aspects of the self are evoked by different individual and different group settings that are present in our environment.

In considering the self in context, perhaps the most fundamental context is one's culture. It would be naïve to ignore consideration of cultural views of the self in a discussion of how an individual develops. For example, Jen (2013), a Chinese novelist, noted that Asian culture is not centered in self-experience. Rather, an "interdependent" self is created by parenting that focuses on social context. Hence a person steeped in an Asian upbringing is less likely to focus on the self-construct apart from its cultural and familial milieu.

After this detour into the problem of the self in contemporary thinking, let us return to the *person* because most assuredly the self is not the same thing as the person. Much of the writing about the self is linked to the subjective experience of reflecting on one's inner nature. However, one can contrast the self-as-experienced with the self-as-observed by others.

The way that one is perceived by others allows for a fuller definition of the person. For example, when one appears on videotape, it is rare for an individual to react positively to how he or she appears and sounds on the video. The vast majority of people are somewhat shocked by what they see on video in contrast to how they imagine they appear and sound. Reactions such as the following are common when psychiatric residents view a video of themselves interviewing a patient. Common reactions are the following: "I don't look like that!" or "My voice doesn't sound like that!" Those in the same seminar will often disagree with the concerned colleague by making corrective comments such as, "Oh yes, you actually do look like that and sound like that." In fact, a debate could be conducted regarding whether the self as subjectively experienced is more valid than the self observed by others. Clearly both are important to a comprehensive view of the *person*. We simply do not see ourselves like others see us no matter how hard we try.

While an individual has difficulty ascertaining how others view him or her, it is also true that others cannot see how we feel inside from the observer's *outside* perspective. Hence a key point is that knowing who the *person* is requires an *integration of the inside and outside perspective*. In psychoanalysis a critically important aspect of the working through process involves the analyst's shift from a first person perspective, provided by the patient, to a third person perspective emanating from the analyst (Goldberg 1999). In other words, therapists must empathically validate the patient's "I" experience, while also bringing to bear their own outside experience as an observer.

Obstacles to integrating psychiatric and psychoanalytic thinking

While psychiatric trainees need to learn that a crucial aspect of diagnosis is understanding the person with the illness, there are obstacles to that perspective. For many years the official diagnostic nomenclature of the American Psychiatric Association separated out an axis of personality disorders from another axis of diagnostic syndromes such as anxiety, depression, schizophrenia, etc. While the intent was to assure that a clinician diagnosing a patient would consider the personality dimensions of that patient, a clinician was prone to ignore the personality disorder axis altogether. A frequent observation on reviewing patient charts was that an Axis I syndrome diagnosis was noted, but under Axis II for personality disorders, the word "deferred" would appear. The assumption was that at a later point the personality of the patient might be considered more thoroughly. However, the word "deferred" could easily have been replaced by "ignored."

In my many years of teaching psychiatric residents, a common experience was for the trainee to use the following phrase: "I think this patient has some Axis II stuff." This language could be translated in the following way: "the patient is obnoxious, difficult, angry, manipulative, or otherwise unpleasant." Hence the separation of personality disorder from syndrome in psychiatry led to a shorthand view that a patient with a diagnosis on Axis II was antisocial, difficult, demanding or unpleasant. These broad brushstrokes used to describe personality overlooked the fact that dimensions of personalities, such as dependency, fear of disapproval, perfectionism, and other areas were common elements of professionals like physicians themselves. In other words, the distinction between the severe personality disorders and the personality characteristics of neurotically organized individuals was blurred. The "Axis II" label became a pejorative adjective. Moreover, it led to an artificial distinction between Axis I and Axis II in which the "person" was deemed not relevant to Axis I diagnoses. Many psychiatrist trainees didn't recognize the distinction between a *personality disorder*, on the one hand, and the *person*, on the other. Even with the discontinuation of the Axis I/Axis II distinction in the latest edition of the diagnostic nomenclature (DSM 5 2013), the dualistic thinking continues.

Who is the person?

The foregoing overview of the problems inherent in integrating the notion of the *person* into present day psychiatry, suggests that it is difficult to provide a facile categorization for a construct like the *person*. Psychiatry has moved in a direction of rapid diagnosis based on symptom check lists and a view that it is too time consuming to study what is unique and idiosyncratic about the patient. The diagnostician in contemporary psychiatry is looking for how patients are *similar*, i.e., how they have common symptoms that gain them entry into a diagnostic category, rather than how they are different from others.

Incorporating the notion of the "person" into the teaching and practicing of psychiatry to make it a truly psychodynamically based specialty, involves a time-consuming process of considering a number of different determinates that go into an understanding of who the patient is (Gabbard 2014):

1   The subjective experience of one's self based on a unique historical narrative that is filtered through the lens of specific meanings to the patient;

2   A set of conscious and unconscious conflicts (defenses), representation, and self-deception;
3   A set of internalized interactions with others that are unconsciously re-enacted;
4   One's physical characteristics;
5   One's brain is a product of genes and interaction with environmental forces and the creation of neural networks by cumulative experience;
6   One's cultural/religious and social affiliations;
7   One's cognitive style and one's cognitive capacities.

I wish to emphasize the inclusion of cognitive capacities and the integration of genetic factors with environmental forces are essential in this list of the determinants of personhood. In the contemporary mental health scene, psychoanalytic thought must be integrated with biological forces when diagnosing the patient. A psychiatric diagnosis that ignores biology can be problematic. While analysts are prone to complain that psychiatry is subject to biological reductionism, analysts can be accused of being *psychoanalytically* reductive as well. After all, there is no psychology without biology.

Case example

While the consideration and integration of the various factors that are involved in defining a person may seem overwhelming, the clinician must always approach the task with the expectation that the diagnostic understanding will be partial in the initial phases of treatment. One continues to alter the understanding of the patient based on new material that emerges in the course of treatment. A case example may illustrate how one integrates some of the factors in a diagnostic assessment:

> Ms. A was a 44 year old teacher who presented to treatment because of a recurrent depression that responded only partially to medication, feelings of self-depreciation, and a wish to improve her sexual desire in her marriage. She said that her husband was a good man, and therefore she pretended to enjoy sex to please him. In fact, she had never had sexual desire throughout her life.
>
> In her first session I asked her to sit wherever she liked, and she chose the chair that was farthest from my own chair. She asked me if I knew about the culture of the Hopi Indians. I told her I did not have much information about that culture but would like to hear what she had to say.

Although she was not a product of the Hopi culture, she had studied the culture and informed me that a popular Hopi saying was that, "Each person finds the most appropriate seat for him or her when entering a room." She soon told me her horrific childhood history of having had an incestuous relationship with her father from the age of 6 to 12. She found the incestuous experience intercourse unbearably traumatic and said that she often found herself depersonalizing, floating above the bed and dissociating herself in such a way that she could view the abuse as occurring to "that girl down there" rather than to her. She kept the experience secret as she felt she could not discuss what was happening with her mother or with a friend. At one point she tried to tell a nun who taught her class in the Catholic school she attended, and the nun told her, "You must never speak of this again. You will burn in hell if you do." As a result, she developed a conviction that she was thoroughly bad.

As I got to know her, I recognized that her absence of sexual response or desire contributed to an ascetic self-view as one who does not need pleasure. She developed an identity as a self-disciplined long distance runner who could take self-punishment with a stoic attitude. In this regard, one could integrate the psychological and the biological using research on the impact of childhood sexual abuse. Heim et al. (2013) studied a group of adult women who had been sexually abused as children and compared them to a control group who had not been abused. They found that exposure to childhood sexual abuse is specifically associated with cortical thinning in the area of the genital representation field within the primary somatosensory cortex. The MRI scanning clearly showed this thinning in the portion of the brain associated with sexual feelings. In other words, the neuroplasticity associated with development appeared to protect the child from the sensory processing of specific abuse experiences but contributed to a deadening of the sexual response in adult life. While at some level she understood that this was a situation that was unlikely to change, she felt to be a good wife she should try to be more responsive to her husband. This absence of sexual response could be viewed as a deficit condition because of the neurological modification associated with childhood sexual abuse. If it were viewed as a psychological conflict, then the patient might be expected to change this aspect of herself and feel like a failure for not being able to do so. Moreover, it might have contributed to her conviction that she was bad or defective in some way. This view was reinforced by her religious/cultural factors in childhood, at least from her perspective, when the nun told her she must be secretive about what had happened to her. She then developed an altruistic devotion to teaching children and providing loving care for her two boys.

Ms. A lived with the expectation that lightning would strike at any moment. Like many victims of childhood trauma, she harbored an assumption that positive expectations of others are dangerous as they might at any moment be shattered by aggression from others. Indeed, she tended to redirect her aggression towards her parents by her intense self-denigration. She also needed interpersonal distance, as shown in her choice of seating in my office. Finally, she had a tenacious clinging to suicidality as an escape hatch from intolerable situations even though she did not act on the suicidal thoughts.

In summary, the patient's sense of herself as a person in my own observations as a psychoanalytically trained psychiatrist trying to evaluate her was that she had a confluence of early environmental factors and biological factors that led her to feel defective. She needed to come to terms with what was truly her fault versus those issues over which she had no control. The treatment plan had to take into account the limits of what one could expect given the alterations of the cortex from the abuse.

Treatment implications of diagnosing "the person"

One implication of this approach to diagnosis that integrates psychoanalytic and psychiatric thinking is that we do not treat disorders in isolation. We are always treating a *person* with a disorder and this notion needs to be center stage in our planning. It is also true that the *person* of the therapist must be taken into account. Treatment is not simply a series of procedures that are geared to a specific diagnosis. We know that the therapeutic relationship appears to be far more important than a specific technique in predicting outcome (Horvath 2005; Zuroff & Blatt 2006). The person of the therapist may be a good fit or a poor fit with the *person* of the patient. There is no doubt that the therapeutic alliance or therapeutic relationship may be enhanced if the fit is good and made more challenging if the fit is less than optimal.

One corollary to this notion of the importance of the therapeutic relationship is the capacity for the therapist to be flexible and shift his or her approach based on the patient's response. There is some preliminary research suggesting that the flexible shifting of the therapist's approach in response to the *person* of the patient is associated with better outcomes (Stiles 2009; Owen & Hilsenroth 2014). The notion of optimal responsiveness appears to have an impact on outcome, meaning that the therapist who adjusts to what the patient needs may form a better therapeutic relationship that helps the patient improve as a result of the therapy process. Similarly, one study (Owen & Hilsenroth 2014) found that the therapists who are flexible in the use of technique within a given treatment had better outcomes across their caseload compared to therapists who are much less flexible with their interventions. Moreover, recent research in the area of "therapist effects" suggests that the characteristics of individual therapists have a great deal to do with outcomes across the various psychotherapeutic techniques (Stiles 2009). Therapists with the best outcomes adjust their approach based on their understanding of the particular patient's needs in the context of the treatment. The optimally responsive therapist is constantly monitoring his or her impact on the patient and modifying the approach so that it is as helpful as possible to a particular patient's needs as well as the patient's idiosyncratic ways of accepting help. In brief, therapeutic action must always take into account the unique features of the therapeutic dyad.

There are a variety of reasons that the "person" is being ignored and neglected in contemporary psychiatry. Psychoanalytic thinking has had a decreasing influence in recent decades, and it is far easier for some clinicians to think productively in terms of biological symptomatology matched to the appropriate pharmacologic agent. There is also a longing for simplicity—accompanied by a hate of complexity—in many practitioners. Recognizing the patient in all of his or her complexity requires greater time and greater flexibility in the clinician. Moreover, there is the simple fact that getting to know the *person* takes time, and as we all know, time is money. Technology has also contributed to the current resistance to seeing the uniqueness of the patient. The electronic medical record now appears to have exceeded the patient in importance in some settings. One may be required to enter a detailed note for every visit, encroaching on the time of face-to-face contact with the patient where one can listen and empathize. Finally, getting to know the *person* may be unsettling to the clinician. Facing a disturbed patient with a complex clinical picture may overwhelm someone who is required to see four patients in an hour.

In closing, we must keep in mind that bringing back the *person* to the diagnostic process in psychiatry involves a way of thinking that is time-consuming. Nevertheless, it is ultimately more satisfying than a brief symptom checklist. Clinicians must let the patient tell his or her story in the time that is required. To some extent we must let the patient supervise us and lead us in the directions of his or her own uniqueness, even if the direction is counter to what we are developing in our own private formulation. We must constantly be thinking of integrating the biological, the psychological, and the social-cultural aspects of the patient. This task requires multiple visits over time and cannot be quickly accomplished in one initial interview.

References

Gabbard, G. O. (2014). *Psychodynamic psychiatry in clinical practice* (5th ed.). Washington, DC: American Psychiatric Publishing.

Goldberg, A. (1999). Between empathy and judgment. *Journal of the American Psychoanalytic Association, 47*: 351–365.

Guntrip, H. (1968). *Schizoid phenomena object-relations, and the self.* New York: International Universities Press.

Heim, C. M., Mayberg, H. S., Mletzko, T., Nemeroff, C. B., & Pruessner, J. C. (2013). Decreased cortical representation of gential somatosensory field after childhood sexual abuse. *American Journal of Psychiatry, 170*: 616–623.

Horowitz, R. I., Cullen, M. R., Abell, J., & Christian, J. B. (2013). (De)personalized medicine. *Science, 339*: 1155–1156.

Horvath, A. O. (2005). The therapeutic relationship: Research and theory. An Introduction to the special issue. *Psychotherapy Research, 15*: 3–7.

Jen, G. (2013). *Tiger writing: Art, culture, and the interdependent self.* Cambridge, MA: Harvard University Press.

Kernberg, O. F. (1982). Self, ego, affects and drives. *Journal of the American Psychoanalytic Association, 30*: 893–917.

Mitchell, S. A. (1991). Contemporary perspectives on self: Toward an integration. *Psychoanalytic Dialogues, 1*: 121–147.

Mauron, A. (2001). Personal identity. *Science, 291*: 831–832.

Nagel, T. (1986). *The view from nowhere.* New York: Oxford University Press.

Owen, J., & Hilsenroth, M. J. (2014). Treatment adherence: The importance of therapists' flexibility in relation to therapy outcomes. *Journal of Counseling Psychology, 61*: 280–288.

Schafer, R. (1989). Narratives of the self. In A. M. Cooper, O. F. Kernberg, & E. S. Person (Eds.), *Psychoanalysis: Toward the second century* (pp. 153–167). New Haven, CT: Yale University Press.

Stiles, W. B. (2009). Responsiveness as an obstacle for psychotherapy outcome research: It's worse than you think. *Clinical Psychology in Scientific Practice, 16*: 86–91.

Strawson, G. (2009). *Selves: Revisionary metaphysics.* Oxford, UK: Clarendon Press.

Sutherland, J. D. (1980). The British object relations theorists: Balint, Winnicott, Fairbarin, Guntrip. *Journal of the American Psychoanalytic Association, 28*: 829–860.

Zuroff, D. C., & Blatt, S. J. (2006). The therapeutic relationship in the brief treatment of depression: Contributions to clinical improvement and enhanced adaptive capabilities. *Journal of Consulting and Clinical Psychology, 74*: 130–140.

CHAPTER TEN

The second edition of the *Psychodynamic Diagnostic Manual (PDM-2)*

Sensible diagnoses for sensitive clinicians

Vittorio Lingiardi

In the field of psychodynamics, "diagnosis" is a controversial word. As Nancy McWilliams (2011) notes, for some therapists it is even a "dirty word" (p. 7). The publication of the first edition of the *Psychodynamic Diagnostic Manual* (PDM Task Force, 2006) has provided an exciting opportunity for a passionate and respectful debate between research-oriented scholars and psychoanalytic colleagues in clinical practice. Irwin Hoffman (2009), for example, critiques the manual, suggesting that virtually any use of categorisation in relation to patients is a "desiccation" of human experience. Hoffman views the *PDM* as merely giving lip service "to humanistic, existential respect for the uniqueness and limitless complexity of any person" (p. 1060). In response, Eagle and Wolitzky (2011) argue that "limitations and inevitable oversimplifications" are intrinsic to "any classification system" (p. 803), but human experience is not "desiccated" when researchers view it through a diagnostic lens and try to measure it. They suggest that a constructive way to bridge the gap between science and analytic work is to do better, more creative, and more ecologically valid research. Many other authors have participated in this debate (see, e.g., Aron, 2012; Fonagy, 2013; Hoffman, 2012a, 2012b; Safran, 2012; Vivona, 2012).

The purpose of this chapter is to introduce readers to the second edition of the *PDM* (*PDM-2*) (Lingiardi & McWilliams, 2017) and to present it in light of the perspective on psychodynamic diagnosis that I have developed in dialogue with colleagues (see also Lingiardi, Holmqvist, & Safran, 2016).

In his *General Psychopathology* Karl Jaspers (1913) claims that "Every diagnostic schema must remain a tiresome problem for the scientist" (p. 615) (*Alle Diagnosenschemata müssen für den Forscher eine Qual Bleiben*). This statement has taught me a great deal. In the original quote, the German word *Qual* is used where "tiresome" has been used here; *Qual* literally means "torment/agony", and in fact, being faithful to the original version, I think that for researchers and clinicians, diagnosis should be a "torment". There is always a tension between the need to connect a patient to a general category and, at the same time, connect the patient to her/his unique qualities – "the impossible science of the unique being", as Roland Barthes (1980, p. 71) would say.

When I speak to a patient with a "narcissistic", "obsessive", or "paranoid" personality (just to name a few diagnoses), I see her/him as inevitably belonging to an *ideal* configuration of symptoms and structures – a diagnostic gestalt that is not perfectly inherent in the person in front of me but can represent a clinical treasure for understanding and treatment. At the same time, I speak of the *unique* way that she/he faces the symptoms and the dynamics of narcissism, paranoia, or obsession. This is why – in our clinical activity, teaching, and supervision – we must try to achieve and maintain a binocular vision that incorporates both the inclusiveness of the "diagnostic label" and the exclusivity of the "case formulation". In my opinion, this is also the only way that the diagnostic process can be rescued from the Scylla of bureaucratic compilation and the Charybdis of self-referential jargon. Both of these mortify the clinician's professional identity and dim or distort the practitioner's ability to detect and describe a patient's characteristics and mental functioning. As a consequence, they jeopardise the clinical relationship.

The quality of a diagnosis is determined by its clinical application as an overall synthesis of a patient's difficulties and resources and an effective index for identifying a suitable therapeutic approach to evaluating changes over time. Separating the diagnostic label from its embodied potential targets may risk imitation of the idiot who, when the wise man points at the Moon, looks at the finger.

To be useful to the clinician, a diagnostic system must:

- consider psychopathology in the context of personality;
- conceive symptoms together with functioning;

- be positioned within the life cycle (e.g., relating to infancy, childhood, adolescence, adulthood, or later life);
- consider the subjective experience of symptoms;
- take into account the relational elements of the act of diagnosing;
- enhance the role of the clinician's subjectivity in the diagnostic formulation;
- contemplate the specificity of the idiographic case formulation, in addition to the synthetic value of the diagnostic label;
- grasp not only the patient's maladaptive aspects, but also her/his resources; and
- connect with research and clinical activity, in order to promote deeper training.

For years, clinical psychologists, in particular those with a dynamic theoretical orientation, underemphasised or neglected the impact of the *DSM* on their diagnostic views. In the 20 year gap between the *DSM-IV* (APA, 1994) and the *DSM-5* (APA, 2013), two exciting diagnostic proposals emerged from a psychodynamic background: the Shedler-Westen Assessment Procedure (SWAP) (Shedler, 2015; Westen & Shedler, 1999a, 1999b, 2007) and the *Psychodynamic Diagnostic Manual* (*PDM*) (Lingiardi & McWilliams, 2017; PDM Task Force, 2006). The SWAP and the *PDM* were the first to systematically finalise a psychodynamic nosography, starting with an integration of clinicians' diagnostic expertise and researchers' methodological skills. Further, these models value aspects of the diagnostic dimension that were previously neglected, such as the role of therapists' emotional responses (e.g., boredom, impotence, protection, hostility, etc.) to different types of patients (e.g., Betan, Heim, Zittel Conklin, & Westen, 2005; Colli, Tanzilli, Dimaggio, & Lingiardi, 2014; Gabbard, 2009; Gazzillo et al., 2015; Lingiardi, Tanzilli, & Colli, 2015; Røssberg, Karterud, Pedersen, & Friis, 2007; Tanzilli, Muzi, Ronningstam, & Lingiardi, 2017).

Reviewing the *PDM-1*, Widlöcher and Thurin (2011) note the emphasis on the transition "from the nosographic to the psychopathologic" and underline as the main goal of the manual not the correction of traditional international psychiatric classifications but etiology, multifactoriality, and pathogenesis.

This chapter is dedicated to the most recent edition of the *PDM* and the potential insights to be gained from the prominent position given to diagnosis in this new model.

The first edition of the Psychodynamic Diagnostic Manual:
Context, birth, and aims

In the last three decades, the most frequently used diagnostic systems have seemed to disregard or underemphasise the subjective experience of patients, since the usual methodologies of "descriptive" or "categorical" psychiatry have not been considered capable of reflecting the complexity of pathological and non-pathological human conditions. Patients in the same diagnostic category, with similar symptoms, may vary widely in their subjective experience, and such variations have implications for treatment. For the above cited reasons, and during a critical period for psychiatric taxonomy, the scientific community witnessed the birth of the first edition of the *Psychodynamic Diagnostic Manual* (PDM Task Force, 2006), steered by Stanley Greenspan, Nancy McWilliams, and Robert Wallerstein, and sponsored by five psychoanalytic and psychodynamic associations: the American Academy of Psychoanalysis and Dynamic Psychiatry, the American Psychoanalytic Association, the Division of Psychoanalysis (39) of the American Psychological Association, the International Psychoanalytical Association, and the National Membership Committee on Psychoanalysis in Clinical Social Work.

The *PDM* is a diagnostic manual that emphasises who a person *is*, rather than the disorder she/he *has*. The descriptive psychiatric model makes nosology more research-friendly, but it may also lead clinicians to underestimate the value of (or even fail to recognise) idiographic clinical information. The *PDM* brings a valuable perspective to this nosographic panorama in its attempts to broaden the horizon and facilitate clinical–diagnostic dialogue in the scientific community (Gershy, 2016). Indeed, it is interesting to observe that even the *DSM-5* identifies the *PDM* as a complementary framework, as written in its *Pocket Guide to the Diagnostic Exam* (Nussbaum, 2013):

> *ICD-10* is focused on public health, whereas the *Psychodynamic Diagnostic Manual* (PDM) focuses on the psychological health and distress of a particular person. Several psychoanalytical groups joined together to create *PDM* as a complement to the descriptive systems of *DSM-5* and *ICD-10*. Like *DSM-5*, *PDM* includes dimensions that cut across diagnostic categories, along with a thorough account of personality patterns and disorders. *PDM* uses the *DSM* diagnostic categories but includes accounts of the internal experience of a person presenting for treatment.

(pp. 243–244)

In 2013, an exciting reference to the *PDM* was published on the American Psychoanalytic Association website. A statement from this piece is now included in the introduction to the second edition of the *PDM* (see also Lingiardi & McWilliams, 2015):

> The *DSM-5*, published by our colleague organization the American Psychiatric Association, has been met with both praise and criticism. Like its predecessors, this fifth edition of the *Diagnostic and Statistical Manual* will be widely used in the mental health field to classify mental disorders according to diagnoses based on descriptive criteria. There is a place in the field for classifying patients based on descriptions of symptoms, illness course, and other objective facts. However, as psychoanalysts, we know that each patient is unique. No two people with depression, bereavement, anxiety or any other mental illness or disorder will have the same potentials, needs for treatment or responses to efforts to help. Whether or not one finds great value in the descriptive diagnostic nomenclature exemplified by the *DSM-5*, psychoanalytic diagnostic assessment is an essential complementary assessment pathway that aims to provide an understanding of each person in depth as a unique and complex individual and should be part of a thorough assessment of every patient. Even for psychiatric disorders with a strong biological basis, psychological factors contribute to the onset, worsening, and expression of illness. Psychological factors also influence how every patient engages in treatment; the quality of the therapeutic alliance has been shown to be the strongest predictor of outcome for illness in all modalities. *For information about a diagnostic framework that describes both the deeper and surface levels of symptom patterns, as well as of an individual's personality, emotional and social functioning, mental health professionals are referred to the Psychodynamic Diagnostic Manual.*

While the *DSM* categorises commonalities among people (by recording a pool of symptoms that can be "recognised" in a particular patient), the *PDM* describes the specificities that make each person unique. Its purpose is thus to foster the integration of nomothetic understanding and idiographic knowledge. Rather than presenting a "taxonomy of diseases", the *PDM* is a "taxonomy of people" who are individually understood through the perspective of lifespan development, from infancy and early childhood through childhood and adolescence, to adulthood and later life. For a long time, identification of the directly observable features of a disorder was the only clinical means of differentiating one disorder (or in some cases, one person) from another; though this method was intended to help clinicians and researchers organise a certain chaos inside psychopathological expressions, it led to greater problems, rather than resolutions. Currently, assessing a patient's personality and mental functioning (including her/ his strengths), in addition to comprehensively describing her/his psycho-pathology and functioning, seems more effective and accurate for treat-ment planning.

Westen, Novotny, and Thompson-Brenner (2004) found that treat-ments focusing on isolated symptoms or behaviours (rather than on per-sonality, emotional themes, and interpersonal patterns) are not effective in sustaining even narrowly defined changes. In recent years, several reliable ways of measuring complex patterns of personality, emotion, and interpersonal processes – the active ingredients of the therapeutic relationship – have been developed. These include, among others, the Shedler–Westen Assessment Procedure (SWAP-200; Westen & Shedler, 1999a, 1999b), on which we have drawn extensively; the Structured Interview of Personality Organization (STIPO), developed by Kernberg's group (Clarkin, Caligor, Stern, & Kernberg, 2004); the Operational-ized Psychodynamic Diagnosis (OPD) system (OPD Task Force, 2008; Zimmermann et al., 2012); and Blatt's (2008) model of anaclitic and intro-jective personality configurations.

The *PDM-1* comprised three main sections: 1) "Adult Mental Dis-orders"; 2) "Child and Adolescent Mental Health Syndromes" (which included "Infant and Early Childhood Disorders"); and 3) "Conceptual and Empirical Foundations for a Psychodynamically Based Classification System for Mental Health Disorders". Except in the evaluation of infants and preschoolers, for which other parameters were provided, clinicians were advised to assess the following dimensions in their patients: per-sonality patterns and disorders (P-Axis); profile of mental functioning (M-Axis); and symptoms pattern and subjective experience (S-Axis).

The manual opened with the section relating to adults. Here, the P-Axis and M-Axis were the first to be diagnosed. The S-Axis, describ-ing patients' symptoms and syndromes and their subjective experi-ence of these, was the final dimension, completing the patient's clinical picture. These three axes were equipped with case formulations to demonstrate the application of the diagnostic system to a real clinical population.

The child and adolescent section, in contrast to the adult section, opened with the M-Axis and followed this with the P-Axis (this is because the personality style of the young patient was considered more emergent than structured) and the S-Axis. Assessment of infants and those in early childhood was also included in this section.

The final section in the manual included a collection of conceptual and research foundations for a psychodynamically based classification system. It described the empirical research literature that supported the *PDM*'s historical and conceptual foundations of psychodynamic diagnosis and psychotherapy research.

Despite the limitations of the decision to self-publish the manual and Greenspan's death soon after its publication, the *PDM-1* was quite successful. In the United States and Europe, the manual achieved considerable sales, even outside the professional field. On 24 January 2006, the *New York Times* dedicated a special article to the *PDM* with the headline: "For therapy, a new guide with a touch of personality"; in 2011, the *Journal of Personality Assessment* also dedicated a special issue to the *PDM*. In 2006, before its publication, 5,000 copies had already been sold on Amazon, alone. Reflecting on the success of the *PDM*, Paul Stepansky (2009, p. 66) writes:

> To achieve commercial success of this order, the 'psychoanalytic' appellation must be diluted to 'psychodynamic', and the psychodynamic 'terms' and 'concepts' offered in a user-friendly format intended to broaden rather than supplant other diagnostic frameworks. This is the very formula that has made the recently self-published *Psychodynamic Diagnostic Manual*, collectively authored by an Alliance of Psychoanalytic Organizations, a stunning success, with sales, as of March, 2008, of over 20,000 copies.

At the IPA Congress in Chicago in 2009, it became clear that the *PDM* had also achieved a foothold in European psychoanalysis. The manual had been welcomed and reviewed in Italy (Del Corno & Lingiardi, 2012), Germany (OPD Task Force, 2001), Spain and Portugal (Ferrari, 2006; Ferrari, Lancelle, Pereira, Roussos, & Weinstein, 2008; Rosenthal, 2008), Turkey (Dereboy, 2013, personal communication), and France (Widlöcher, 2007; Widlöcher & Thurin, 2011). However, Italy had responded to the manual over and above the other countries. Here, the words of Nancy McWilliams (2016), the historical soul of the *PDM*, are best placed to capture the manual's past, present, and future:

> With Greenspan's death, I thought the *PDM* would die as well. Most of the *PDM-1* Steering Committee members were elderly, and those under age 70 were saying they did not want to devote the rest of their career to the *PDM*, which had been entirely a labor of love [. . .]. I was among those. I did not expect anyone to emerge who would take on the project of a revised *PDM* [. . .] Vittorio Lingiardi contacted me unexpectedly, emphasizing the need for a second edition.

The second edition of the PDM

Nancy McWilliams and I started updating the *PDM* in 2012. The support we received from Nancy Greenspan, the faithful caretaker of her late husband's legacy, and Jim Nageotte of Guilford Press, whose suggestions improved the final manuscript, were invaluable. Again, Nancy McWilliams (2016) says:

> Our first job was to obtain the support of all the organizations that sponsored the original *PDM*, which turned out to be easy. Our second was to obtain support from some additional organizations, including the International Association for Relational Psychoanalysis and Psychotherapy, and the Italian Group for the Advancement in Psychodynamic Diagnosis. [. . .] Then we sought people to head task forces. Not so easy, but again, we found many energetic, highly qualified, and hard-working individuals willing to donate most generously their time and effort [. . .] Then we approached Guilford Publications in the United States and Raffaello Cortina Publisher in Italy. Both were immediately enthusiastic about publishing *PDM-2*.

The decision to update and revise the *PDM-1* was reinforced by the feedback of mental health professionals. We intended to incorporate this feedback in a second edition, with the aim of enhancing its empirical rigour and clinical utility, preserving its strengths, and editing it weaknesses (e.g., Clarkin, 2015; Lingiardi & McWilliams, 2015, 2018; Lingiardi, McWilliams, Bornstein, Gazzillo, & Gordon, 2015). Relative to the first edition, the *PDM-2* is more grounded in systematic research, with special regards to the application of the SWAP-200, and it confronts the diagnostic descriptions offered by the *ICD-10* and *DSM-5*.

The *PDM-2* proposes a synergistic description of the three main lines around which diagnosis moves: personality patterns, mental functioning, and the descriptive and subjective experience of symptoms. It draws on Freud's original conception of the continuity of mental functioning, with clinical nuances described to greater or lesser degree within the spectrum of normal to abnormal, healthy/adaptive to ill/maladaptive, and borderline to psychotic levels of neurotic constellations.

For the revision, seven task forces were organised, each under the leadership of two editors:

1   Adulthood: P-Axis (Nancy McWilliams & Jonathan Shedler); M-Axis (Vittorio Lingiardi & Robert Bornstein); and S-Axis (Emanuela Mundo & John O'Neil);

2   Adolescence: MA-Axis (Mario Speranza & Nick Midgley); PA-Axis (Johanna Malone & Norka Malberg); and SA-Axis (Mario Speranza);

3   Childhood: MC-Axis (Norka Malberg & Larry Rosenberg); PC-Axis (Norka Malberg, Larry Rosenberg, & Johanna Malone); and SC-Axis (Norka Malberg & Larry Rosenberg);

4   Infancy and Early Childhood (IEC: Anna Maria Speranza & Linda Mayes);

5   Later Life (Franco Del Corno & Daniel Plotkin);

6   Assessment within the *PDM-2* Framework (Sherwood Waldron, Robert Gordon, & Francesco Gazzillo); and

7   Case Illustrations and *PDM-2* Profiles (Franco Del Corno, Vittorio Lingiardi, & Nancy McWilliams).

The second edition maintains the structure of the *PDM-1*, with the chapters dedicated to personality syndromes organised around level of personality organisation and personality style/type. Level of personality organisation refers to severity of dysfunction, ranging from healthy to neurotic, borderline, and psychotic levels. Style/type identifies clinically familiar motifs that cut across the level of personality organisation and do not inherently connote health or pathology. Adolescents' and children's personalities are mainly considered in terms of emerging patterns and/or difficulties.

The section on mental functioning is dedicated to a detailed description of overall mental functioning (see below), and encourages the assessment of particular areas of mental functioning. Complementary to the P-Axis, the M-Axis enriches the assessment of personality by considering the specific functions that contribute to a particular patient's personality organisation.

The main focus of the section dedicated to symptom patterns is their description in terms of affective dynamics, mental content, somatic states, and associated relationship themes.

The evaluation of any single axis (P as Personality, M as Mental Functioning, and S as Symptom Patterns and their Subjectivity) follows a different order in adult patients, relative to other age groups. In adults, personality is assessed first, whereas in children, adolescents, and elderly patients it is evaluated after mental functioning. The reason for this is that, for adults, personality is conceived of as quite stable and thus a primary frame in which symptoms arise; in children, adolescents, and the elderly, however, it is typical for developmental issues and mental states related to age to take priority in clinical evaluations.

The section on infancy and early childhood (IEC) follows a multi-axial approach that differs from the other sections due to its 0–3 peculiarities. The approach includes functional emotional developmental capacity (Axis II), regulatory-sensory processing capacity (Axis III), relational patterns and disorders (Axis IV), and other medical and neurological diagnoses (Axis V) as determinant components of a diagnosis (Axis I). This section has undergone significant change since the *PDM-1*, and it now includes various assessment tools, such as user-friendly scales to enable clinicians to formulate a clinically relevant profile of an infant or child.

Several other important changes, updates, and reformulations have been introduced in the *PDM-2*. With regards to the P-Axis (for a wider perspective, see also McWilliams, Grenyer & Shedler, 2018), for example, a new psychotic level of personality organisation has been included in light of clinical, theoretical, and empirical contributions that support the clinical evidence of this concept. For example, it has been demonstrated that some patients who have never met a clear diagnosis of psychosis may nonetheless manifest psychotic states associated with primitive defences, inadequate reality testing, lack of differentiation between representations of the self and others, and low discrimination between fantasy and external reality under the pressure of specific dynamics. Seasoned therapists have long reported that they understand their most disturbed patients to be organised at a psychotic level, even when those patients have never had a diagnosed psychotic illness. Clinical explorations that assume a psychotic range of functioning include the writings of Bion (1967), Kernberg (1984), McWilliams (2015), Rosenfeld (1987), Steiner (1993, 2011), and others. In addition, the P-Axes have been integrated and revised according to indications derived from measures such as the SWAP-200 and the SWAP-II, including their adolescent versions (Lingiardi, Gazzillo, & Waldron, 2010; Lingiardi, Shedler, & Gazzillo, 2006; Shedler, 2015; Westen, DeFife, Malone, & DiLallo, 2014; Westen & Shedler, 1999a, 1999b, 2007; Westen, Shedler, Bradley, & DeFife, 2012; Westen, Shedler, Durrett, Glass, & Martens, 2003).

As regards the M-Axis (see also Lingiardi, Colli, & Muzi, 2018), the number of mental functions has increased from nine to twelve, which now include capacity for regulation, attention and learning; capacity for affective range, communication and understanding; capacity for mentalisation and reflective functioning; capacity for differentiation and integration; capacity for relationships and intimacy; self-esteem regulation and quality of internal experience; impulse control and regulation; defensive functioning; adaptation, resiliency and strength; self-observing capacities (psychological mindedness); capacity to construct and use internal standards and ideals; and meaning and purpose. A Likert-style scale associated with each mental function enables practitioners to assess a patient's mental profile.

Finally, the S-Axis has been reformulated according to in-depth comparisons with the *DSM-5* and *ICD-10*. Clinical and empirical studies support exhaustive explanations of "affective states", "cognitive patterns", "somatic states", and "relationship patterns". Accordingly, this section more thoroughly depicts both the subjective experience of the patient and the likely countertransference reactions of the treating clinician. It also outlines psychological experiences that may require clinical attention (e.g., conditions relating to culture, gender identity, sexual orientation, and minority status) in order to illustrate the way in which certain states may affect the expression of symptom patterns when related to experiences such as bullying and stigmatisation.

The *PDM-2* splits the first edition's section on "Child and Adolescent Mental Health Disorders" into two distinct sections relating to the child (aged 4–11) and the adolescent (aged 12–19), respectively. This decision was made because it seemed clinically unsophisticated to suggest similar levels, patterns, and functioning in a 4-year-old child and a 14-year-old adolescent.

The "Infancy and Early Childhood" section includes detailed considerations of developmental lines and homotypic/heterotypic continuities of early infancy, childhood, adolescence, and adult psychopathology, in line with empirical and clinical literature (see, e.g., Costello, Mustillo, Erkanli, Keeler, & Angold, 2003; Speranza & Fortunato, 2012). In addition, the editors have given more attention to the quality of primary relationships (between a child and caregivers), family systems and their characteristic relational patterns, attachment patterns and their possible connections to both psychopathology and normative development, and contributions from theoretical, clinical, and empirical investigations into infant research and attachment theory (see Cassidy & Shaver, 2008).

The *PDM-2* includes three new chapters: "Later Life", "Tools for Assessment", and "Case Illustrations and PDM-2 Profiles". The inclusion of a chapter on later life makes the *PDM-2* the first classification system with distinct treatment of the geriatric life stage. The hope is that this will contribute to a greater sensitivity in mental health towards older adults. Many of the contributions in this section are based on clinical observation, as there is a notable paucity of studies about this stage of life and its outstanding connotations for psychological treatment. The "Tools for Assessment" chapter illustrates both *PDM* and non-*PDM* derived instruments. Among the *PDM-2* derived instruments, the main tool is the Psychodiagnostic Chart-2 (PDC-2; adult version by Robert Gordon and Robert Bornstein) with all the PDC versions for different age groups included in the manual. Regarding the other (non-*PDM* derived) tools, the chapter describes many more or less known and popular empirical instruments that may be useful for patient assessment (such as the SWAP, STIPO, MMPI, TAT, and Rorschach test). One of the aims of this chapter is to improve the dialogue between clinical practice and research (see also Hilsenroth, Katz, & Tanzilli, 2018).

Finally, the "Case Illustrations and PDM-2 Profiles" chapter aims at demonstrating the pertinence of the *PDM-2* diagnostic model and helping readers enhance and improve the structure of their formulations. Brief explanatory vignettes appear throughout the manual, but this final section includes complete clinical cases that exemplify the manual's approach.

The *PDM-2* omits a substantial part of the *PDM-1*: the "Conceptual and Empirical Foundations for a Psychodynamically Based Classification System" section that concludes the manual. The literature that appeared in this section has been integrated into relevant sections of the *PDM-2*.

A historical opportunity

By embracing the complexities of human experience in its healthy and disturbed features and by returning to the core of subjective phenomenology and its underlying dynamics, the *PDM-2* could serve as a holistic diagnostic tool. Greenspan thought it could help therapists to

> understand their patients more fully. [. . .] We've seen interest from people in anthropology, sociology, educators, legal scholars and people in the justice system. [. . .] It's broadened the purview of psychology to reach into all the related disciplines that deal with human beings.
>
> (Packard, 2007, p. 30)

He also believed it could be a beneficial source for not only psychodynamically oriented clinicians, but also behavioural, cognitive, humanistic, family-systems, and biologically oriented therapists.

The *PDM-2*'s multidimensional approach aims at providing a comprehensive profile of an individual's mental inner life; in this way, it is a landmark framework that registers the intricacies of each patient's functioning and ways of engaging in the therapeutic process. This diagnostic perspective will, in turn, affect treatment planning. Traditional therapeutic outcomes, such as stability of self-esteem, self and object constancy, flexibility of coping strategies, affect tolerance, sense of agency, resilience, reality testing, and the capacity to think about the self and others in complex and subtle ways, might be difficult to evaluate in terms of symptoms, but they are often significant to patients and more connected to enduring, stable change and the prevention of future psychopathology (Shedler, 2010; Shedler & Westen, 2004; Waldron, Moscovitz, Lundin, Helm, & Jemerin, 2010; Wampold, 2013; Westen, Gabbard, & Blagov, 2006).

For many years, I have led the training of clinical psychologists at my university. Throughout this time, I have realised that many young colleagues feel lost in a biomedical diagnostic world and keenly feel the lack of a more psychologically articulated diagnostic system. Too often they feel compelled to "choose" between oversimplified diagnostic labels and idiosyncratic, unreliable, and "local" diagnostic languages and procedures. Moreover, they miss the dynamic and intersubjective aspects of diagnosis. In their view, the traditional approach to diagnosing – a challenging and thought-provoking process – makes little sense and is a routine – (and often boring) activity.

In attempting to return the patient to the centre of diagnosis, the *PDM* has the potential to expand symptom checklists and delve into the deeper complexities of individuals. We hope that the *PDM-2*, in taking on the "torment" of diagnoses, may lead to a fruitful tension between idiographic and nomothetic knowledge, to enriched clinical work that views each patient within a larger family of people with similar characteristics and difficulties, and – last but not least – to clinicians' renewed pleasure in diagnosing, embracing it as a lively act that is significantly different from reliance on anonymous and repetitive bureaucratic models and unreliable, idiosyncratic, and unvalidated subjective measures.

References

American Psychiatric Association (1994). *Diagnostic and statistical manual of mental disorders* (4th ed.). Washington, DC: American Psychiatric Association.

American Psychiatric Association (2013). *Diagnostic and statistical manual of mental disorders* (5th ed.). Washington, DC: American Psychiatric Association.

Aron, L. (2012). Rethinking "doublethinking": Psychoanalysis and scientific research – An introduction to a series. *Psychoanalytic Dialogues*, 22(6): 704–709.

Barthes, R. (1980). *Camera lucida: Reflections of photography.* New York: Hill & Wang.

Betan, E., Heim, A. K., Zittel Conklin, C., & Westen, D. (2005). Countertransference phenomena and personality pathology in clinical practice: An empirical investigation. *American Journal of Psychiatry, 162*: 890–898.

Bion, W. R. (1967). *Second thoughts.* London: Karnac.

Blatt, S. J. (2008). *Polarities of experience: Relatedness and self-definition in personality development, psychopathology, and the therapeutic process.* Washington, DC: American Psychological Association.

Cassidy, J., & Shaver, P. R. (2008). *Handbook of attachment: Theory, research, and clinical applications* (2nd ed.). New York: Guilford Press.

Clarkin, J. F. (2015). A commentary on "The *Psychodynamic Diagnostic Manual, Version 2 (PDM-2)*": Assessing patients for improved clinical practice and research. *Psychoanalytic Psychology, 32*: 116–120.

Clarkin, J. F., Caligor, E., Stern, B. L., & Kernberg, O. F. (2004). *Structured interview of personality organization (STIPO).* Unpublished manuscript, Personality Disorders Institute, Weill Cornell Medical College, New York.

Colli, A., Tanzilli, A., Dimaggio, G., & Lingiardi, V. (2014). Patient personality and therapist response: An empirical investigation. *American Journal of Psychiatry, 171*: 102–108.

Costello, E. J., Mustillo, S., Erkanli, A., Keeler, G., & Angold, A. (2003). Prevalence and development of psychiatric disorders in childhood and adolescence. *Archives of General Psychiatry, 60*: 837–844.

Del Corno, F., & Lingiardi, V. (2012). The *Psychodynamic Diagnostic Manual (PDM)* in the U.S.A. and in Europe: Between commercial success and influence on professionals and researchers. *Bollettino di Psicologia Applicata, 265*: 5–10.

Eagle, M. N., & Wolitzky, D. L. (2011). Systematic empirical research versus clinical case studies: A valid antagonism? *Journal of American Psychoanalytic Association, 59*(4): 791–817.

Ferrari, H. (2006). Book reviews: *Psychodynamic Diagnostic Manual. Vertex, 17*: 356–361.

Ferrari, H., Lancelle, G., Pereira, A., Roussos, A., & Weinstein, L. (2008). *El Manual Diagnostico Psicoanalìtico. Discusiones sobre su estructura, su utilidad y viabilidad. Reportes de Investigatiòn, 1, Universidad de Belgrano.* Retrieved from www.ub.edu.ar/investigaciones/ri_nue-vos/1_rep1.pdf

Fonagy, P. (2013). There is room for even more doublethink: The perilous status of psychoanalytic research. *Psychoanalytic Dialogues, 23*: 116–122.

Gabbard, G. O. (2009). Transference and countertransference: Developments in the treatment of narcissistic personality disorder. *Psychiatric Annals, 39*: 129–136.

Gazzillo, F., Lingiardi, V., Del Corno, F., Genova, F., Bornstein, R. F., Gordon, R., & McWilliams, N. (2015). Clinicians' emotional responses and *Psychodynamic Diagnostic Manual* adult personality disorders: A clinically relevant empirical investigation. *Psychotherapy, 52*(2): 238–246.

Gershy, N. (2017). Psychodynamic case formulation: A roadmap to protocol adaptation in CBT. *Psychoanalytic Psychology, 34*(4): 478–487.

Hilsenroth, M., Katz, M., & Tanzilli, A. (2018). Psychotherapy research and *Psychodynamic Diagnostic Manual (PDM-2)*. *Psychoanalytic Psychology, 35*(3): 320–327.

Hoffman, I. Z. (2009). Doublethinking our way to "scientific legitimacy": The desiccation of human experience. *Journal of American Psychoanalytic Association, 57*(5): 1043–1069.

Hoffman, I. Z. (2012a). Response to Eagle and Wolitzky. *Journal of American Psychoanalytic Association, 60*: 105–120.

Hoffman, I. Z. (2012b), Response to Safran: The development of critical psychoanalytic sensibility. *Psychoanalytic Dialogues, 22*(6): 721–731.

Jaspers, K. (1913). *Allgemeine Psychopathologie [General Psychopathology]*. Berlin: Springer-Verlag. (Tr. Eng. Johns Hopkins University Press, Reprint edition, November 1997).

Kernberg, O. F. (1984). *Severe Personality Disorders: Psychotherapeutic Strategies*. New Haven, CT: Yale University Press.

Lingiardi, V., Colli, A., & Muzi, L. (2018). A clinically useful assessment of patients' (and therapists') mental capacities: M Axis implications for therapeutic alliance. *Psychoanalytic Psychology, 35*(3): 306–314.

Lingiardi, V., Gazzillo, F., & Waldron, S. (2010). An empirically supported psychoanalysis: The case of Giovanna. *Psychoanalytic Psychology, 27*(2): 190–218.

Lingiardi, V., Holmqvist, R., & Safran, J. (2016). Relational turn and psychotherapy research. *Contemporary Psychoanalysis, 52*(2), 275–312.

Lingiardi, V., & McWilliams, N. (2015). *The Psychodynamic Diagnostic Manual. Second Edition (PDM-2)*. *World Psychiatry, 14*(2): 237–239.

Lingiardi, V., & McWilliams, N. (2017) (Eds.). *The Psychodynamic Diagnostic Manual. Second Edition (PDM-2)*. New York: The Guilford Press.

Lingiardi, V., & McWilliams, N. (2018). Introduction to the Psychoanalytic Psychology Special Issue. The *Psychodynamic Diagnostic Manual (PDM)*: Yesterday, today, tomorrow. *Psychoanalytic Psychology, 35*(3): 289–293.

Lingiardi, V., McWilliams N., Bornstein, R. F., Gazzillo, F., & Gordon, R. (2015). The *Psychodynamic Diagnostic Manual* version 2 (*PDM-2*): Assessing patients for improved clinical practice and research. *Psychoanalytic Psychology, 32*: 94–115.

Lingiardi, V., Shedler, J. & Gazzillo, F. (2006). Assessing personality change in psychotherapy with the SWAP-200: A case study. *Journal of Personality Assessment, 86*: 36–45.

Lingiardi, V., Tanzilli, A., & Colli, A. (2015). Does the severity of psychopathological symptoms mediate the relationship between patient personality and therapist response? *Psychotherapy, 52*: 228–237.

McWilliams, N. (2011). *Psychoanalytic diagnosis: Understanding personality structure in the clinical process* (rev. ed.). New York: Guilford Press.

McWilliams, N. (2015). More simply human: On the universality of madness. *Psychosis: Psychological, Social and Integrative Approaches, 7*: 63–71.

McWilliams, N. (2016). *The long journey of psychodynamic diagnosis: The PDM-2 between diagnostic accuracy and clinical complexity.* Conference held in Genoa, Italy, Palazzo Ducale, September 15, 2016.

McWilliams, N., Grenyer, B., & Shedler, J. (2018). Personality in *Psychodynamic Diagnostic Manual (PDM-2)*: Controversial issues. *Psychoanalytic Psychology, 35*(3): 299–305.

Nussbaum, A. M. (2013). *The pocket guide to the* DSM-5 *diagnostic exam*. Washington, DC: American Psychiatric Publishing.

OPD Task Force (Eds.) (2008). *Operationalized Psychodynamic Diagnosis – OPD-2: Manual of diagnosis and treatment planning*. Cambridge, MA: Hogrefe & Huber.

Packard, E. (2007). A new tool for psychotherapists. Five psychoanalytic associations collaborate to publish a new diagnostic manual. *Monitor, 38*. Retrieved from www.apa.org/monitor/jan07/tool.aspx

PDM Task Force (2006). *Psychodynamic Diagnostic Manual*. Silver Spring, MD: Alliance of Psychoanalytic Organizations.

Rosenfeld, H. (1987). *Impasse and interpretation*. London: Routledge.

Rosenthal, R. J. (2008). Psychodynamic psychotherapy and the treatment of pathological gambling. *Revista Brasileira de Psiquiatria, 30*, 41–50.

Safran, J. D. (2012). Doublethinking or dialectical thinking: A critical appreciation of Hoffman's "doublethinking" critique. *Psychoanalytic Dialogues, 22*(6): 710–720.

Røssberg, J. I., Karterud, S., Pedersen, G., & Friis, S. (2007). An empirical study of countertransference reactions toward patients with personality disorders. *Comprehensive Psychiatry, 48*: 225–230.

Shedler, J. (2010). The efficacy of psychodynamic psychotherapy. *American Psychologist, 65*: 98–109.

Shedler, J. (2015). Integrating clinical and empirical perspectives on personality: The Shedler-Westen Assessment Procedure (SWAP). In S. K. Huprich (Ed.), *Personality Disorders: Toward Theoretical and Empirical Integration in Diagnosis and Assessment*. Washington, DC: American Psychological Association.

Shedler, J., & Westen, D. (2004). Dimensions of personality pathology: An alternative to the five-factor model. *American Journal of Psychiatry*, *161*: 1743–1754.

Steiner, J. (1993). *Psychic retreats: Pathological organizations in psychotic, neurotic, and borderline patients*. London: Routledge.

Steiner, J. (2011). *On seeing and being seen*. London: Routledge.

Speranza, A. M. & Fortunato, A. (2012). Infancy, childhood and adolescence in the diagnostics of the *Psychodynamic Diagnostic Manual* (PDM). *Bollettino di Psicologia Applicata*, *265*: 53–65.

Stepansky, P. E. (2009). *Psychoanalysis at the Margins*. New York: Other Press.

Tanzilli, A., Muzi, L., Ronningstam, E., & Lingiardi, V. (2017). Countertransference when working with narcissistic personality disorder: An empirical investigation. *Psychotherapy*, *54*: 184–194.

Vivona, J. (2012). Between a rock and hard science: How should psychoanalysis respond to pressures for quantitative evidence of effectiveness? *Journal of the American Psychoanalytic Association*, *60*(1): 121–129.

Waldron, S., Moscovitz, S., Lundin, J., Helm, F., & Jemerin, J. (2010). Evaluating the outcomes of psychotherapies: The Personality Health Index. *Psychoanalytic Psychology*, *28*: 363–388.

Wampold, B. E. (2013). The good, the bad, and the ugly: A 50-year perspective on the outcome problem. *Psychotherapy*, *50*(1): 16–24.

Westen, D., DeFife, J. A., Malone, J. C., & DiLallo, J. (2014). An empirically derived classification of adolescent personality disorders. *Journal of the American Academy of Child and Adolescent Psychiatry*, *53*(5): 528–549.

Westen, D., Gabbard, G. O., & Blagov, P. (2006). Back to the future: Personality structure as a context for psychopathology. In R. F. Krueger, & J. L. Tackett (Eds.), *Personality and Psychopathology* (pp. 335–384). New York: Guilford.

Westen, D., Novotny, C. M., & Thompson-Brenner, H. (2004). The empirical status of empirically sup- ported psychotherapies: Assumptions, findings, and reporting in controlled clinical trials. *Psychological Bulletin*, *130*, 631–663.

Westen, D., & Shedler, J. (1999a). Revising and assessing Axis II, part I: Developing a clinically and empirically valid assessment method. *American Journal of Psychiatry*, *156*: 258–272.

Westen, D., & Shedler, J. (1999b). Revising and assessing Axis II, part II: Toward an empirically based and clinically useful classification of personality disorders. *American Journal of Psychiatry*, *156*: 273–285.

Westen, D., & Shedler, J. (2007). Personality diagnosis with the Shedler-Westen Assessment Procedure (SWAP): Integrating clinical and statistical measurement and prediction. *Journal of Abnormal Psychology*, *116*: 810–822.

Westen, D., Shedler, J., Bradley, B., & DeFife, J. A. (2012). An empirically derived taxonomy for personality diagnosis: Bridging science and practice in conceptualizing personality. *American Journal of Psychiatry*, *169*: 273–284.

Westen, D., Shedler, J., Durrett, C., Glass, S., & Martens, A. (2003). Personality diagnoses in adolescence: *DSM-IV* Axis II diagnoses and an empirically derived alternative. *American Journal of Psychiatry, 160*: 952–966.

Widlöcher, D. (2007). *Le Manuel Diagnostique Psychodynamique.* Du nosographique au psychopathologique. Pour la recherche. *Bulletin de la Fédération Française de Psychiatrie, 52.* Retrieved from www.psydoc-france.com

Widlöcher, D., & Thurin, J.M. (2011). *Le Manuel Diagnostique Psychodynamique*: Integrer dans une perspective nosologique les apports d'une psychopathologie dynamique. *Psychiatrie Française, 42*: 7–18.

Zimmermann, J., Ehrenthal, J. C., Cierpka, M., Schauenburg, J., Doering, S., & Benecke, C. (2012). Assessing the level of structural integration using *Operationalized Psychodynamic Diagnosis* (OPD): Implications for DSM-5. *Journal of Personality Assessment, 94*(5), 522–532.

CHAPTER ELEVEN

The structural interview

Otto F. Kernberg

W hat follows is an overview of the diagnostic method we have developed at the Personality Disorders Institute of the Weill Cornell Medical College to facilitate the descriptive, structural, and dynamic diagnosis of patients with personality disorders. In our work with severe personality disorders we have developed an overall structural concept of the nature of this psychopathology, and a system of classification related to their structural characteristics, and relevant for the prognosis and treatment of these conditions (Kernberg, 1984; Yeomans, Clarkin, & Kernberg, 2015). The present day DSM-V classification of personality disorders is undergoing significant changes (American Psychiatric Association, 2013). Major controversies in this field are reflected in the dialectics of the present classification system of personality disorders in the DSM-V system as contrasted to the proposed alternative method of classification of personality disorders in Section 3 of the DSM-V system. The latter method we believe, represents a significant progress in the understanding of the essential nature of personality disorders, and, in fact, approaches clearly our own findings and conclusions that underlie our conceptualization of this field.

The method for diagnosing personality disorders that we have proposed and that is synthesized in what we have called the structural interview should facilitate the diagnosis of individual personality disorders throughout their entire spectrum of severity. It is eminently compatible with the descriptive classification of personality disorders regardless of whatever classifying system is utilized. In addition, however, this method, should permit to highlight what we have called the underlying structural characteristics of severe personality disorders, that is, typical clinical manifestations of each of them that reflect habitual ways of processing and organizing psychological experiences. Finally, this method conveys prognostic and therapeutic implications for the personality disorders that are diagnosed.

The term "psychological structure" refers to habitual ways of organizing experience and behavior that serve defensive functions against unconscious conflicts, and constitute compromise formations between powerful emotional needs and fears that oppose them. The essential structures that differentiate personality disorders and permit their classification in terms of their severity include personal identity, that is, the extent to which there is available an integrated concept of self and the capacity for establishing integrated concepts of significant others; the predominant constellation of defensive operations, which differentiates defensive operations centered upon the mechanism of repression or maintenance of unacceptable mental contents out of consciousness, in contrast to defensive operations centered on splitting or primitive dissociation, that is, the avoidance of intolerable conflict by mutual separation or isolation of intolerable emotional contents; and reality testing, that is, the capacity to differentiate self from non-self, intrapsychic from external stimuli, and the capacity to maintain empathy with ordinary social criteria of reality.

These three structural characteristics, namely, identity, defensive organization, and reality testing permit the classification of personality disorders into two major groups: first, neurotic personality organization, characterized by a solid establishment of normal identity, defensive operations centered around repression, and excellent reality testing. The second group, of severe personality disorders or borderline personality organization, is characterized by the lack of an integrated identity or "identity diffusion," defensive operations centered on splitting mechanisms, and frailty of reality testing, in the sense of the loss of the finer capacity of tactful differentiation of subtle social stimuli and interactions, while still maintaining intact the essential criteria of reality testing mentioned before. These, then, are the fundamental psychic structures the diagnosis of which is facilitated by structural interviewing. Additional psychological structures evaluated in the structural interview include the quality of relationships with others or "object relationships" in psychoanalytic object relations theory terminology; the integration of an internal system of ethics or value systems in contrast to the disposition for anti-social behavior; and the nature of the elaboration and control of negative affect systems or aggression. In addition, specific abnormal psychic structures characterize particular personality disorders, such as, very importantly, the development of pathological narcissism, and the description of these psychological structures overlaps with that of the specific personality disorders.

The method of structural interviewing that I shall describe permits the diagnosis of the personality disorders of the DSM-V and ICD-10 systems as well as the diagnosis of the structural characteristics proposed in the DSM-V alternative classification of personality disorders. This alternative model includes as central criteria the degree of severity of pathology of the self and of the relations with significant others, and it should clearly convey the general severity of the personality disorder that has been diagnosed. As mentioned before, this diagnostic method we have proposed should not only facilitate the diagnosis of the specificity of the personality disorder and its severity, but also convey therapeutic implications and the prognosis for psychotherapeutic treatment of these patients.

The structural interview, in fact, is a classical mental status examination enriched by an initial, major addition of a set of inquiries geared to clarifying the symptoms and the nature of the personality disorders. The interview starts with the diagnostician's greeting the patient, and letting the patient know all he knows about the patient through other sources and previous information the patient has communicated to him. This may vary from only knowing the patient's name and perhaps age, to abundant information that the diagnostician has received before seeing the patient. In the latter case he would let the patient know that he has received all this information, has been able to study it or not, and now would like to invite the patient to respond to a set of early questions that the diagnostician then expresses.

These initial questions are: What brings you here? What is the nature of your difficulties? What do you expect from treatment? And finally, where are you now?

These four questions, formulated within variations typical for any diagnostician are presented in sequence, all at once, and they have the purpose of indicating to the diagnostician the basic views and intentions of the patient as well as carrying out a mini-mental status examination. In fact, the capability of attending to these four questions, understanding them, remembering them, and answering them meaningfully implies that the patient is conscious, able to listen and to understand, has available short term memory, the capacity for formulating responses and for conveying them at an appropriate level of abstraction. The patient's incapacity to respond to these questions may reflect disturbances in attention, consciousness, memory, intelligence, or the presence of a psychotic distortion of the perception of the present reality, the interview, or the nature of the questions. In short, any gross incapacity to respond to these questions may alert the diagnostician to the possible presence of a mentally organic or psychotic condition that would orient the following inquiry into the direction of a traditional or classic mental status examination.

If, to the contrary, the patient is able to respond to those four questions, that response, as a minimum, will involve information about one or many symptoms that bring him to see a specialist in psychological difficulties. The diagnostician's response to the patient's capacity to provide adequate responses to this first set of four questions then consists in proceeding with the following inquiry, focused on the patient's functioning in his present life's situation, the major content of the structural interview under these circumstances.

First, the diagnostician now explores all the symptoms that the patient has conveyed to him. We try to obtain as complete as possible a list of physical symptoms, psychological symptoms, difficulties in daily functioning, and interpersonal difficulties. At a certain point, the diagnostician is able to ask "is there anything else that you have not been able to mention so far, or would you be perfectly alright if you didn't have any of all the symptoms that you have mentioned so far?"

By then asking more regarding detailed information about selected symptoms mentioned by the patient, we try to carry out an immediate differential diagnosis, for example, between the different conditions characterized by anxiety, or the differentiation of depression, and the motivation behind suicidal ideation, intention, or behavior. We try to transform all the "technical lingo" with which the patient may respond to our questions, in an effort to retranslate such "technical" descriptions into the direct feelings and experiences that the patient has sensed. In short, the objective is to obtain a complete set of present symptomology, as much as the patient is able to convey, with an early effort to carry out the differential diagnosis of some frequent, salient symptoms.

This inquiry regarding the patient's symptoms may take a relatively brief time or up to an hour of raising questions, depending on the nature of the case. The general principle is to take all the time that is needed to obtain a complete inventory of symptoms.

A second level of inquiry now focuses on the patient's present life experiences. Patients may spontaneously start talking about important experiences in their past that they believe are relevant for what is happening to them now, or regarding which they have been told by other professionals that they are relevant for what their present difficulties are. We try to listen patiently to this information a sufficient time to be able to tell the patient, "this seems to be important and we shall have time to return to it, but now I would like to return to what is going on presently in your life." And we proceed by telling the patient "I'm interested to find out how you are functioning in the most important aspects of your present life, which means, in the areas of work or profession, regarding your love life and sexual experiences, your social life and areas of your independent creative functioning and employment of your free time." "To begin with, I would like to know more about your work or profession."

This question opens up a series of related questions about the nature of the patient's work, his functioning in his work, the extent to which the patient has difficulties in his work, his working up to his capabilities, the relationship the patient has with co-workers, superiors, and subordinates, the extent to which his present work corresponds to his education, aspirations, and capabilities. We try to find whether work is gratifying or frustrating, and to what extent the patient's functioning in this area has suffered because of other symptoms or difficulties. We are trying to obtain, in short, as detailed information as necessary to be able to answer the question, whether this is an area in which the patient is not functioning optimally, and what is the nature of the difficulties, both in his technical functioning and in the interpersonal relations carried out in the context of his work situation, that represent significant problems. In the case of students, of course, the same type of questions are posed regarding their functioning in their studies, their success or failure at school, their relationship with colleagues, teachers, the extent to which they are able to live up to their responsibilities or not, and the extent to which extra-curricular activities or problems not related to school or school relations are influencing or interfering with school work.

We then explore the patient's functioning in love and his sexual life. This is an area that diagnosticians often feel inhibited from exploring fully, and our experience is that the more the diagnostician feels comfortable with exploring this area of the patient's functioning, the easier it is for the patient to provide information in this regard. Obviously, the patient's gender and age have to be taken into consideration in raising questions in this area. We are interested if the patients has been in a stable love relation or not and in either case, what his difficulties have been in the relationship or in establishing a relationship. We are interested whether the patient has been able to establish stable love relations or not, whether he presents serious inhibition in this regard or sexual promiscuity, and, obviously, whether his orientation is predominately heterosexual or homosexual. We try to find out whether the patient loves his or her partner, whether the patient has been has been able to fall in love (the incapacity to falling in love is a significant symptom of narcissistic personalities), and the extent to which emotional investment, idealization, and tenderness are going hand and hand with the patient's sexual interest and activities, or, to the contrary, to what extent there exists disassociation between the patient's objects of sexual interest and objects of emotional idealization of a love relationship.

We are interested in exploring inhibitions both in the capacity to love and in the capacity to establish or not a love relationship, and in the capacity to engage or not in sexual activities, to what extent sexual intercourse is normal or troubled by some degree of sexual difficulty or inhibition. The nature of the psychological difficulties with love objects or sexual partners, the internal sense of freedom to engage in such relationships versus severe inhibition are an important subject of this interview. We also try to find out to what extent the patient is able to masturbate, whether this is a satisfactory activity or whether the patient has problems regarding masturbation, and the extent to which the total amount of sexual activities seems to correspond to the patient's age and development or to what extent there seems to be either a significant inhibition in the total sexual activity, or an abnormal intensity combined with a high degree of dissatisfaction in this area.

We then explore the patient's social life and the field of his particular creative interest in any area not related to his work. First of all, we try to find out, how does the patient relate to friends and family? Does he have a social network, close friends over many years that are an important source of gratification and stimulation in his social life, niche or social network to which he belongs? Is he comfortable with his social life? What is the relationship between the patient and the immediate members of his family, his parental couple and their generation, his children and their generation? To what extent is there any inhibition or sense of imposition of social involvement that constitutes a burden to the patient? We try to find out what important conflicts or inhibitions, preferences and distaste are expressed in his daily relations with family, friends, and acquaintances.

Again, the questions will vary with age and social background of patients, but the extent to which there are flexible and free interactions with others, significant problems in such interactions, inhibitions or frustrations, should become evident at this point. Then we inquire about any particular interest the patient may have in whichever area he is interested: sports, politics, science, art, religion, inventive pursuits in the technical, scientific or spiritual realm, the extent to which the patient can dedicate himself enthusiastically to something not directed at personal success or prominence, but where the motivation resides within an intrinsic interest in the subject proper.

The structural interview then approaches a third major level of inquiry, the presence of an integrated, normal identity, or the presence of the syndrome of identity diffusion. This is a crucial dimension that differentiates higher level of personality disorders, that is, neurotic personality organization, from the area of severe personality disorders or borderline personality organization (Kernberg, 2006). At this point of the interview we have already achieved a reasonable awareness of the patient's daily personal life, the most important persons who are part of his life, and we now ask the patient to describe two or three of the persons with whom he is closest at this time, persons with whom there is the highest level of present relationship and mutual engagement. We ask him to describe, first, one of these persons more in detail, and then one other, or two other people. We ask the patient to give us, in the course of a few minutes, a brief description of what seems to him most important in that particular person, what differentiates that person most significantly from other people, what is it that the patient might convey to us so that we can construct an image of that person in our minds, and then we listen to this description.

Persons with normal identity, that is, a normal integration of the concept of self, and a normal integration of the concept of significant others (the definition of normal identity integration) should be able, with some effort on their part, to describe such a person they are very close to, in ways that give us a specific image that may differentiate that person in our mind. In contrast, in the case of identity diffusion, with a lack of integration of the concept of self and lack of integration of the concept of significant others, patients are unable to do what we ask, and convey a chaotic, contradictory description of such other persons, or a highly conventional, superficial one, that does not permit the interviewer to develop any particular specific image of that person. Or else, the patient may even declare his incapacity to provide such a description.

After having raised this question regarding two or three persons, the interviewer should be able to detect whether, indeed, there is a serious difficulty on the part of the patient to describe another person in sufficient clarity and depth for the interviewer to obtain a differentiated individualized picture. We then move on to tell the patient, we would now like him to describe himself as a specific person, trying to covey to us in a few minutes what he would think is essential in his personality, the most important aspects of his personality that would give us an idea of what makes him a unique person, different from anyone else. The question about the description of the self is posed only after having asked him to describe significant others, so as to use that effort to describe others as a learning process, which the patient can then apply to himself.

Again, patients with normal identity integration, and with some self-reflective effort, are able to describe themselves in terms of some important central traits they feel jointly represent a picture of what makes them different from other persons, convey what is unique about them, what might permit the interviewer to have a better knowledge and understanding of who they are. When that is a successful effort, it indicates the capacity for experiencing an integrated self, and that is an essential component of normal self-identity. The incapacity to do this would again signal identity diffusion. Identity diffusion, in short, is constituted by the lack of the capacity to convey an integrated concept of self and an integrated concept of significant others, signaling the presence of borderline personality organization, the presence of some constellation of severe personality disorder.

This is perhaps the most difficult element in the assessment involved in structural interviewing. A practical way to train students in the capacity to process this inquiry appropriately, is to suggest to them to carry out structural interviewing with a significant number of patients who have been diagnosed with severe personality disorders, for example, within a population of inpatient personality disorders, and then raise the same questions, carry out the same inquiry with members of the students' social group (who, presumably, mostly will not be constituted by patients with severe personality disorder, and thus permit learning to evaluate the difference between the expression of normal identity and that of identity diffusion.

If the patient presents normal identity and indications of a significant personality disorder, it probably is one of the neurotic levels of personality organization, particularly, an obsessive–compulsive, hysterical, or depressive – masochistic personality disorder. In contrast, with the presence of a syndrome of identity diffusion, the patient probably suffers from a severe personality disorder, particularly, a borderline personality disorder, histrionic personality disorder, narcissistic personality disorder, antisocial personality disorder – if his temperamental predisposition is mostly extroverted, or else with introverted temperament, most probably a schizoid, schizotypal, hypochondriacal or paranoid personality disorder.

The fourth level of inquiry, finally, covers the presence or absence of reality testing. Reality testing is an enormously important symptom that separates personality disorders from atypical psychotic and organic mental disorders, thus representing the boundary between personality disorders and other areas of major psychiatric disorders that may imitate but not constitute personality disorders proper. It is a relatively simple inquiry, as contrasted with the inquiry of identity diffusion, and of great clinical value in difficult diagnostic cases. Reality testing consists in the capacity to differentiate self from non-self, intrapsychic from external origin of perceived stimuli, and it signals the capacity for maintaining empathy with ordinary social criteria of reality. Practically, reality testing is lost in the case of patients who present hallucinations and delusions, but is maintained in cases who present obsessive ideas, overvalued ideas, pseudo-hallucinations and illusions. Pseudo-hallucinations, illusions, and overvalued ideas also may be present in psychotic illness, but only hallucinations and delusions are definite indications for loss of reality testing.

It is important to keep in mind that there are patients who, without presenting obvious indications of hallucinations nor delusions, nevertheless, may have lost the capacity for reality testing, signaling what may be called psychotic personality structure in the sense of loss of differentiation between intrapsychic and external reality. These are patients who impress us with some strange, exotic, weird, idiosyncratic aspects of behavior that seem clearly or even vaguely discrepant with ordinary social interactions such as the one activated in the diagnostic interview. They impress the interviewer as "flaky," very often without the possibility of specifying what makes the patient appear so strange. In any case, it is that subjective experience of the interviewer that, at this advanced point of the interview, should guide him to assess to what extent there is something strange or weird in the patient's behavior, in the patient's affect, in the patient's thought content or in the formal aspects of the patient's language and thinking.

If we detect any such peculiar aspect in the patient's presentation, at this point we would confront the patient in a tactful way with the fact that we observed something that seems to us strange in the interaction with the patient, and would like to know whether the patient can understand that that aspect of his behavior, or affective expression, or thinking had seemed strange to us. We tell the patient what it is that seemed strange to us, and ask him how he would explain that this seemed strange to us. If reality testing is maintained, the patient will be able to understand what seemed strange to us, applying his understanding and empathy with ordinary criteria of social reality to clarify it. Under these circumstances, the patient will try to reflect on what we have observed, and give us an explanation that will make that which seemed at first strange to us more understandable. The patient will signal that he can see that this behavior seems strange and needs to be explained in the light of ordinary social reality.

If, to the contrary, the patient is expressing a psychotic experience, conviction, or perception related to that particular behavior, affect, or thought content, he will feel threatened or challenged by our question. That will determine an increase in the degree of anxiety regarding the interview, and possibly cause a greater disturbance in his relation with us. Here the indication is that the patient does not preserve empathy with ordinary social criteria of reality: he is being challenged, and may feel criticized or attacked unfairly, reacting correspondently to our inquiry.

Indication of loss of reality testing indicates psychotic functioning and should trigger in the interviewer the decision to pursue the interview in terms of a standard mental status examination of criteria that, so far, have not been explored systematically. This includes, to begin with, the description of the patient's distorted behavior, distorted affect, and/or distorted thought content or formal organization of language. Then, it should include a systematic analysis of the sensorium, of memory and intelligence, with a careful inquiry regarding previously not perceived positive indications of psychosis, specifically, hallucinations and delusions.

To the contrary, if realty testing clearly is maintained, the patient's pathology can assuredly be diagnosed as a personality disorder. The severity of this disorder will be determined by the presence or absence of normal identity. The information the patient has given us about his present life situation, his present interpersonal functioning in the area of work or profession, love and sex, social life and creativity will have provided us with important indicators of the predominant constellation of pathological character traits reflecting his personality disorder. This description will lead us to the particular personality disorder within the neurotic or borderline level of personality organization.

In fact, within the broad spectrum of personality disorders that fall within the area of borderline personality organization, this method may differentiate patients who, in spite of the presence of identity diffusion are still able to work, to maintain a relatively stable if conflictual intimate relationship, and participate in a social life environment, as presenting a higher level of functioning within borderline personality organization. In contrast, complete breakdown in the capacity for work or profession, in the capacity to maintain a stable intimate relationship, and severe distortion or withdrawal from social life will indicate a lower level of functioning within borderline personality organization.

In general, in addition to the syndrome of identity diffusion, the severity of the distortion of object relations, the presence of antisocial behavior, and the expression of intense, pathological aggressive interactions indicate the more severe level of borderline personality organization. The most severe level of personality disorder is represented by the antisocial personality disorder that evinces the worst prognosis for any psychotherapeutic approach (Hare, 1999; Kernberg, 1984, 1992; Stone, 2009).

This completes the outline of the structural interview, the clinical method we have developed to diagnose the nature, severity, and prognosis of personality disorder by means of an enrichment and modification of the standard mental status examination. It has been proven as effective clinically, while not being a useful research instrument in this form. We have modified this interview into a specific structured interview, the structured interview for personality organization (STIPO), a validated and reliable instrument for the diagnosis of personality disorders that, in contrast to the clinical structural interview, is a useful research instrument although it does not have the flexibility and immediate clinical usefulness of structural interviewing (Hörz et al., 2012).

References

American Psychiatric Association. (2013). *Diagnostic and Statistical Manual of Mental Disorders: DSM-V*. Washington, DC: American Psychiatric Publishing.

Hare, R. D. (1999). *Without conscience: The disturbing world of the psychopaths among us*. New York: Guildford Press.

Hörz, S. Clarkin, J. F., Stern, B. L., Caligor, E. et al: (2012). The structural interview of personality disorders (STIPO). In R. Levy, J. Ablon, & M. Karchele (Eds.) *Psychodynamic psychotherapy research* (pp. 571–592). New York: Springer.

Kernberg, O. F. (1984). *Severe personality disorders: Psychotherapeutic strategies*. New Haven, CT: Yale University Press.

Kernberg, O. F. (1992). *Aggression in personality disorders and perversion*. New Haven, CT: Yale University Press.

Kernberg, O. F. (2006). Identity: Recent findings and clinical implications. *Psychoanalytic Quarterly*, 75: 969–1044.

Stone, M. H. (2009). *The anatomy of evil*. Amherst, NY: Prometheus Press.

Yeomans, F. E., Clarkin, J. F., & Kernberg, O. F. (2015). *Transference focused psychotherapy for borderline personality disorders: A clinical guide*. Washington, DC: American Psychiatric Publishing.

CHAPTER TWELVE

Clinical picture as an open window

From symptoms to a phenomenological-dynamic stance on the patient's world[1]

Mario Rossi Monti and Alessandra D'Agostino

Diagnosis between public and private

Today it is possible to give a psychiatric diagnosis by relying on a series of standardized and empirically validated procedures. The Diagnostic and Statistical Manual of Mental Disorders – now in its fifth edition (APA, 2013) – and the SCID-CV-5 are the most popular diagnostic tools. To these, we can add the AMDP-System (*Arbeitsgemeinschaft für Methodik und Dokumentation in der Psychiatrie*) (1981), now in its eighth edition, and other diagnostic manuals inspired by psychoanalysis such as the Operationalized Psychodynamic Diagnosis OPD-2 (2008) or the PDM Psychodynamic Diagnostic Manual (2006), whose second edition is forthcoming. While on the one hand we can count on a number of codified and standardized diagnostic procedures, on the other it is hard to believe that in their daily work therapists slavishly follow these standardized procedures. For example (and thankfully), live clinical assessment does not follow the decision tree procedures as outlined in the DSM or other standardized procedures. At this level, the diagnosis seems to be the outcome of a naive and fuzzy process that is strongly influenced by personal training, theoretical models, and also by one's masters as well as by experience gained on the field. This nuanced and vague procedure consists of a set of attitudes, questions, opinions and exploratory moves that gradually come to form a well-tested, personal and private repertoire: each therapist develops his or her own in order to navigate the mind of the patient and answer a series of questions. Such questions may range from the most classic and reductive ones (*What is the disorder here?*) to more complex ones such as: *Where is this patient speaking from?* – or rather: *What kind of world does this patient inhabit? From what place is he speaking? How does he see himself and others? And himself in relation to others (and vice versa)?* And again: *To whom is he speaking?* And also: *What is it like to hear his voice coming from a world so different from mine?* Only later, when he has gained some knowledge of the patient with the help of his personal and private repertoire, the therapist may try to place what he has learned from his contact with the patient in the context of a standardized framework. The material he has collected, all that he has focused on and experienced within the personal and private dimension of the clinical encounter, is now formatted through a codified procedure, thereby acquiring a public and official dimension.

What happens inside the no man's land of the clinical encounter, the first clinical evaluation or the descriptive diagnosis that – according to the DSM-5 – should be part of a "case formulation assessment"? Is it possible to say something more precise about what happens when the therapist is trying to find his way in his relationship with the patient without the help of decision trees or standardized grids? Can we identify some landmarks in these 'amoeboid' exploratory moves that do not follow a standardized but rather a fuzzy logic? This essay will address the problem of diagnosis as understood not only as a *noun* or *name* ('diagnosis') but also as a *verb* ('diagnosing'): We will attempt to argue that a 'diagnostic space' opens up thanks to an *oscillatory state of mind* (Modell, 1990) taking place at the intersection of different ways of looking 'through' the symptom. This state has often been described through the metaphor of 'binocular vision' (Bion, 1961). Binocular vision is acquired when, having pointed the binoculars toward a specific object, one tries to adjust the two eyepieces to integrate the two perspectives and thereby acquire depth perception. While on the one hand this procedure is certainly useful to avoid making a superficial diagnosis, on the other it seems to give the illusion that it is possible to reach a final integration and a stable, in-depth and defined view on the object. In the context of a diagnosis, however, it would be more appropriate to see such integration only as an ideal destination. In this sense, depth perception should never be achieved once and for all. On the contrary, rather than on a *binocular* vision, the function of diagnosis should be based on a certain degree of *cross-eyed* vision, so to speak: this would allow one to focus on a particular object and capture some of its aspects while at the same time leaving other aspects of the same object out of focus, in a process of continuous and almost endless adjustment. In this continuous focusing (as when microscopists gradually focus on different layers of an object), the diagnosis as a name is turned into a process or verb ('diagnosing') and then again back into a name, and so on, in a spiral sequence that accompanies the entire course of treatment.

Diagnosis: name or verb?

The word 'diagnosis' indicates both the destination and the process of investigation that leads to assign a name to a clinical picture when theory-laden events clump around a specific label. On the one hand, therefore, we have the diagnosis as *name* or *denotation*, and, on the other, as *process* or *verb* (Rothstein, 2002; Sadler, 2005). As a name, the diagnosis is a necessarily very condensed and impersonal description/display of psychopathological facts, which holds together and conveys a constellation of generic data. It represents a sum of our knowledge about a particular state of mind, and its main purpose is to convey as much information as possible in the most concise possible way (Stanghellini & Rossi Monti, 2009). By gathering the available data under a specific umbrella-term, the diagnosis provides additional information about the location of this syndromic framework within a classificatory systematics. To the diagnosis as name applies what Wilfred Bion (1963) has written about the nature and function of the 'name': the name is an invention to make it possible to think and talk about something before it is known what that something is. The name is simply the first step of a process (the diagnostic process) in which the rest of the time, Bion argues, should be spent in trying to understand what that name actually means and to which aspects of the person's existence it refers.

Diagnosis, however, is not only a static name. It is also and above all a dynamic process (the 'diagnosing') that unfolds over time, a process that intertwines closely with the therapeutic process and orients its development. Indeed, if at the beginning of a therapeutic relationship it is important to understand whether a person suffers or not from a Major Depressive Disorder or a Borderline Personality Disorder, soon the therapist's questions change. Instead of asking whether this particular person is depressed or not, the therapist now wonders *how* this particular person experiences his or her depression. *How* is this depressed person depressed? Or even: *how* is this borderline person borderline? From a recognition and delineation of the clinical picture, in the course of treatment the diagnosis gradually turns into a reformulation and description of how the manifestations of mental illness are shaped over time in relation to the specific personality traits of the subject. From this point of view, the diagnosis should be seen as a compass to consult at the beginning of a journey so as to find the right direction and chart a course. However, in order to monitor and recalculate the route, it is necessary to consult this compass repeatedly during the journey. Something similar often happens with the (slightly annoying) function 're-calculate route' in our modern automotive navigation systems, which forces us to constantly rethink our itinerary. This function is of great importance for the diagnosis and is inseparable from the cross-eyed gaze that feeds the diagnostic process, a process during which the therapist runs the constant risk of remaining trapped in his or her first diagnostic hypothesis. Indeed, in the formulation of a psychiatric diagnosis the danger of dogmatism and reification is always present. To reify the diagnosis means to think that by knowing the diagnosis one also knows the patient. It is no coincidence that already in 1764 Immanuel Kant warned the doctors of the mind that to invent a new word does not mean to understand a disease. It would be even worse to think that by knowing the word one can also understand the person!

To sum up, we could argue that every diagnosis has both merits and flaws: its main merit is to help the therapist to orient himself and focus on an established set of ideas; its main flaw is exactly the same: to focus on an established set of ideas, thereby often 'nailing' a person to his or her diagnosis once and for all (Racamier, 1992). In this sense, as Karl Jaspers wrote (1913), it is absolutely true (no matter how paradoxical this may sound) that the diagnosis should be the last, not the first concern of the psychopathologist. However, the diagnosis as a *function* and as a *process* ('diagnosing') should begin immediately and unfold over the entire course of the treatment. Each diagnosis, therefore, is a bit like a tailor-made garment that never fits the patient's body perfectly and permanently. It is as if the tailor invited the customer for an endless series of fittings with the excuse of having to continually adjust and rearrange a garment that never fits the customer's features faultlessly.

It is precisely because of this situation that, strangely enough, a therapist might be perfectly able to identify the symptoms of depression, arranged for example according to scales of quantitative evaluation, but totally unable to question their meaning (Fédida, 2001). It is not at all certain, in other words, that a therapist capable of using the diagnosis as a 'name' will also be able to use it as a 'verb', i.e. to switch from an objectifying and static to a dynamic and evolutionary use of the diagnosis. A dynamic use should take account of the fact that patients change over time, both in the sense that they gradually show different aspects of themselves and are subject to transformations. From this point of view, a great deal of attention should be paid to the proposal developed among others by Wigman et al. (2013), according to which the diagnosis should be seen as a process that has at least two sides or dimensions: *clinical staging* and *profiling*.

The first dimension (clinical staging) identifies the nomothetic component of diagnosis and takes into account the fact that in the early stages of disorder its symptomatic expression is more diffuse and generic. With the progression of the disorder, however, such expression becomes more specific and symptoms tend to crystallize into more particular and pronounced syndromes. The second dimension (profiling), instead, stands for the ideographic component of diagnosis and takes into account the fact that, due to the great heterogeneity of clinical pictures observable within the same diagnostic category, individual differences increase as the disorder progresses. This approach is in stark contrast with the static and fixistic perspective developed by DSM, which concerns almost exclusively patients in whom the psychopathological expression has taken the stable form typical of the most serious mental illnesses in their advanced stages.

Three modes of looking through

The term 'diagnosis' literally means 'to know through'. In the diagnostic process, therefore, the gaze of the therapist 'looks through' the phenomena. If one can certainly argue that the diagnosis is a way to name and identify a *clinical picture*, at the same time one must be aware that this *picture* is also a *window* overlooking the inner world of the patient, his experiences, his history and so on. It is a matter of looking *through* a *picture* so as to see it also as a *window*. Something similar happens in many of Magritte's paintings, where, according to the logic of *mise en abyme*, a window opens on another window in an endless sequence. To clarify the twofold nature of diagnosis as a picture and a window I will refer to a famous painting by Pablo Picasso depicting a dove flying with a twig in its beak. This immediately points to the dove as a symbol of peace. However, this *picture* can also be thought of as a *window* on Picasso's inner world and personal history. As the great art historian Ernst Gombrich (1958) reminds us, Picasso's father was a rather mediocre painter: his name was Don Pepe Ruiz and he was the curator of the municipal museum of Malaga. His favorite subjects were pigeons and rabbits. At some point Pablo chose to change his last name and adopted that of his mother (Picasso). Thinking back to his childhood years, he used to visualize his father's paintings disseminated in the family residence: paintings hanging in the dining room, animal hair and feathers, hundreds of pigeons, hares and rabbits. As a child, he recalled, when left alone at school, he used to fall into a state of real terror. Paralyzed by fear, he would cling to his father and try to seize some of his belongings: the walking stick, the paint brushes, and most of all a stuffed pigeon that he always carried with him as a model for his paintings. Keeping some of his father's belongings as hostages, little Pablo would feel a bit safer: he was certain that his father would come back to pick him up. Thus, the dove as a symbol of peace appearing in the *painting* by Pablo Picasso is at the same time a *window* on the inner world, the personal history and the significant relationships of Pablo *Ruiz* Picasso. On the one hand, the dove is immediately inscribed in a constellation of shared meanings that refers to peace as a value; on the other, the dove refers to a series of idiosyncratic personal layers that are a part of Picasso's history and experience. The dove is placed exactly at the intersection between a *picture* and a *window*.

Similarly, we could conceive psychiatric diagnosis as a device capable of outlining a clinical *picture*. So, for example, drawing on the DSM case studies, a patient who has trouble falling asleep, wakes up too early in the morning and shows suicidal ideation, loss of interest in life, serious weight loss, fatigue, and great difficulty in concentrating seems to fit the clinical picture of a Major Depressive Disorder. Currently, this particular *picture* belongs to a constellation of meanings shared by psychiatric nosology. At the same time, however, this picture is also a *window* that – as when one looks inside a well – allows a glimpse of the inner world of the patient and provides the opportunity to explore the personal meaning of his or her condition. What kind of 'pigeons' will the therapist be able to spot by looking out of the patient's window? We do not know. The answer can come only through a prolonged therapeutic relationship, one in which the therapist does not confine himself to a diagnosis 'as a name', but keeps searching for a 'diagnosing' that can unfold throughout the entire course of treatment. To make a diagnosis, in this sense, means to 'look through' an object, namely to look at the disease through the symptoms. However, the diagnosis as a form of 'looking through' can adopt at least three different epistemological stances:

1   A first configuration of the diagnosis as 'looking through' points to the ability to look through the symptoms established by the current nosology, and on such basis, identify the disorder, or even the disease:

through the symptoms I identify the disorder. In a conception of the diagnosis as a locus of tension between a picture and a window, one could say that in this case by looking through the dove one can recognize the disorder. In this first configuration, the therapist looks at the phenomena *from the front* and aims at the identification of *'the what'*. The operations implemented here are the objectification, the reduction, and the description of the symptoms from the outside in a third-person perspective. This is the typical configuration of psychiatric diagnosis in its medical version as promoted by the various DSM, grounded on the logic of what is normally called (a bit hypocritically) 'atheoretical' description. This description relies fundamentally on the idea that the symptom is the product of a subpersonal dysfunction and represents a useful mark for the diagnosis of a disease.

2   A second configuration of the diagnosis as 'looking through' has to do with the ability to look at the symptoms as experiential data and subjective feelings of discomfort inducing a person to ask for help: through these symptoms, the therapist gains access to the characteristics of such person as a whole and to the personological matrix inscribed in his or her experiential world. In other words, *through the symptoms I get to know the person*. If we conceive the diagnosis as a locus of tension between a picture and a window, we could say that in this case by looking through the dove, so to speak, we find a window that improves our knowledge of the person in which these phenomena take place. In this second configuration, the clinical gaze focuses on what lies *behind* the phenomena and aims at formulating hypotheses about their *reasons* (*'the why'*).

The operations carried out in this case are the explanation and the identification of the causes and/or reasons, again from a third person perspective. This configuration of the diagnosis belongs to the psychoanalytic tradition. A classic example of this approach is Freud's seduction theory in the etiology of hysteria. A more recent one is trauma theory in the etiopathogenesis of Borderline Personality Disorder. In an extraordinarily evocative simile, Félix Guattari (1986) has compared the symptoms to birds that come to knock at the window with their beak. Something strange and unexpected is out there: what to do? Drive the birds away? Approach them so as to get to know them? Perhaps, the most important thing to do is to retrace their journey and understand where they came from. On that basis, one can also conceive of a way to receive their transformative message and reinterpret it in an evolutionary sense. Every symptom has a history and refers to a concatenation of meanings; at the same time, it begs to be heard and sheds light on the future.

3   A third configuration of the diagnosis as 'looking through' concerns the possibility of learning more about the symptoms by looking through the person as both their author and bearer: *through the person I get to know more about his or her symptoms*. In a conception of the diagnosis as a locus of tension between a picture and a window, one could say that in this case by tuning into how that person 'looks at the dove' one comes to a better understanding of the nature and personal meaning of such dove. In this third configuration the clinical gaze tries to go deep *into* the phenomena and aims at the identification of *'the how'*.

The operations carried out in this case are the immersion in the phenomenon, the exploration of the lived subjectivity of the patient, and the 'explication' as understood by Paul Ricoeur (1970): an unfolding of subjective experiences according to a meaningful narrative. It is a matter of painstakingly browsing through the experiences of the subject, as when one peals an onion, in an attempt to organize them according to a pattern. In this case, the description of phenomena is given 'from the inside' and is based on the possibility to 'interrogate' the symptom and establish a real dialogue with it. Here the goal is a first-person description as a first step to the co-construction of a second-person narrative negotiated with the therapist (Fuchs, 2010).

This configuration of the diagnosis coincides with Kraus' notion of phenomenological diagnosis (1994), which aims at describing the form of lived experience characterizing the patient's relationship with himself and the world. Unlike the symptomatological one, which is "morbus-oriented", this is a "person-oriented" diagnosis, one more attentive to experiences than symptoms. Its goal is to identify the "psychopathological organizers" (Rossi Monti & Stanghellini, 1996: 196), understood as synthetic schemes of understanding conferring unitary meanings to groups of pathological phenomena co-occurring in the same person. These sets of psychopathological experiences or *Gestalt* are endowed with a specific internal coherence and function as meaningful organizers of an entire clinical picture, a bit like what happens with the theme of decomposition and formlessness in the world of the obsessive person or that of guilt in the world of the melancholic person. After all, as Parnas and Henriksen (2014) have emphasized, our patients do not bring us a series of isolated symptoms corresponding to a specific anatomical and physiological substrate; on the contrary, they bring us *Gestalt* of experiences, feelings, phrases, beliefs and actions interconnected and closely related to their biography.

Let us clarify this with an example: Laura, a twenty-three-year-old girl, asks for help because lately she has been tormented by the fear of 'losing a space where to feel safe'. In these circumstances, she experiences a sense of suffocation and fast heartbeat. In her neighborhood, which is constantly invaded by hordes of tourists, she feels 'overwhelmed by people' and confused by all their different languages: 'in the middle of the city I feel lost', she says. As she walks, she often lurches and feels unstable. Often, she goes on, 'I feel like I'm going crazy and I'm afraid I might start screaming in the middle of the street'. According to a diagnostic configuration of the first type – which observes the phenomena *from the front* – these symptoms clearly fit the clinical picture of Panic Disorder. However, by following a diagnostic configuration of the second type – which focuses on what lies *behind* the phenomena ('*the why*') – it is possible to explain the onset of panic, for example, with the fact that very recently Laura went to live by herself.

By looking 'through' the symptoms it is possible to get to know the person and make assumptions about where these symptoms 'come from'. Until a few months ago Laura was living in the outskirts of the city with her parents. Now she lives alone, in the city center. What are we dealing with here? Separation anxiety? A traumatic event? A reactivation of a set of conflicting feelings about the relocation process? Or about the separation from her parents? Or about her relationship with a particularly vexing and cumbersome father? By relying on the third type of diagnostic configuration – which attempts to go deep *into* Laura's clinical picture and focus on *how* she experiences her symptoms – the therapist will try, together with Laura, to handle each of her experiences as a package to unwrap and open in order to 'leaf through' its possible meanings. Thus, as the therapist gradually gets to know Laura better, he gathers more material and comes to understand that Laura is afraid of being touched by others: 'If someone touches me I'm afraid he will invade me . . . as if there was an alien force seizing and pulverizing what is mine, as if when I get in contact with others something of mine is stolen, and I lose something.' In public spaces, she says, 'I feel as if I am transparent . . . I'm afraid my ideas might enter the minds of others [and vice versa] . . . I feel deprived of immune defenses and build myself a shield so as to say: no one can touch me.' Thus, if one ventures into Laura's panic one discovers a person who feels exposed, vulnerable, with no immune defenses, transparent, besieged by feelings that penetrate and confound her. In the world of Laura each contact is an invasion. She feels prey to outside forces that take away something of herself. She experiences a constant feeling of hemorrhagic loss and feels that her head is 'split' so that ideas (hers and/or others') enter or exit out of her control. What we find in Laura's panic, therefore, is a sense of annihilation of the self, which is something quite different from the most typical forms of panic attacks, where the subject, terrified, goes through – so to speak – a somatic storm of panic that, like a bolt from the blue, throws him or her in anguish and in a state of fear of imminent death. In the case of Laura, we are dealing with a person who feels shaken to her foundations and sees the fundamental structures of her existence called into questions. The feeling of having a skin around her that defines, separates and protects her from others, the ability to formulate thoughts in her head with the absolute certainty that they are sealed by a membrane that protects them from others – all these certainties are shattered. The psychopathological organizers around which this particular condition is structured are the permeability of the boundaries of the self; its psychodynamic organizers are transitivism and appersonation (Federn, 1952).

Why is it important to focus on these organizers and on the dimension of the *how*? First of all, because they help to understand how the person experiences his symptoms. Second, because they help to put into words the terribly distressing experience that the patient is experiencing first-hand and in so doing they turn it into the subject of a dialogue.

The three configurations that we reviewed are not organized in a hierarchy but should rather be viewed as three concomitant and competing ways of 'looking through' – as the constitutive elements of the slightly cross-eyed gaze characterizing the diagnostic process. Each of them plays an essential role in the diagnostic process and only by taking all three of them into account through an oscillatory state of mind (Modell, 1990) one can reach a diagnosis in its fullest sense: a living and dynamic diagnosis (Foresti & Rossi Monti, 2010).

The (fruitful) ambiguity of the clinical process – Danilo Cargnello has written (1999) – lies in the perennial oscillation between *facing something* (i.e. the symptom, the syndrome, the disorder, the illness) and *being-with someone*. The diagnosis as a *name* and as a *process* is located at a crossroads and must be constantly maintained in a state of tension. This tension gives life to the diagnosis and prevents it from turning into a fixed entity, a sort of inescapable fate or even a tombstone. A diagnosis that extinguishes any further possibility of knowledge represents an obstacle to the therapeutic relationship. It is vital for the therapist to preserve the ability to be amazed by the observed phenomena: the diagnosis should function as a kind of flywheel capable of powering the therapist's drive to understand and turn this understanding into a crucial step in the construction of the therapeutic relationship. Karl Jaspers' words (1913) – a real warning to all those who are going to perform a diagnostic procedure – should be taken precisely in this sense: every diagnostic schema must remain a tiresome problem for the clinical researcher.

Note

1 An earlier version of this paper was published in *The Psychoanalytic Review*, 105(2), 209–222, 2018.

References

AMDP-System (1981). *Arbeitsgemeinschaft für Methodik und Dokumentation in der Psychiatrie*. Berlin: Springer.

APA (2013). *DSM-5. Diagnostic and statistical manual of mental disorders*. Washington, DC: American Psychiatric Association.

Bion, W. R. (1961). *Experiences in groups*. London: Tavistock Publications.

Bion, W. R. (1963). *Elements of psycho-analysis*. London: William Heinemann.

Cargnello, D. (1999). Ambiguità della psichiatria. *Comprendre. Archive International pour l'Antropologie et la Psychopathologie Phénoménologiques, 9*: 7–48.

Federn, P. (1952). *Ego psychology and the psychoses*. New York: Basic Books.

Fédida, P. (2001). *Des bienfaits de la dépression: Éloge de la psychothérapie*. Paris: Odile Jacob.

Foresti, G., & Rossi Monti, M. (2010). *Esercizi di Visioning: Psicoanalisi, psichiatria, istituzioni*. Roma: Borla.

Fuchs, T. (2010). Subjectivity and intersubjectivity in psychiatric diagnosis. *Psychopathology, 43*: 268–274.

Gombrich, E. H. (1958). Psychoanalysis and the history of art. In B. Nelson (Ed.) *Freud and the twentieth century* (pp. 182–293). London: Allen & Unwin.

Guattari, F. (1986). *Les années d'hiver*. Paris: Barrault.

Jaspers, K. (1913). *General psychopathology*. Manchester, UK: Manchester University Press, 1968.

Kant, I. (1764). Essay on the illness of the head. In *Anthropology, history, and education*. Cambridge, UK: Cambridge University Press, 2007.

Kraus, A. (1994). Phenomenological and criteriological diagnosis: different or complementary? In J. Sadler, O. Wiggins, & M. Schwartz (Eds.) *Philosophical perspectives on psychiatric classification*. Baltimore, MD: John Hopkins University Press.

Modell, A. (1990). *Other Times, other realities. Toward a theory of psychoanalytic treatment*. Cambridge, MA: Harvard University Press.

OPD Task Force (Eds.) (2008). *Operationalized Psychodynamic Diagnosis OPD-2. Manual of Diagnosis and Treatment Planning*. Cambridge, MA: Hogrefe & Huber.

Parnas, J., & Henriksen, M. G. (2014). Disordered self in schizophrenia spectrum: A clinical and research prospective. *Harvard Review of Psychiatry*, 22(5): 1–14.

PDM Task Force (2006). *PDM. Psychodynamic Diagnostic Manual*. Silver Springs, MD: Alliance of Psychoanalytic Organizations.

Racamier, P. C. (1992). *Le Génie des origines*. Paris: Payot.

Ricoeur, P. (1970). Qu'est-ce qu'un texte? Expliquer et comprendre. In R. Bubner (Ed.) *Hermeneutik und Dialektik, vol. 2* (pp. 181–200). Tubingen: JCB Mohr.

Rossi Monti, M., & Stanghellini, G. (1996). Psychopathology: an edgeless razor? *Comprehensive Psychiatry*, 37(3): 196–204.

Rothstein, A. (2002). Reflections on creative aspects of psychoanalytic diagnosing. *Psychoanalytic Quarterly*, 71: 301–326.

Sadler, J. Z. (2005). *Values and psychiatric diagnosis*. Oxford, UK: Oxford University Press.

Stanghellini, G., & Rossi Monti, M. (2009). *Psicologia del patologico: Una prospettiva fenomenologico-dinamica*. Milan: Cortina.

Wigman, W., van Os, J., Thiery, E., Derom, C., Collip, D., Jacobs, N., & Wichers, M. (2013). Psychiatric diagnosis revisited: Towards a system of staging and profiling combining nomothetic and idiographic parameters of momentary mental states. *PLOS ONE*, 8(3): 1–8.

CHAPTER THIRTEEN

The importance of psychodynamic diagnosis in patients with severe mental illnesses

Humberto Lorenzo Persano

Introduction

Psychoanalysis is a complex discipline which has made a significant contribution to the realms of psychiatry. Some of its most profound influences were a method of research on the human mind and a method for psychotherapeutic treatment (Reiser, 1989). Psychoanalysis also offers several theories that can be applied to gain a deeper insight and understanding of psychopathology.

In this chapter, I shall address some of the main contributions that psychoanalysis has made to psychiatry, particularly in the field of diagnosis, and I will do so from a psychodynamic perspective. I shall also focus on the way these approaches could be applied to the treatment of patients with severe mental illnesses.

I will begin by introducing some remarks on the points of convergence and controversy that may arise from the different approaches that psychiatry and psychoanalysis have, and the ways in which these disciplines can reinforce one another.

The relationship between psychoanalysis and psychiatry has been regarded, since the very beginning, as rather controversial. Freud pointed out that there were strong differences among psychoanalytic and psychiatric perspectives, because while in psychiatry we do not make any inferences about the meaning of symptoms, in psychoanalysis this is a common practice (Freud, 1915). There have been periods of time when psychoanalysis and psychiatry mutually reinforced one another, which resulted in rich theoretical exchanges for both fields; nowadays, such exchanges seem to have ceased.

Psychiatry is a branch of medicine. Psychiatrists need to identify symptoms in order to elaborate proper diagnoses, and they resort to recognised therapeutic approaches to decide upon courses of treatment, which are sometimes shared with other branches of medicine (Friedman et al., 2015). Over the past decades, psychiatry has been strongly influenced by neurobiological perspectives and psychopharmacological approaches. Nowadays, we have a better understanding of the way the human brain works and how the brain and the mind are connected; we owe much of this knowledge to the bottom-up epistemological perspective on brain functioning. As useful as this might have been, it is still insufficient to fully understand how the human mind works.

For psychiatrists, particularly those who work in hospitals and/or mental health institutions, it is a mandatory part of their practice to apply recognised psychiatric diagnoses; namely, those diagnoses that were reached through consensus among the psychiatric and medical communities around the world. Currently, there is a tendency that favours diagnosing according to standard classifications that can be found in different, renowned manuals, mainly the Diagnostic Statistical Manual (DSM-V) for American psychiatrists and the International Classifications of Diseases (ICD-10) for other regions of the world. These manuals take on a descriptive perspective, but they lack a psychopathological point of view.

Psychoanalysis as a theory of the mind belongs to the realm of psychology, and it had a very strong influence on the field of psychiatry from the early 1950s until the late 1980s. This influence was present on psychiatric diagnosis and on the choice of therapeutic approaches. The training of psychiatrists in this period embraced psychoanalytic concepts of mind functioning and psychotherapeutic approaches. This was mainly due to the influence exerted by the leading psychiatrists of the time who were trained as psychoanalysts in psychoanalytic institutes. This group of dynamic psychiatrists were members of the main boards at universities. They introduced significant changes into academic psychiatry and they had a great influence on the training of psychiatric residents. Precisely, by teaching what the mind really is, how it is structured, and how unconscious contents can be expressed through psychopathological symptoms, they were teaching residents to identify defence mechanisms and how to perceive them during interviews or psychotherapeutic sessions. Such influences played a key role in understanding transference and counter transference processes during the psychiatric interview and during the psychotherapeutic processes.

Other important issues that those psychiatrists learned to recognise when treating patients were the role of the psychic conflict theory, the developmental theory of mind, and the object relations theory in the realm of psychopathology (Frosh, 1990). These concepts had also been reached through the psychoanalytic training during their own practice in the psychiatric ward. These topics turned out to be crucial for understanding how the human mind works according to top-down epistemological perspectives.

Nowadays, things have changed dramatically in psychiatry. Only a few recognised psychiatric training institutions adhere to these psychoanalytic perspectives and transmit this knowledge to their residents.

The human mind has not changed dramatically over the past decades; what has changed drastically is how relevant the mind has become to psychiatry and, more specifically, to conceptualisations in this field. This paradigmatic shift can be attributed to different causes. Some of them can be traced to changes in the policies of mental health institutions and boards, others to the influence of economic agendas of both insurance and pharmaceutical companies. Last, but by no means a less relevant issue, is the lack of interest on the part of psychoanalytic societies and institutes in showing how useful psychoanalytical concepts are, and how they can be incorporated into the work of psychiatric and mental health institutions. In my opinion, this is mainly due to the fact that psychoanalysis is also a profession, i.e. a way of making a living (Reiser, 1989), and not all psychoanalysts are involved in working at mental health and/or medical institutions. On the contrary, most of them seem to be worried about issues concerning their own psychoanalytic work in their private practice. We should also consider that not all psychoanalysts devote themselves to research and research-related issues. Research is indispensable for both medicine and psychiatry: therapeutic approaches and diagnosis need to be based on evidence. As it has become clear, psychoanalysts seem to have disregarded the importance of evidence in their everyday practice. However, this huge amount of knowledge which belongs to the psychoanalytic domain is useful and should be applied to the clinical, theoretical and therapeutic psychiatric and medical approaches to the mental health system.

Psychoanalytic diagnosis

As I have mentioned before, psychoanalysis has contributed to improving our knowledge on how the mind works and the ways in which its mechanisms can be revealed. This knowledge could be used to gain a deeper understanding on the structure of the mind and how is it that psychic changes occur during psychotherapeutic processes.

There are several components of psychoanalytic diagnosis that uniquely belong to psychoanalysis as a discipline of the human mind. But, what is exactly psychoanalytic diagnosis, and how can we profit from it during psychiatric interviews? First, we should consider that in making a psychoanalytic diagnosis, we are not categorising or "labelling" patients; rather, we are conceptualising what is happening inside their minds and in their lives in order to choose the best treatment possible for them (Bernardi, 2010).

The psychiatric clinical interview is the most powerful diagnostic and therapeutic tool that can be used by psychiatrists in clinical psychiatry. There is a foundational work on this matter, published by Sullivan in the United States in the 1950s (Sullivan, 1954), and there were other approaches to the topic in South America by Rolla (1981) and most recently by Bernardi and colleagues as a systematic research tool (Bernardi et al., 2016).

There was an outstanding contribution on the topic of psychic organisation made by Kernberg in the US in the 1960s, in which he describes structural diagnosis (Kernberg, 1967). As you can read in another chapter in this book, Kernberg pointed out that personality organisation level can be diagnosed by means of three main and specific domains of psychic structure, namely the hierarchy's level of defence mechanisms, identity integration of self and object representations, and reality testing as an ego function. In the 1980s, Kernberg devised the structural interview, which is used for psychoanalytic diagnosis purposes in psychiatric clinical settings and for distinguishing among neurotic, borderline and psychotic personality organisation levels (Kernberg, 1984). The structural interview is an excellent clinical and research tool to be used in clinical psychiatric inpatient units as well. Kernberg, Clarkin and their collaborators from The Personality Disorders Institute at Cornell University also operationalised their contributions to psychoanalytic diagnosis through the semi-structured STIPO interview and the self-report structured IPO interview. These interviews can also be used for clinical research purposes both in medicine and psychiatry. They include diagnosis of control aggressive behaviours and integration of superego through the moral values domain, and the STIPO also allows to diagnose internalised object relation representations. This thorough research, carried out over decades, enabled Kernberg's group to design proper psychotherapeutic interventions for borderline personality organisations, which were well-documented and compiled in a transference focused psychotherapy (TFP) clinical guide (Yeomans, Clarkin, & Kernberg, 2015).

Psychoanalytic diagnosis also gathers other important aspects such as type of psychic conflicts, the level of predominant anxieties (i.e. castration, separation or dissolution anxieties). In order to properly diagnose any resistances that may emerge during psychotherapy processes, it is crucial to identify the predominant hierarchy of defence mechanism levels. There are important research tools for identifying them: DMRS (defence mechanisms rating scale) in clinical interviews or DSQ (defence style questionnaire) as a structured self-report interview. It is also essential to identify the level of sublimation capabilities as well the impulse control capacity, as it will allow us to recognise how the ego is functioning. Reality testing is a pivotal ego function that allows us to differentiate psychotic from non-psychotic patients. The relationship to reality, the subjective sense of reality, and an individual's adaptation to reality, are all essential domains that will help us identify psychotics and people who suffer from severe personality disorders (Frosch, 1983).

Another important issue is the subjective experience of symptoms. The capacity for mentalisation, which includes the symbolisation process, is also crucial. In addition, the capacity for affect regulation, emotion control, and the capability to evaluate how people can feel their own feelings are indispensable in making psychoanalytic diagnosis.

Other important aspects to be considered in psychoanalytic diagnosis are the transference and counter transference phenomena and the level of regression shown during interviews and psychotherapeutic processes, as well as the empathy that patients show when we suggest psychotherapeutic treatment.

We can observe and listen to a patient and we can diagnose what is going on in their mind. This can be achieved through a single psychoanalytical structural interview or during an entire diagnostic process, but this kind of mental diagnosis can only be carried out by mental health professionals who have been rigorously trained in the domain of psychoanalytic diagnosis.

The reader can understand, at this point, that this complex, yet fundamental, knowledge can only be gained through a deep and systematic psychoanalytic training of psychiatrists, both for diagnostic purposes and for the choice of psychotherapeutic approaches.

Some psychoanalysts have been involved in research projects and some of us have worked in operationalising the psychoanalytic diagnosis into detailed manuals, such as the Operationalized Psychodynamic Diagnosis – OPD-2 (OPD Task Force, 2008) and, more recently, the new version of The Psychodynamic Diagnostic Manual – PDM-2 (Lingiardi, & McWilliams, 2016).

Although the reader can find more detailed information on these manuals in other chapters, I will briefly summarise the contents of the OPD-2 (Cierpka et al., 2007); (Bernardi, 2010). It focuses on five dimensions:

Axis 1 – Experience of illness and prerequisites for treatment; which involves subjectivity, personal and environmental resources for psychic change.

Axis 2 – Interpersonal relations; which involves the enactment of dysfunctional relational patterns.

Axis 3 – Conflict; which also implies level and relation to emotional subjective experience.

Axis 4 – Structure; which explores what the psychic structure is and how it is conformed.

Axis 5 – Syndromes; according to chapter V of ICD-10 psychiatric classification of mental diseases.

The PDM-2 uses a multidimensional approach to describe the details of each patient's functioning and it suggests ways of engaging in the therapeutic process. It attempts to provide a comprehensive profile of an individual's mental life, and to do so it focuses on three levels: Axis P focuses on personality organisation and personality disorders; Axis M focuses on mental functioning, and Axis S focuses on the subjective experience of symptomatic patterns (Lingiardi et al., 2015).

To reach a psychoanalytic diagnosis it is necessary to maintain a balance between the free listening of the patient's mental contents and his/her speech as well as the objective evaluation of the different dimensions of the patient's mental functioning. It is of utmost importance to understand what happens to the patient in real life and what is the connection between the patient's symptoms and the environmental triggering factors. At the same time, we need to monitor our own counter transference feelings and observe as a third person the enactment of activated relational patterns and their shifts in the context of the interview.

Contributions of psychoanalytic diagnosis to clinical psychiatry

I have been involved in both psychiatric and psychoanalytic practice for more than three decades and my own experience in mental health units at psychiatric hospitals allows me to hold an intimate dialogue connecting both disciplines, psychiatry and psychoanalysis. In addition, I am frequently involved in discussions with other colleagues from mental health teams. This, combined with my duties at university and in academic psychiatry, has enabled me to merge and articulate different points of view expressed by a multiplicity of perspectives originating from the different disciplines which are involved in mental health systems.

As psychoanalysts, we have a vast experience listening to patients. Furthermore, as psychiatrists, we are also very experienced in observing behaviours, actions and manners of our patients. The combination of psychiatric and psychoanalytic training is a wonderful experience and people who work in both fields can greatly profit from the overlapping of such fields: they have a deeper knowledge of mental illnesses, which is crucial for comprehending severe mental disorders and psychopathology.

As I have mentioned before, the structural interview is a magnificent tool that combines knowledge from both disciplines. I would like to illustrate how this type of interview could help us in making differential diagnosis in patients with severe mental illnesses.

I will begin by introducing a clinical vignette from a patient who went into a psychiatric hospital as she experienced depressive symptoms with psychotic-like features.

Miss C. was a young woman who had recurrent visual hallucinations about her cousin who had committed suicide some time ago. Miss C. believed that her cousin had appeared before her at different places in her own home. She claimed that this cousin was her soulmate, that they had had a very strong friendship in their adolescence. Miss C. could not accept her loss and believed her cousin was still alive. The psychiatrists and psychologists in our team were very confused about her condition because she had a sympathetic adaptation to reality in other issues and her depression did not look like a typical affective illness. She was treated following a psychopharmacological approach with antidepressants and atypical antipsychotic drugs but she did not improve, which led the team to ask for my supervision. We decided to perform a structural interview and we asked for her permission to record it on video, as well as her informed consent to use such material for teaching purposes. The benefits of relying upon a structural interview are not limited to the diagnostic process, but they extend to the therapeutic process as well. It is a powerful device that may allow us to understand how patients who suffer from severe mental illnesses can improve their mental functioning.

According to Kernberg, when we carry out a structural interview we must ask, at the initial phase, which are the main symptoms or conditions that the patient suffers and what is the significance or implications that these symptoms have on the patient's life. We should also ask about the expectations that the patient has about the treatment itself.

Miss C. said that she had sought help because the mental professionals treating her had doubts about her condition; consequently, she had agreed to another consultation with a senior psychiatrist. I told her that I would be talking to her for diagnostic purposes only, so as to decide on the best strategies and course of treatment for her. The whole interview lasted about one hour and 15 minutes. In the initial phase, she talked about her symptoms and she was utterly convinced that her visual hallucinations were real. During the initial and middle phases of the structural interview I made many clarifications about her symptoms. Miss C. also talked about having "magic", premonitory thoughts; she said that she could anticipate some real-life events and mentioned that her family thought she had special abilities, a clairvoyance. During the interview, she said that she would like to transform the external reality through her job in mass media, and was convinced that she could do it. When I asked her if she could explain how she could do it, she used rationalisation defence mechanisms and answered that mass media could change people's thinking. Although she was well adapted to reality and showed social skills for working and studying, Miss C. had a tendency to understand reality in a special way, which generated an increasing doubt in me that made me question her sense of reality. This special focus on reality issues was carried out to differentiate between a psychotic organisation and a lower level of borderline personality organisation.

At this point I would like to focus on her psychotic symptoms. She had visual hallucinations, but these symptoms were incongruent with her emotional face expressions, which were vivid and not rigid or frozen as is often the case in psychotic patients. Her answers and way of speaking were clever. When I asked her about her self and object mental representations, she defined herself in a contradictory way. When I confronted these split aspects of herself, she responded in a positive emotional way and she showed insightful integration.

From the middle phase of her structural interview on, Miss C. became tearful and anguished. She talked about her cousin's funeral. She said that she had not been able to see his body because the coffin was closed, and therefore she had doubts about his death. At that stage, I decided to confront her with her "cousin alive" hallucination. I asked her *"If your cousin is your best friend, why does he appear in your kitchen, at such a distance from you? Why doesn't he come closer to you?"*. She answered *"I don't know"*. I told her *"You must choose an option: either your cousin is not alive, which means that you have wishful illusions of him being present, or else he is still alive but he does not love you as much as you believe".* She became very weepy and replied *"It may have been an illusion; his image was not clear at all".* I would like to explain that while it is very common to use clarifications and confrontations during structural interviews, interpretations are not. I made an interpretation. For diagnostic purposes, it was imperative to differentiate between a psychotic personality organisation and a borderline one. This was crucial because it would define the strategy of interventions. I added *"I think you want to keep a good memory of your cousin; if you choose to accept his death, you can keep a good image of him. Otherwise, you will have to accept that he is not your best friend".* Miss C. burst into tears and said her cousin had committed suicide. She also remembered another traumatic family loss, the death of another, younger cousin who had passed away in a fire. She talked about mourning and her difficulties in accepting loss. The interview ended with reflections about the way in which she could process and deal with her family losses and how she could go on talking about these issues in the course of her psychotherapeutic treatment.

This clinical vignette is useful for understanding the psychodynamics of reality testing, sense of reality and adaptation to reality in patients with severe mental illnesses. From a psychiatric diagnosis perspective, Miss C. suffered from delusional and hallucinatory phenomena. However, she also showed symptoms of depression. Her diagnosis fulfilled the criteria for a mood disorder with incongruent psychotic features. The initial psychopharmacological treatment had been correct; nevertheless, Miss C. did not show signs of improvement. The clinical discussion had to contemplate a delusional disorder with depressive symptoms and changes in the psychopharmacological approach would have led to increasing the doses of antipsychotics. However, her personality organisation did not meet a permanently distorted reality testing criteria.

The psychoanalytic diagnosis allowed us to understand how reality testing had dynamically changed in the transference process of the structural interview; this feature, though uncommon in psychotic patients, appears frequently in borderline personality organisations with symptoms of psychoticism.

Another important issue is the power of the psychotherapeutic interventions, and in this particular case, the power of a mutative interpretation which allowed Miss C. to make a shift in her mental functioning.

After these interventions, Miss C. started talking about mourning, and after that she showed a historicity process about her role in her family. By idealising her clairvoyance, her family environment had not helped her to cope with reality. This led Miss C. to maintain archaic defence mechanisms such as omnipotence, splitting of self and object mental representations, rationalisation and primitive denial.

Nevertheless, in another context (namely, the structural interview), she managed to shift her psychic functioning after several interventions. As Busch has expressed, during a psychoanalytic process the patient is introduced to (and develops) new perspectives, which contribute to the building of new knowledge and allow the patient to reach a new state of mind (Busch, 2014).

According to Freud, once Miss C.'s mental functioning was changed; she was able to inhibit the regression phenomenon (previously expressed through her hallucinations) and she could avoid regression into the psychic apparatus' perceptual pole (Freud, 1950 [1895]).

The empathy Miss C. felt during the structural interview for her own feelings and thoughts and for her reactions to psychoanalytic interventions, is another important issue because it made us think about possibilities for psychic change and psychoanalytic treatment (Bolgnini, 2004). This empathy also allowed her to apply for psychotherapy.

In my professional practice, I ask myself many times what happens to patients who are treated by psychiatrists who are only trained in a neurobiological domain. These patients challenge us into categorising them into multiple psychiatric diagnoses or treating them in novel ways. When making a psychoanalytic diagnosis, we can greatly improve our approaches as well as the patient's quality of life; thus, psychoanalysis becomes essential when we work in psychiatry. In the case presented earlier, it became clear that psychoanalytic interventions can bring about significant changes in the dynamics of the mind's functioning.

I would like to continue by discussing the importance of unconscious psychic contents when working with patients who suffer from severe mental illnesses. I will introduce a discussion on bipolar disorders that contemplates both psychiatric and psychoanalytic perspectives, as these two disciplines have overlapping views on the same phenomenon.

Bipolar disorder, and bipolar I disorder especially, is a clinical condition that is studied by clinical psychiatry only. Recommendations for its treatment have focused mainly on pharmacological approaches. Although psychoanalysts were involved in understanding manic depressive illness around the early and mid-twentieth century, lately psychoanalysis has made no significant contribution to this affective condition. The neurobiological knowledge about bipolar conditions was the only significant advance, made two decades ago. Still, I would like to introduce a discussion on this topic, followed by the analysis of another clinical vignette on a patient suffering from bipolar disorder.

Mr. M., a man in his thirties who presented a bipolar I diagnosis, had been hospitalised several times for his condition. He had been admitted to emergency psychiatric units for excited furious manic episodes and had also experienced rapid cyclic type bipolar episodes. Aggressive behaviours, flying thoughts, delusions inspired on religious themes and hallucinatory phenomena were evident during his psychotic manic episodes, and he had also shown depressive episodes. During the stages of calm and recovery, he used to work properly, spent time looking after his children, and, according to his wife, he was a very kind man.

Some years ago, I treated him as an inpatient in a psychiatric hospital. During manic episodes, he was treated with antipsychotics and lithium as a mood-stabilizer for long periods. During his last crisis and hospitalisation, he suffered from another manic aggressive episode. In one of our sessions we had a long conversation about his life and, in a very intimate confession, he revealed that he had been sexually abused during his infancy.

Mr. M.'s parents usually left him under the supervision of his sister, who was a prostitute and often left her little brother unattended in the brothel, exposing him to very dangerous situations. Mr. M. kept this a secret to avoid exposing the truth about his sister and also because he did not want to acknowledge his sexual abuse, due to his feelings of shame. At this stage of the session, he started crying and behaving like an unprotected child. His authoritarian temper had shifted and he was transformed into a tearful, childish, fragile man who showed deep feelings for having been neglected by his family. Then, he recognised that those memories of sexual abuse were the triggering factors behind the aggression that surfaced during his manic episodes. When he was a child, while he was being abused, he talked and prayed to God asking for help. During his psychotic episodes, he said he heard God's voice and believed he could talk to God; he had sensory hallucinations of being struck by lightning, and interpreted these as God's influences. During his psychotic episodes, Mr. M. lost his reality testing and became a bipolar I manic type patient.

This clinical vignette illustrates how the unconscious mental contents invaded his mind functioning with primitive thoughts, disturbing his psychic structure and forcing him to function in a psychotic condition. This condition was aggravated by feelings of fear, anger and sadness which could not be felt, but could only be expressed through primitive emotions of fear, anger and sadness. He also exhibited primitive motor discharge behaviours. According to Freud, pain passes along all pathways of discharge in the psyche, as though there had been a stroke of lightning (Freud, 1950 [1895]). Mr. M. could not talk about his painful experiences; he had painful memories of having experienced sexual abuse, but these memories became psychotic thoughts and aggressive behaviour. He had attempted to cope with them through primitive and distorted psychic mechanisms, and probably they corresponded to very primitive ways of neural connections in the brain's working. As it happens in fight behaviours, primitive reptilian fear and anger emotions are activated, and the latter suppresses the activity of the seeking system (Panksepp, 1998).

This vignette also helps us realise how relevant psychoanalytical perspectives can be in clinical psychiatry, even when working with patients with severe mental disorders who suffer from psychotic episodes (Freeman, 1988). Discovering the unconscious mental contents, even in patients with severe mental disorders, reveals the underlying meanings of their symptoms. When he acknowledged his painful memories, Mr. M. improved his mental functioning and condition, transforming painful experiences into painful thoughts. The transformation of his sensory mental experiences into mental painful memories was the first sign of an incipient psychic change.

Conclusions

Dialogues between psychoanalysis, psychiatry and medicine remain essential. Psychoanalysts need to borrow new discoveries on brain functioning from other disciplines, so that they can keep the dialogue between the brain, the mind and the body, fluid. Freud had the idea that the human mind is an emergent expression of the whole nervous system, which has emerged as an evolutionary consequence of life (Freud, 1950 [1895]). Today, we know that the human mind emerges from a countless number of neural connections that allow the display of what was defined as a synaptic self – our neural connections determine who we are, that is to say, our brains become who we are (LeDoux, 1996). This point of view belongs to an emergent evolutionary monistic epistemological perspective in science. This was also Freud´s conception of the human mind. If we adhere to this view, then the dialogues between psychoanalysis and psychiatry become important and valuable, as both disciplines are benefited. Seen from a bottom-up perspective, applying neurosciences to the field of psychiatry allows us to introduce new biological treatments, but this is insufficient to grasp the mind in all its complexity. Psychoanalytic diagnosis from top-down strategies enables us to interpret psychopathological clinical conditions better and, as such, it becomes useful for planning treatments (McWilliams, 1994).

Both clinical vignettes show how knowledge in both psychiatry and psychology leads to a better understanding of a patient's condition and treatment. In the first case, a young woman with psychotic-like symptoms recovered her reality testing during a psychoanalytical structural interview which had enormous consequences for her treatment and the strategy behind it. Furthermore, it also enhanced her insight and her future life possibilities and envisioning. In this particular case, antipsychotic drugs did not improve her condition but psychoanalytic interventions throughout this interview did.

In the second case, we encountered an inpatient, a man in his thirties, with bipolar I psychiatric diagnosis who discovered during his psychotherapeutic sessions what was the triggering factor behind his rapid cycling manic type bipolar episodes. He had been sexually abused during his childhood, a traumatic and painful experience that he had been unable to share before. Antipsychotics and lithium were a substantial part of the treatment for his condition. However, listening to his sexual abuse history turned out to be crucial to have an insight into why his symptoms had surfaced. The fact that he could elaborate on what sexual abuse was for him, his subjective feelings, allowed him to put an end to his hospitalisations for furious mania illness. Probably, these memories had persisted in his mind firing repetitive neural circuits as a kindling phenomenon, and for this reason he had required mood-stabilizer drug treatment. Having someone listening to him allowed him to have a new perspective on his own symptoms, making psychic change possible.

Psychoanalysis may help psychiatry in revealing intimate and unconscious mental contents of patients however severe their symptoms may be, even if their conditions require hospitalisation as part of the treatment. By applying psychodynamic diagnosis, psychiatrists may gain knowledge about different mental functioning, mental dynamics and unconscious contents, thus improving the psychotherapeutic approach.

Even though psychiatry and psychoanalysis are two separate and different disciplines, they have a common goal: to improve a patient's quality of life. We should be aware of the points of contact that exist among them and the contributions that each discipline can make to clinical settings, but we should not lose sight of the fact that even when we apply common strategies for patients' illnesses, symptoms remain unique expressions of each patient's life history.

References

Bernardi, R. (2010). DSM-V-OPD-2 y PDM: Convergencias y divergencias entre los nuevos sistemas diagnósticos psiquiátricos y psicoanalíticos. *Revista de Psiquiatria del Uruguay, 74*(2): 179–205.

Bernardi, R., Varela, B., Miller, D., Zytner, R., De Souza, L., & Oyenard, R. (2016). *La Formulación Psicodinámica de Caso: Su valor en la práctica clínica*: Montevideo, Grupo Magro Editores, 2016.

Bolognini, S. (2004). *Psychoanalytic empathy*. London, Free Association Books.

Busch, F. (2014). *Creating a psychoanalytic mind: A psychoanalytic method and theory*. New York: Routledge.

Cierpka, M., Grande, T., Rudolf, G., von der Tann, M., Stasch, M., & The OPD Task Force (2007). The operationalized psychodynamic diagnostics system: Clinical relevance, reliability and validity. *Psychopathology, 40*(4): 209–220.

Freeman, T. (1988). Appendix: The psychoanalytic examination of a psychotic state. In *The psychoanalyst in psychiatry* (pp. 166–183). London: Karnac.

Freud, S. (1950 [1895]). Project for a scientific psychology. In *The standard edition of the complete psychological works of Sigmund Freud, volume I* (pp. 281–397). London: The Hogarth Press.

Freud, S. (1915). Introductory lectures on psycho-analysis. Lecture XVI psycho-analysis and psychiatry. In *The standard edition of the complete psychological works of Sigmund Freud, volume XVI* (pp. 243–256). London: The Hogarth Press.

Friedman, R. C., Alfonso, C. A., & Downey, J. I. (2015). Psychodynamic psychiatry and psychoanalysis: Two different models. *The American Academy of Psychoanalysis and Dynamic Psychiatry-Psychodynamic Psychiatry, 43*(4): 513–522.

Frosch, J. (1983). The ego position vis-à-vis reality. In *The Psychotic Process* (pp. 269–355). New York: International University Press, ed. 1981.

Frosch, J. (1990). *Psychodynamic psychiatry: Theory and practice, volume I, part I* (pp. 21–233). Madison, CT: International University Press.

Kernberg, O. F. (1967). Borderline personality organization. *Journal of the American Psychoanalitical Association, 15*(3): 641–685.

Kernberg, O. F. (1984). The structural interview. In *Severe personality disorders: Psychotherapeutic strategies* (pp. 27–51). New Haven, CT: Yale University Press.

LeDoux, J. (1996). *Synaptic self: How our brains become who we are*: New York: Penguin Books, 1994.

Lingiardi, V., McWilliams, N., Bornstein, R. F., Gazzillo, F., & Gordon, R. M. (2015). The psychodynamic diagnostic manual version 2 PDM-2, assessing patients for improved clinical practice and research. *Psychoanalytic Psychology, 32*(1): 94–115.

Lingiardi, V., & McWilliams, N. (2016). *Psychodynamic diagnosis manual 2nd edition –PDM-2*. Berkeley, CA: The Guilford Press.

McWilliams, N. (1994). *Psychoanalytic diagnosis: Understanding personality structure in the clinical process*. New York: The Guilford Press.

OPD Task Force (2008). *Operationalized psychodynamic diagnosis – OPD-2: Manual of diagnosis and treatment planning*. Cambridge, MA: Hogrefe & Huber.

Pankseep, J. (1998). *Affective neuroscience: The foundations of human and animal emotions*. New York: Oxford University Press.

Reiser, M. F. (1989). The future of psychoanalysis in academic psychiatry: Plain talk. *Psychoanalytic Quarterly, 58*: 185–209.

Rolla, E. H. (1981). *La entrevista en psiquiatría, psicoanálisis y psicodiagnóstico*. Buenos Aires: Ed. Galerna.

Sullivan, H. S. (1954). *The psychiatric interview*: Oxford, UK: Norton & Co.

Yeomans, F. E., Clarkin, J. F., & Kernberg, O. F. (2015). *Transference-focused psychotherapy for borderline personality disorder: A clinical guide*: Washington DC: American Psychiatric Publishing.

CHAPTER FOURTEEN

Self-disorders in psychosis
A possible integrative concept of phenomenology and psychoanalysis

Bent Rosenbaum, Mads Gram Henriksen
and Borut Škodlar

Introduction

Psychoanalysis has never been very receptive to the philosophy of phenomenology – and vice versa. Nonetheless, both psychoanalysis and phenomenology share a critical attitude toward mainstream psychiatry and especially its need to limit itself to a narrowly defined medical speciality, with an emphasis on "a-theoretical" categories of discrete, atomic-like symptoms and signs that are clustered together in different syndromes without any conceptual considerations about their organizing Gestalts. In different ways, these disciplines are today seen as outsiders in the psychiatric discourse formations. The underlying forces in these processes of rejection are based on differences of philosophical cultures, language differences (especially German, French, English/American – the latter being dominant in psychiatry within the last 4–5 decades) as well as on differences in theories, concepts and methods of investigation developed within psychiatry. While psychoanalysis and phenomenology are critical towards mainstream psychiatry, they also share a strong focus on the experiential dimensions of mental problems.

Yet, the relation between psychoanalysis and phenomenology appears difficult on several issues, anchoring theoretical conceptualizations. We shall list a few:

- The understanding of the Unconscious and unconscious processes of the mind
- The understanding of intersubjectivity and the structure of the subject-other-Other
- The understanding of development of the self/ego
- The understanding of thinking and symbolization as related to the experience and integration of here-and-now in relation to there-and-then
- The understanding of 'listening to listening', and intervening as a possible transforming process, both unconsciously and consciously.

What does the phenomenological and psychoanalytical psychiatrist listen for and what kind of listening is implied in the concept of *gleichschwebende Aufmerksamkeit* (evenly hovering attention) that they both exert? How do they investigate the speech and bodily presence of the patient? When, how and for what reasons do they intervene?

Despite possible differences, we think that in the field of psychosis some co-constructions between psychoanalysis and phenomenology may take place, and we shall highlight some possible shared aspects. First, we present the phenomenological account of schizophrenia and explore a vignette. Second, we turn to psychoanalytic views on schizophrenic psychosis, also including a detailed vignette. Finally, we propose some recommendations from psychoanalysis and phenomenology to improve the psychiatric care and treatment of persons in psychotic states of mind.

Phenomenology, self, and psychosis

From a phenomenological perspective, the self is not an ontologically independent entity, below or beyond the stream of consciousness, and although the self cannot show up as an 'object' we can direct our attention towards, it is also not considered entirely absent. By contrast, phenomenologists claim that the self manifests itself pre-reflectively as a certain configuration of experience. For example, when I listen to a melody, move my arm or entertain a thought, I am – without ever reflecting upon it – implicitly (or pre-reflectively) aware that I am the one who listens to the melody, moves the arm or entertains the thought. In fact, it is this pre-reflective self-awareness that renders self-reflection possible (e.g., Sartre 2003, p. 9). We are here dealing with a feature of consciousness without which there would be no subjective experience. In the phenomenological literature, this feature is described as the first-personal givenness of experience, i.e. all experience manifests in the first-person perspective as 'my' experience, articulating the 'ipseity', 'mineness' or 'for-me-ness' of experience (Sartre 2003, p. 126; Zahavi 2014, p. 19). More recently, this ubiquitous first-personal feature of experience has been referred to as the 'minimal self' (Zahavi 2005; 2014).

Parnas and Henriksen distinguish between two mutually implicative aspects of the minimal self, i.e. a 'formal' and an 'affective' aspect (2016, p. 84). The formal aspect depicts the invariant first-personal character of experience, which remains identical through changing experiences and modalities of consciousness, namely that all experience is given to me in my first-person perspective. The affective aspect of the minimal self articulates an enduring, elusive, and yet absolutely vital feeling of 'I-me-myself' (e.g., Sass and Parnas 2003, p. 428f; Hart 2009, p. 310), which permeates the experiential life and imbues the first-person perspective with an inchoate sense of singularity or proto-individuation (Parnas & Henriksen 2016, p. 84). In the phenomenological tradition, this persistent sense of self-presence is perhaps best understood as an incessant, immanent auto-affection, a 'self-sensing of self' (*se sentir soi-même*), as Henry (1973) puts it. However, as Hart (2009) notices, this feeling of 'I-me-myself' (or self-presence) is paradoxical: it is 'propertyless' and yet foundational of our identity. It constitutes the 'foundation' upon which much more rich and sophisticated forms of selfhood such as personality, narrativity, and social identity are constructed throughout life, especially through interactions with others, not least caregivers in childhood, and cultural and symbolic objects.

According to an influential approach in phenomenological psychopathology, a generative trait-feature of schizophrenia is a disturbance of 'ipseity' or 'minimal self', namely, the so-called *ipseity disturbance model* (Sass and Parnas 2003; Cermolacce et al. 2007; Nelson et al. 2014). In other words, in schizophrenia, we are dealing with a self-disturbance that is far more fundamental than any 'self-related' problems or difficult behaviours or characterological traits that may be encountered in disorders outside the schizophrenia spectrum, e.g., mood, anxiety, and personality disorders. In these disorders, the minimal self is never at stake – a claim consistently supported by systematic, phenomenologically informed empirical studies (for a review, see Parnas & Henriksen 2014). According to this approach, patients with schizophrenia may also experience difficulties at more complex levels of selfhood (e.g., impaired social functioning, incoherent personal narrative, and memory loss) but these difficulties are considered largely consequential to the disturbance of minimal self.

But how precisely is the minimal self supposed to be disturbed in schizophrenia? According to Parnas and Henriksen (2016), the formal aspect of the minimal self, i.e. the first-personal character of experience, remains largely unaffected – e.g., a patient, who reports that someone is inserting malicious thoughts into her head or controlling her bodily movements, is not in doubt that she is the one who experiences having thoughts inserted or her body steered. By contrast, the affective aspect of the minimal self, i.e. the sense of self-presence, is threatened and unstable in schizophrenia, causing an incomplete saturation of experiential life (ibid., p. 83ff.) that may render self-ascription problematic and enable a distance to emerge between the experiencing (noetic) self and its noematic elements. A profound self-alienation may grow from within the disturbed subjectivity, allowing, e.g., one's own thoughts to be experienced as increasingly alien to the degree that the patient no longer recognizes the alien thoughts as her own thoughts. The failing of the 'self-sensing of self' de-structures the field of immanence, affecting its very limits, e.g., the self/non-self boundary, and may facilitate an affection of 'another presence' within the very intimacy of one's sphere of ownness (Henriksen & Parnas 2014, p. 545). In premorbid and prodromal stages of schizophrenia, the wavering sense of self-presence may bring about a variety of anomalies of self-experience (Parnas et al. 2005). In psychosis, the sense of another presence may often materialize into a persecuting, influencing or hallucinatory Other, which due to its origin and continual links to the de-structured immanence typically is felt as 'hyper-proximate' by the patients (Charbonneau 2004) and retains a peculiar subjective or solipsistic quality (Sass 1994).

Case presentation

The patient is a 32-year-old male who has be in treatment since 2008, occasionally requiring hospitalization.

The central problem for the patient is an inability to engage and remain in relationships with others. From age 8, he has always felt *shameful* and felt *uneasy whenever he was exposed*. He could not adapt to these interactions with others and felt *as if he didn't exist*. He stopped communicating with others, hoping that they would then notice his presence. Until the age of 18, he believed it was genetically determined, since his father was also very silent and withdrawn. He later decided to study communication at university, but dropped out after a year.

He feels uncomfortable in the presence of others. Whenever he enters a room or approaches others, he feels as if he *radiates negative energy* and others get affected by it. He also feels boring as a companion, and he feels that he never shows any emotions. When interacting with others, he observes minute processes. He is mostly attentive to his potential responsibility in them, which is hypertrophied. He feels that starting a conversation with someone implies taking over responsibility for the relationship, especially for the next step. Because he feels paralysed at the same time, he doesn't dare to even start a conversation. The scenarios, which are constructed in his head before any relationship even takes place, completely block him.

For him, women are something one experiences from television, not something natural. Talking to them feels unnatural and, in front of them, he feels as absolutely nothing. He decided long ago that he is nobody.

Due to all these processes at play inside him, he is confronted with a constant *fear of appearing strange and inappropriate* in the eyes of others. This is another reason why he does not give any initiative to meeting others. He has a problem calling anybody to meet him etc. Whenever he is among other people, he feels the pressure of their expectations.

The only two positive characteristics he feels that he possesses are creativity and humour. He wanted to talk like philosophers, e.g. Sartre, in order to rise above the triviality of everyday-ness. Once when he travelled in India he felt unburdened; but back in Slovenia, he became anxious again. There are these unwritten rules that everybody knows unconsciously but that he cannot grasp. Finally, he feels *different bodily sensations*, like muscular twitches, flows of energies, stomach aches and uneasiness, a heightened sense of hearing, undefined noises etc., which he tends to relate to forces outside him, influencing him, and he notices connections that are plotted against him.

In psychotherapy, he prefers the therapist to talk impersonally about the processes, mechanisms etc. If the therapist says he would like to help him, he gets anxious and uneasy. He feels as if he has no grounding. He cannot build hope and is thus in *despair* because he doesn't see any solution to his problems and does not hope for any. He has endorsed suicidal thoughts since he was 19 and has previously attempted suicide. He feels *imprisoned in himself*, overwhelmed by doubts and even more by involuntary inhibition. With everything he wants and tries to start, he feels a strong counter-impulse that prevents him from pursuing the things he wants.

His psychotic themes revolve around mystical-religious experiences with paranoid and grandiose features. Before being hospitalized for the first time, he travelled to India. There he was in touch with a certain Indian 'mystic', who told him that he has spiritual talents and will be an important spiritual figure in the future. Much later after the hospitalization, he explained to us that he is often in touch with this mystic, who sends him messages through the *cenesthetic experiences and muscular twitches*. If he thinks spiritually inappropriate thoughts, he receives the twitches to remind him of his nature. He has often felt that somebody is *playing games with him*.

In the year when his therapist (BŠ) was abroad, he gradually felt more intensive somatic sensations and *feelings*, which evolved into *two internal systems*: one was connected to the digestive apparatus and stood for mundane matters, and the other was connected to the respiratory apparatus and stood for spiritual matters. It further evolved to the *feeling of being Jesus*.

Lately, he feels that the *devil is taking control over him*. He is afraid how this process will end. Increasingly, he feels under the devil's influence and if he refuses him, his feeling of emptiness or nothingness will remain. When, in the past, he was under the influence of God, he refused Him and neglected his own divine mission, which resulted in the automatism of denying the good.

Psychoanalysis and psychosis

Within psychoanalysis many theories have been proposed to explain the phenomenology and development of the psychotic states of mind (Frosch 1983; Robbins 1993; Rosenbaum 2005; de Masi 2009; Harder & Rosenbaum 2015). They all assume that the main disturbances lie beyond the failure of repression (that usually maintains the stability of the neurotic structure), and that the main disturbances are linked with processes in the basis of the psychic apparatus affecting the development of self and the structure of the ego in its relationship to the frustrating and traumatic impact of the world. In modern psychoanalysis, the anchoring of the structures of representations and symbol-formation may be seen as a function of primal repression. The primal repression anchors the structure and functions of Unconscious–Preconscious–Conscious and its ways of relating to the world, and it serves the integration of primary and secondary processes (Freud). It anchors the transformations of raw sensory impressions into thoughts and thinking (Bion terminology), and it is an aspect of a successful outcome of the paternal metaphor (Lacan terminology), where the knotting of signifier and signified is accomplished and speech becomes thematically and narratively coherent. It forms nodal points in the unconscious network of representations and in the traces of memory. If this anchoring system has not been installed safely in the development of the individual or if it has been foreclosed for other traumatic reasons, then primordial features of the mind may dominate and take over.

Certain characteristics are (to a different degree) prominent in the clinical work:

- Withdrawal of psychic investment in external reality – causing break-downs of the testing of one's thoughts and fantasies related to perceptions and understanding of external reality, and also leading to a (defensive) non-interest in the social world and a (hypersensitive) preoccupation with thoughts and fantasies;
- Attacks on the drive towards mutuality of being oneself in relating to others leading to disrupting the boundaries between 'I' and the world;
- States of non-integration of self/other/Other, me/not-me, thoughts/ feelings, inside/outside, absence/presence;
- Anxiety and aggression directed towards external and internal reality to the extent that being conscious about this is painful, intolerable, and unbearable;
- A disorganised answer to the danger that thoughts and memories may entail when they cannot be symbolised and be integrated in the symbolic order (and thus acquire a common sense status), leading to vulnerability of uncontrolled anxiety.

In psychotic states of mind, these (overlapping) characteristics dominate the person's psychic attitudes towards others, and especially the person's expectations about the others' desires and demands toward oneself. They are the manifestations of the severe disturbances of the processes of symbolization and intersubjectivity. Elements of language may be treated as unconscious presentations, without any rational communicational background or coherence. Communication and thinking – thinking about oneself related to the world or about oneself positioned in a past–present– future process of development – become fundamentally destabilized. Vagueness, incoherence, and private language, as well as feelings of non-existence or ambivalence in the person's expressions of his or her ideas, may thus become prominent.

Psychoanalytically informed psychotherapy in psychiatry

The inseparable bond and dialectic relation between cure and research ('heilen und forschen', cf Freud, 1926) is the basis of psychoanalysis as a science. The above conceptualizations are all derived from, or shall be understood in relation to, psychic phenomena as they are observed and experienced subjectively by patient and analyst/therapist. Thus, psychoanalysis as a science is based in the intersubjective field of subject and Other: body–mind–world, subject–other, subject–group and subject–discourse.

In meeting the patient, a relevant question for the psychiatrist should always be: how can the patient learn from the experience of the therapeutic relation, and how can the patient, in this process of learning, develop a more integrated view of oneself and others?

Moments of curative progression are marked by non-linearity, and the therapist's capacity for listening and intervening in language (whether spoken or silent language) can never be predicted in details or completely rehearsed beforehand. Nevertheless, some principles for intervention can be proposed, and in a prospective, comparative, quasi-randomized research project (Rosenbaum et al., 2012; Rosenbaum, 2015; Harder & Rosenbaum, 2015), the following guidelines were stated:

- Establishing a working alliance that functions even in periods marked by the patient's ambivalent, confusing or negative attitude (negative transference) towards the therapist. The therapist needs to manifest a creative mind, sufficiently calm and balanced so that the patient may feel a secure attachment;

- Using the dynamics of the therapeutic relationship and setting to understand communication processes in other relationships outside the psychotherapy setting. The kind of interventions employed for the promotion of this kind of understanding should finally lead to getting in touch with internal, traumatically disrupted thoughts and emotions, that in the working-through phase of therapy can be interpreted in such a way that vulnerable and painful aspects, usually leading to psychotic breakdowns, can be integrated in a more healthy way;

- Keeping in mind the role and influence of the counter-transference on the therapist's understanding and responses. Being aware as therapist that even though you are experienced and an authority qua therapist, you are never a total master of the curative processes, and sometimes the patient may even be able to 'diagnose' your countertransference manifestations which you should be open to and make use of in a creative way;

- Emphasizing the patterns of conflicts and primitive defence mechanisms, and by doing this helping the patient to understand that defence mechanisms are necessary part of one's personality and that they are helpful in many aspects of life, and destructive in other aspects;

- Recognizing and respecting in the therapist's clarifications, confrontations, and interpretations, the coexistence of both psychotic and non-psychotic aspects of the patient's personality (Bion 1957);
- Acknowledging in the interventions that mental functioning develops in a dialectic of different levels, i.e. 'turning the raw sense impressions into thoughts' and 'thoughts into thinking' (Bléandonu 1994, p. 146). Empathizing with this development enables the patient to deal with emotional experiences in a more adaptive way, and it should help the patient to make sense of and better understand his/her feelings, attitudes and subjective intentions in concrete interpersonal relationships;
- Helping the patient to recover from the psychosocial losses related to his or her suffering from psychosis by, in a trusting manner, reformulating the patient's story of development with elements of hope and realistic optimism, counterbalancing the patient's negative and self-denigrating attitude;
- Including an array of supportive (modified psychoanalytic) techniques in the here-and-now interactions of the sessions: clarifications, affirmations, and suggestions; holding and containing the patient's painful state of mind; maximizing adaptive strategies, encouraging patient's activities; helping the patient to understand how psychotic mechanisms work psychologically in the individual and in specific interactions with others, and how other people might be expected to react (common sense reactions).

Case (extracts from therapist's report)

A young female nurse writes to a psychiatrist (BR) about her feelings of having thin-skin, feelings of falling apart side by side with experience of 'self-centred chaos' and taking colour from others that she is together with. She also has particular feelings about words: they are felt as dangerous, as if they have been melted in a black pot and unexpectedly turned into shapes of reality, or they may disintegrate and fall totally apart.

Her father was a captain in the army and he wanted her to be boy-like. He punished her and wanted her to avoid sex while he, at the same time, said that had she not been his daughter he would have had sex with her. In her mind, the patient had killed the father several times together with other persons whom she found intrusive and abusive. 'I have an inner cemetery where I can allocate people whom I dislike'. Sometimes she could fear that the killing had taken place in reality and not only inside her mind.

Her mother had, in her view, an esoteric appearance, living in her own fairy-tale like world, telling the daughter to rely on a fairy-tale, fictive, inner friend who should take care of her when the mother vanished from her mother-role into narcissistic self-occupation. She connects that with her own feelings of non-existing. No secure-attachment relations existed in her world.

Approximately two-and-a-half years into a psycho-analytic psychotherapy, the theme of trust became explicit. She said to me: 'During the first year you were an eyebrow, and then you became a doctor with a white coat and shortly after a doctor. But I am not sure that I will ever be able to experience you as a person.'

I hesitated in my response with many questions in my head: 'What is an eyebrow able to perceive and say, and does it have the capacity for listening?' 'What is the symbolic meaning of an eyebrow for this patient – if it has any?' 'How could I understand the sequence of the doctor in a white coat and then one without a coat?'

Countertransference thoughts rotated around the following: Did I, despite my assumed analytical listening attitude, raise the feelings in her that I was a person with a non-listening, authoritarian, paternalistic attitude? Or was the transformation from 'with white coat' to 'without coat' an indication that she experienced me as moving from a super-ego position – punitive or controlling – towards a more caring object raising sensual feelings in her? Or, was her utterance an indication of pain from her side, telling me that regardless of how much progress we would be able to make, I should anticipate and accept a limit? Did she tell me that she could not imagine any way out of the claustrum in which she was chained and that any push toward this would possibly be an all-absorbing catastrophe?

I ended up saying that I felt that as an eyebrow I may have observed many things, but I might not have been able to listen properly to her – and I wondered what she had permitted me to see and say from that perspective. She responded by saying that my words made her think of an episode after she had moved away from home when she had returned to visit her parents for a dinner. The main course was roast lamb cutlet from which 'the bone stood out as a penis without the foreskin'. She had to leave the dinner immediately. She believed her mother understood her reaction since her mother 'was made of that stuff dreams were made of'.

For a moment I was stuck in the countertransferential split between on one side being able to empathize with her fear of being attacked by some penetrating stimuli, impressions or words – father's gaze or voice, memories from childhood or youth, my attitude – against which she could not defend herself, and on the other side her striving towards a state of integrating different emotions and, by means of the therapy, finding an object that she could trust.

In another session, she told me that she wanted to find a man who did not scare her or demand too much of her. She had not been lucky in previous relationships with men, though had had two children with one of them. The act of sexuality could be very frightening to her since she might experience her labia enlarge to the extent that they would fill the whole room in which the act took place, and she would then feel suffocated. In several sessions, I had experienced her in hallucinatory states of mind. She once saw a man wearing a big black plastic bag and immediately believed that this bag contained her two children chopped into small pieces. She looked at the street sign and the words were cut up into small fragments. She remembered occasions when her children were babies, and it was hard for her to have them close to her body, because she could feel as if they crept under her skin, or ate her breast.

She thought that some of the difficulties with her relationship to men had their origin in her father's ways of behaving when she was a baby. In one of her memories her father would lift her in the air when she was six months old and was not wearing a nappy, and he would place her behind on his nose while blowing air on her genitals. In a later session she told me that one of his characteristics was his eyebrows.

Concluding recommendations for the field of psychiatry

Both the phenomenological and the psychoanalytic approach recommends that psychiatrists deepen their understanding of the patients' subjective experiences of themselves, others, and the world, including an increased understanding of the patients' anomalous experiences as well as their disturbed common sense understanding of their own and others' experiences. These non-psychotic anomalous experiences, such as very fragile sense of self, inadequate self/no-self boundaries, hyper-reflectivity etc. are overlooked in mainstream psychiatry. Each in its own way, and with a shared interest in the patient's subjective experiences, thus contributes in depth and with seriousness to the idea that it is the *person* with the illness who is the central feature of diagnostic investigation (Gabbard 2019).

As a psychiatrist, one cannot understand psychiatric symptomatology by only registering the presence or absence of symptoms and signs. Symptoms and signs are not unrelated features of psychopathology, but mutually implicative and intertwined aspects of an underlying psychopathological Gestalt. Since the introduction of the polythetic diagnostic criteria in DSM-III (APA

1980), we have lost sight of the synchronic and diachronic psychopathological Gestalts that underlie and unite the clinical manifestations of mental disorders. Anxiety is not just anxiety but may imply different dynamics, different qualities of subjective experiences and lead to different subjective conclusions, depending on the patient and the structure of his/her mental processes, and thus the integrative capacities of the patient's mind (Gabbard 2015). Similarly, hallucinations are not just hallucinations. They may have different qualities: benign vs malign, helpful vs persecuting voices, clearly perceptual vs diffuse sensorial, balancing between one's internal and external reality, being an integrated part of a narrative, or being a thought-related phenomenon with an unclear psychic representation.

Psychiatry may profit from a phenomenological and a psychoanalytic approach, both in the assessment of psychopathology (Nordgaard et al. 2013; Lotterman 2015) and in the successive treatment of the patient – using affirmation and respectful suggestions as well as clarifications, confrontation, and interpreting understanding. From the very first moment, diagnostic assessment must be understood as the beginning of treatment.

Research in psychopathology should encompass more than registration of symptomatology (mainly by psychometric instruments) and reductionistic measurements of quality of life, mental and social functioning, etc. The patients' descriptions of their subjective experiences of symptoms and signs, of psychic change, of changes in the their interpersonal relationships, as well as clarifications of internal and external object relations, should be systematically listened to, understood, and investigated. Finally, neurophenomenology and neuropsychoanalysis add additional insight to 'the person with the illness' but these aspects have not been included in our chapter.

References

American Psychiatric Association (APA) (1980). *Diagnostic and statistical manual of mental disorders, third edition (DSM-III)*. Washington, DC: APA.

Bion, W. R. (1957). Differentiation of the psychotic and non-psychotic personalities, *International Journal of Psychoanalysis*, 38: 266–275.

Bléandonu, G. (1994). *Wilfred Bion: his Life and Works, 1897–1979*. London: Free Association.

Cermolacce, M., Naudin, J., & Parnas, J. (2007). The 'minimal self' in psychopathology: Re-examining the self-disorders in the schizophrenia spectrum. *Consciousness and Cognition, 16*: 703–714.

Charbonneau, G. (2004). Introduction à la phénoménologie des hallucinations. In G. Charbonneau (Ed.). *Introduction à la phénoménologie des hallucinations* (pp. 17–42). Paris: Circle Hermeneutique.

De Masi, F. (2009). *Vulnerability to psychosis*. London: Karnac.

Freud, S. (1926). The question of lay analysis. *SE, Volume XX*: 177–258.

Frosch, J. (1983). *The psychotic process*. New York: International Universities Press.

Gabbard, G. O. (2015). *Psychodynamic psychiatry in clinical practice* (5th ed.). Washington, DC: American Psychiatric Publications.

Gabbard, G. O. (2019). The person with the diagnosis. (This volume)

Hart, J. G. (2009). *Who one is. Book 1. Meontology of the 'I': A transcendental phenomenology*. Berlin: Springer.

Harder, S., & Rosenbaum, B. (2015). Psychosis. In P. Luyten, L.C. Mayes, P. Fonagy, M. Target and S.J. Blatt (Ed.). *Handbook of psychodynamic approaches to psychopathology* (ch. 13, pp. 259–286). New York: Guildford Press.

Henriksen, M. G., & Parnas, J. (2014). Self-disorders and schizophrenia: A phenomenological reappraisal of poor insight and noncompliance. *Schizophrenia Bulletin, 40*: 542–547.

Henry, M. (1973). *The essence of manifestation*. The Hague: Martinus Nijhoff.

Lotterman, A. (2015). *Psychotherapy for people diagnosed with schizophrenia*. London: Routledge.

Nelson, B., Parnas, J., & Sass, L. A. (2014). Disturbance of minimal self (ipseity) in schizophrenia: Clarification and current status. *Schizophrenia Bulletin, 40*: 479–482.

Nordgaard, J., Sass, L. A., & Parnas, J. (2013). The psychiatric interview: Validity, structure, and intersubjectivity. *European Archive of Psychiatry and Clinical Neurosciences, 263*(4): 353–364.

Parnas, J., & Henriksen, M. G. (2014). Disordered self in the schizophrenia spectrum: A clinical and research perspective. *Harvard Review of Psychiatry, 22*(5): 251–265.

Parnas, J., & Henriksen, M. G. (2016). Schizophrenia and mysticism: A phenomenological exploration of the structure of consciousness in the schizophrenia spectrum disorders. *Consciousness and Cognition, 43*: 75–88.

Parnas, J., Møller, P., Kircher, T., Thalbitzer, J., Jansson, L., Handest, P. and Zahavi, D. (2005). EASE: Examination of anomalous self-experience. *Psychopathology, 38*: 236–258.

Robbins, M. (1993). *Experiences of schizophrenia*. New York: Guilford Press.

Rosenbaum, B. (2005). Psychosis and the structure of homosexuality: Understanding the pathogenesis of schizophrenic states of mind. *Scandinavian Psychoanalytic Review, 28*: 82–89.

Rosenbaum, B. (2015). Psychodynamic psychotherapy for persons in states of psychosis: Some research perspectives. *British Journal of Psychotherapy, 31*(4): 476–491.

Rosenbaum, B., Harder, S., Knudsen, P., Koester, A., Lindhardt, A., Valbak, K., & Winther, G. (2012). Supportive psychodynamic psychotherapy versus treatment as usual for first episode psychosis: Two-year outcome. *Psychiatry: Interpersonal and Biological Processes, 75*(4): 331–341.

Sartre, J.-P. (2003). *Being and nothingness*, trans. H. E. Barnes. London: Routledge.

Sass, L. A. (1994). *Paradoxes of delusion: Wittgenstein, Schreber, and the schizophrenic mind.* Ithaca, NY: Cornell.

Sass, L. A., & Parnas, J. (2003). Schizophrenia, consciousness, and the self. *Schizophrenia Bulletin, 29*: 427–444.

Zahavi, D. (2005). *Subjectivity and selfhood: Investigating the first-person perspective.* Cambridge, MA: MIT Press.

Zahavi, D. (2014). *Self and other: Exploring subjectivity, empathy, and shame.* Oxford, UK: Oxford University Press.

PART III

The formative dimension
Teaching and continual education

CHAPTER FIFTEEN

Teaching, training and continual education
Methods and models

Anna Ferruta

Beyond supervision – La mujer que llora: Clinical Group Seminars as Psychoanalytic Experience

Specificities for the psychiatry of Clinical Group Seminars

The instrument of Clinical Group Seminars (CGS) is specifically indicated for the patients treated by psychiatry professionals and institutions. Clinical Group Seminars or Clinical Conferences are a training device made up of a group of professionals (psychiatrists, psychotherapists, postgraduates) and a psychoanalyst leader who meet to work on a clinical case: it is not the analysis of the unconscious dynamics brought into play by the participants at the level of their personal situation nor is it supervision by a more expert psychoanalyst on the clinical material, as takes place in a setting of dyadic supervision.

It is an instrument that activates an analytical way of functioning, particularly useful in situations where, in the treatment relationship with patients who are difficult to reach, there is a block of thought in the patient–therapist relationship and a tendency to take the defining-diagnostic escape route and to apply predefined concepts to a static reality that ends up by representing only one element to be examined (anamnesis, behaviour, diagnosis, therapies etc.).

The seminar represents a mental place that can receive aspects of the mind of a severely affected patient (situations of psychic death, blocked capacities of thinking, loving, working) that the individual mind of the therapist does not have sufficient space to hold, and that induce him symmetrically into being imprisoned in inert, ideological or imitative patterns.

The Clinical Group Seminar is a place where movements of mental freedom that can unblock situations of stalemate in the relationship of the patient with the therapist and/or with the treating institution are activated and allow the formation of new psychic reorganizations.

Its analytic quality is made up of the elements characterizing the method: a well-defined setting (ample space-time, at least two hours so that the group can meet in a condition of freedom that allows movement of thought) and a method based on free associations by the participants and evenly hovering attention by the leader. After an intense interaction of conscious/unconscious communications in the group, the leader has the task of putting together the different aspects of the patient that each person has understood, as in a painting by Picasso: in *La mujer que llora* (*The Weeping Woman*, 1937, Tate Modern) putting together the different facets allows meeting the grief of the woman in her living depth.

Training through the emotional experience

This mental functioning is described by various authors with different, but essentially converging formulations: the *central phobic position* described by Green (2000) as functioning in analysis of patients who repeat rigid mental structures to avoid, through the associative fluctuation, coming into contact with emotions that they are not equipped to deal with; the Bionian *reverie*, reinterpreted by Ferro (2011 often with very audacious passages, as the capacity to dream, with dream-thoughts, unconscious contents that are not accepted (e.g. the news of a tumour by a patient who uses the "reality" of the tumour to block the path to the terrifying "reality" that is emerging in analysis and that can also be referred to the experience of an interpretation experienced as a malignant instead of nurturing proliferating content); and the Bionian container–content relationship understood by Ogden (2004) as a vital process in continuous expansion and change. The expansion of the capacity of the container can take shape in beginning to host heterogeneous associations or noticing apparently insignificant details; the growth of the content is reflected in the expansion of the range and depth of the thoughts and feelings derived from the emotional experience. Container and content are inseparable, in a relationship of reversible figure-background.

The CGS appears as a "playful" container – in Winnicott's (1971) sense: it proposes work by the group which as in a game does not consist only of observing a phenomenon (for example the patient) but of becoming part of the dynamic activated, implementing a participation in the first person in the experience of the group and the therapeutic activity.

Jaak Panksepp (Panksepp & Biven, 2012) highlighted the importance of play in the development of the child, biologically rooted in the primary structures of the BrainMind, those which he indicates as "The fabulous PLAYful circuits of the brain" (*The Archaeology of Mind*, 379).

The playful mode of functioning represents a fundamental training instrument to allow psychiatric therapists to experience their emotions during the group seminar, to be themselves sound boxes of the split or denied emotions of the patient they are talking about and made perceptible through the spokesperson function of the participants in the group.

In its functioning in free associations and hovering attention, the group resumes the functioning of the apparatus to think as oscillation between emotion, action and knowledge, according to the analytic specificity, an oscillation between knowing and becoming, between Bion's K and O (1962). The fundamental need is to widen the playful space in which knowing is also often becoming the object, it is experiencing a process of self-transformation and not only of observation.

A narrative function is activated that finds ways to give shape and meaning to what happens, removing it from the one-way fate of the evacuating action of release, which can be done both by the patients and the therapists. The treating and thinking function is carried out by the group itself to which the clinician who presented the case and the psychoanalyst-leader belong, without charismatic proxies and without extractive intrusions.

From this point of view, the clinical seminar represents an opportunity for transformative learning: it presents the characteristics of a process of supervision because it allows understanding aspects of the patient that have not been picked up by only the individual dimension of the mind; it activates a transformation of the emotional state of the participants who in turn become characters of the inner world of the case presented, functioning as split and denied aspects, not represented by this and challenged by unconscious group dynamics. The transformation concerns the emotional state of the participants as the main source of knowledge and not as use of the seminar in a therapeutic sense: the emotional exposure of each person, willing to function in free association to give their permeability to host the stranger, the other than oneself, to let unknown aspects of the self emerge, must not be abused for purposes of individual analytic interpretations. Verbal communication is at stake not only in its referential meaning, but also in its dramatic and scenic meaning, of becoming someone else, i.e. the character that speaks in the name of denied or split or unrepresented parts of the patient.

An example of a Clinical Group Seminar

The Group is made up of 13 professionals (psychiatrists or psychotherapists) who work in the Psychiatric Services with severe cases and of three psychoanalysts (two of whom lead the group, one records a summary of the work done, which is read at the end of the following session and given to the participants). The time available is two hours. The presenter reads a brief history of the case and the account of two sessions. Then he/she stays silent and the dynamic interaction of the group is developed on the basis of free associations. When the configuration of the case starts to emerge, one of the two leaders proposes a psychodynamic portrait of the patient, as it has emerged from the work of the group mind. Discussion is then opened once again in the group, including the contribution by the leader. At the end, a new name is given to the patient to whom the group work has provided a living affective representation.

The case of F, a 45-year-old man, is presented by a young psychiatrist who works in an outpatient clinic. It is his first meeting with F who has just been discharged from hospital, accepted voluntarily under pressure from his GP, for a persecutory situation that prevents him from sleeping and living (disturbances from the neighbouring Chinese family: he hears a woman, ill-treated by a man, screaming and crying), which he has reported to the police with whom he clashes. In F's history, there is a mother with post-partum depression, sexual abuse by an older boy, unemployment and difficulties in establishing affective relationships. He is HIV positive and suffers from ulcerative colitis.

In the first session, F appears collaborative and evasive (he says that the next day he is leaving for Sicily with friends), autonomous and dependent: he asks for advice on the antipsychotic and anxiolytic medications prescribed to him on discharge from hospital, but states he will not take them because he prefers natural remedies (e.g. the trip to Sicily with friends).

He returns especially from Sicily for the second session.

An extract from the psychiatrist's notes: "I ask him to sit down and I comment: 'So you decided to come, you didn't go to Sicily'; he answers, 'No, I went to Sicily and I came back yesterday because I had the appointment today . . . if I really have to go down this route, then I will.' In my heart I am surprised, I would not have bet that we would have met again and even less that he would have come back especially for the meeting. During the session he did not take off his jacket and I noticed again, as I had the last time, his serious and peering gaze and lively capacity of expression. I begin the session by reconnecting to the end of the previous one and making it clear that I had asked us to meet to evaluate the trend of the therapy. 'I did as you said: half of the one with zeta . . . zapam . . . and that one to sleep' . . . I think he is confused between lorazepam and olanzapine and I explain to him once again that I had prescribed half an olanzapine and one lorazepam. 'Yes, the one with a zed, zapam, zapina, I don't know now . . . I can't remember the name and I haven't got the boxes with me . . . anyway, half of one and the one that makes me sleep . . . Anyway I took it again last might when I came back because I didn't take anything at all when I was away and I was fine . . . friends, quiet evenings . . . everything was fine and I didn't need anything, but anyway, I took the one to sleep last night again.' I cannot understand whether he is really confused or whether he is pretending to be confused, as he has not taken the treatment and that is the only element of evaluation. I do have the perception that for the time being he is measuring up the situation, I am not worried and I decide not to dwell too long on this point. I repeat what he should do and ask him to tell me how the Sicily trip went: 'Ah doctor, very well, it would be the ideal place for me, I would like to live there . . . surrounded by my friends . . . I stayed with this friend of mine who has a lot of physical problems so I went with him, backwards and forwards for exams, check-ups, certificates, poor guy . . . he can't use the car and so I made myself useful . . . we had no times to respect . . . we would wake up when we wanted, we would eat when we were hungry and we always stayed up until one or two in the morning. . . . On New Year's Eve there were eight of us, but all very quiet . . . I really didn't need any drugs . . . not with the peaceful life there . . . and then I came back last night.' I tell him I am surprised as he had warned me that if things went well there he would have stayed there for at least a month: 'Look, we had made this appointment and as I said, if I have to go down this path then I will be glad to do so.' I ask him how things are going in the family: 'Well . . . I would say fine, I've never had any problems with my parents but of course it's not easy at over forty to be without a job and to have to live with your parents . . . anyway now that I'm back I've started to study English, I want to do an exam to get a qualification that gives me greater chances of finding a job . . . so I'm very busy studying . . . of course it's difficult with the racket that comes from the other house . . . all day I can hear that TU-TUM TU-TUM . . . all day long . . . from four in the morning!' I ask him what he hears most: 'From my room, if I put my ear against the wall, I can hear two voices . . . a woman moaning and a man calling her "bitch! whore!" non-stop' (. . .) I tell him that if things are that way about those noises, there is nothing to be done, so the only thing to do is sleep better and distract his attention from it, doing things that interest him such as studying English or looking for a job. I try to explain to him that this is precisely what the pharmaco-logical treatment is for and I suggest going back to the full dosage of the anti-psychotic drug (olanzapine). He accepts and this surprises me. We agree on the next time to meet and say goodbye."

The group work is also oriented towards listening to something that has taken place elsewhere and that has a "traumatic" consistency: mater-nal depression, sexual abuse, casual promiscuous sexuality, etc. The main sensation is that the group moves isomorphically in relation to the experi-ence of the patient who is in the condition of not knowing exactly what is happening inside himself and who therefore pays attention to what hap-pens beyond the wall, to have something to clutch to and not to let himself be submerged by confusion. The hypothesis that starts to appear is that F has until now used isolation as his main defence (for example, the holi-day in Sicily, the voluntary admission to hospital, occasional relationships, especially gay ones) and that now this mechanism is no longer able to protect him and he is seeking new solutions. The project of learning a new language such as English can be understood as a request for help aimed at establishing bonds that allow him to come out of his isolation.

F is terrified by what takes place in the next apartment, but at the same time he cannot take his attention away from the voices and noises that come from the other house, as though on the one hand he were threatened but also attracted and seduced by this strong experience that oppresses him. He is unable to stay away from meetings including intimate ones, with people with whom he does not build up relationships, but from which he nevertheless comes out infected.

The group discusses how an evolution of the patient can be fostered in the treatment and the risk of a stable breakdown into psychosis. The observation is made that F was able to ask for help first from the police and then the Psychiatric Services, and this suggests that inside the therapeutic relationship as well he would be able to communicate his need for containment and protection of the psychotic part and develop a relationship useful for his emotional development.

The new name given by the group to F, Zenzero ("ginger" in Italian) (prompted by the name of the drug that F cannot remember but that starts with a zed and his declaration of loyalty to natural treatments).

The group has analysed the case of its own interactive dynamic which at first listened to what took place outside the relationship with the psychiatrist presenting the case (maternal depression, abuse, etc.) and used it for the purpose of understanding an aspect of F's psychic functioning: to hold onto something strong in the patient's history so as not to drown in confusion was symmetrical to the patient's need for a strong reference outside himself, a reference with a disturbing and annihilating character that invades his fragile psychic life which has little consistency. One alternative to suggest to him is a stable therapeutic relationship open to listening to what F feels in the first person, thanks to a language of which he has little knowledge, the one that combines empathic understanding and personal identification, an English to be learned.

Using the instrument of the Clinical Group Seminar not only in the psychiatric services but also in other fields of medicine (oncology, diabetology, physical medicine and rehabilitation) has been widely experimented, with excellent results, especially in areas where the pathology tends to produce phenomena of prolonged relationships between therapists and patients, with risks of chronicity both in the illness and in the treatment devices. This training approach offers doctors the experience of how to relate to the patient, to understand the emotions that the session arouses and use them as a therapeutic instrument.[1]

This change introduced by psychoanalysis in the conception of the psychic functioning and treatment, a continuous dialectic between the construction of the subject and function of the setting, is reflected in the current development of theories which pay attention to the processes of subjectivation and subjectualization, i.e. the evolution of the subject through experiences of contact with the other, used to build up and expand the self (after Winnicott: Bollas, 1992; Roussillon, 1995; Cahn, 1998); as well as other authors who have opened up the study of the unconscious to group functioning (after Bion: Anzieu, 1985: Kaës, 2007) and those who have studied dissociative mechanisms as a creative aspect of the functioning of the mind (Bromberg, 2011).

Function and characteristics of the setting and active role of the patient in giving flavour and consistency to the representations form an important aspect of the treatment process, which has to go in the opposite direction of avoidance and phobia, but which are often justified as protective measures or as functions of metabolization prepared by the mental activity of the therapist who draws on his unilateral imaginative heritage, overlooking the imaginative capacity of the patient.

The dimensions of the device of the Analytic Group Seminar

One specific added value of the CGS is its feasibility, as it presents a "light" methodology that includes depth and simplicity of the instruments necessary, mainly a group of therapists and a psychoanalyst trained to listen, and uses unconscious mental functioning in groups. Its functioning can be illustrated by these five dimensions: constructing a setting, listening, suffering, associating and configuring.

Constructing a setting

The Analytic Group Seminar has in the construction of a specific setting its fundamental value: all the other activities are suspended, all the therapists available are present and an expert psychoanalyst is ready to listen. A clinical case is presented through the voices and reports of the therapists who are most directly responsible and who have the opportunity to have experience with the subject being discussed. A group dynamic of conscious and unconscious communications is activated.

Creating this "analysing situation" is the first and fundamental function of a psychoanalyst-leader: identifying the optimal conditions of place and time in which this device can take place and function. This device must have characteristics of inflexibility and rigorousness, otherwise the process of openness to listening of what is not known and what cannot be understood with the individual mind in the dyadic relationship does not work.

If the psychoanalyst who leads the group is able to build up the analysing device, a good part of the work has already been done, because the useful daily action is put on standby and for two hours the group members are in a mental condition of listening, to each other and to themselves, to understand and configure what in the action and in the excessively involving relationship is broken up and made less significant.

The setting functions as a condition in which each of the participants in the Seminar unconsciously relocates themselves in the mental position of container of the contents that the patient has put inside them.

Listening

After building up the device necessary for the work of the Clinical Group Seminar, the main role of the expert is to offer analytical listening. The leader must make silence in himself, get rid of "pre-judgements" on the structure where he is, its organization, its methods and therapeutic ideals, and put himself in the position of listening with the greatest mental and emotional openness possible, also hosting his feelings of sympathy, antipathy, indifference, interest, solicited by the different subjects at play and by the stories told. This type of "dramatic" supervision resembles a theatre where you go to be reached by emotions and stories. The role of the leader is to act as container, not so much in the meaning of containment, but in the meaning of a deposit of living and vibrant material waiting to be put into shape.

The listening function of the leader is the central one; it puts his narcissism and that of the therapists to the test, who have to become concave and host in a rich and desiring subjectivity the otherness of subjects marked by encounters with destructive narcissisms.

Suffering

The third dimension to practise has already been preannounced in the description of the function before listening. The leader necessarily has to reach the point of feeling in the first person, the emotional condition described by the therapists who are taking part in the analytic group seminar. He has to reach an acme in which, when he is convinced of having understood, of holding the right solution to offer, precisely at that moment he has to be able to understand that he is suffering the flow of projective identifications that submerge him and that he can use as an instrument to understand the relational context of that moment in the institution where he is.

The function of a psychoanalyst in the Analytic Group Seminar has a specificity of its own, which does not give up the elements of knowledge and science of psychopathology, nor does it renounce putting into play a specific element of the psychoanalytic method: using the emotions suffered to understand, instead of keeping them at bay and rejecting them. It is precisely when the emotions felt by the leader in the group reach an acme of intensity and almost certainty that the time has come to use them to understand, reflect and configure the relationship identified between the subject and the therapeutic group.

Associating

In the psychic space created by the setting and in the dimension of conscious and unconscious emotional activation, communication develops between the participants, based on the method of free associations. The implicit assumption concerns the difficulty for those who are in direct contact with a severely troubled patient, having tried to avoid the formation of blind spots, disturbances of perception and cognition induced by times of excessive almost identifying nearness and by others of excessive defensive distance. The mental work of the group that freely associates consists of the possibility for the participants who do not have direct responsibility for the patient, to allow images, characters and emotions, including unforeseeable and unexpected ones, to surface, which nevertheless have to do with the object under discussion.

In a group context, the emotional responses of the therapists can be a basis on which the knowledge of the way in which the human mind works is founded. That mental function of container-content of which Bion speaks is activated in the group, as a process of thinkability of what is experienced but not yet acceptable and digestible: in the group there emerges a dream-like psychic functioning, in which an excess psychic content overcomes the barrier of deep sleep and generates images and stories that begin to configure it and make it appear on the stage of the subject's mind. Ogden (2004, p. 159) expresses it particularly clearly:

> The notion of container-content refers not to what we think, but to how we think, i.e. to how we elaborate the lived experience and what happens on the psychic level when we cannot achieve psychic work with the experienced one.

Configuring

At this point, the role of the psychoanalyst is to give shape and a container to the flow of knowledge and emotions that have gone through the work of the group, trying to sketch out the relational profile between patient and group that emerged in the interaction between unconsciousnesses.

Configuration has as its object that of describing better how the patient functions psychically, what the typical patterns determining the breakdown moments are and how to use the comprehension of these functionings to travel down the same road together and for psychic growth. The model of intervention of the psychoanalyst is characterized by the "understand/transform" pair, i.e. by the conviction that the understanding that has emerged from the cognitive/emotional participation in the group represents at least in part a transformative experience in itself for all the participants, made up of feeling emotions directly and using them to understand, in a container/content relationship, that identifies new representative containers to give shape and communication to new contents.

This function of processing and emotional-narrative configuration carried out in the Seminar allows the clinician, who at the beginning took on the subject, to communicate the result of the consultancy as a product of a configuration made up of informative data and emotional resonances that refer to the human group both belong to, and not as an arduous message of diagnosis to be got rid of as soon as possible. One tool that has proved valid is concluding the Seminar with the creation of a new name for the patient, the one that has emerged through the work of the group.

In conclusion, the Clinical Group Seminar describes figuratively and scenically situations in which the therapist and the group are blocked (paralysis of the therapeutic device and difficulty in representing and moving affects, thoughts, gestures) and therefore the relational ways through which the psychic functioning can start off again. Moreover, the origins of psychoanalysis bear this mark, situated as they are between the paralysis of the patients in the *Studies on hysteria* (Freud, 1892–95) and the oneiric movement of emotions, figures and thoughts of *The interpretation of dreams* (Freud, 1900).

Note

1 One could object about the difficulties of this work in public and hospital structures. This is why it is interesting to make wider known a project (Astori et al., 2015) that uses CGS and that has lasted for ten years and is still active at the "Carlo Besta" Neurological Institute of Milan, a hospital and research centre. The project concerns the communication of the genetic diagnosis to those requesting the clinical tests relative to hereditary neurological diseases with late development (ALS, Huntington's disease, etc.). This is an instrument that, with appropriate adjustments, is widely used in psychiatry and in groups with doctors of other specializations, such as oncology, diabetology, physical medicine and rehabilitation, (Hautmann, 2007; Ferruta & Galli, 1994, 2010; Foresti & Rossi Monti, 2010) to make an overall diagnosis of the somatopsychic aspects and to give indications on the methods of the doctor–patient therapeutic relationship.

References

Anzieu, D. (1985). *The skin ego*. New Haven, CT: Yale University Press, 1989.

Astori, S., Ferruta, A., & Mariotti, C. (2015). *La diagnosi genetica: un dialogo per la cura*. Milan: Angeli.

Bion, W. R. (1962). *Learning from experience*. London: Heinemann.

Bollas, C. (1992). *Being a character*. London: Routledge.

Breuer, J. & Freud, S. (1892–1995). *Studies on hysteria*, Standard Edition.

Bromberg, P. M. (2011) *The shadow of the tsunami*. New York: Routledge.

Cahn, R. (1998). *L'aventure de la subjectivation*. Paris: PUF.

Ferro, A. (2011). *Avoiding emotions, living emotions*. London: Routledge.

Ferruta, A., & Galli, T. (1994). Il gruppo Balint: difficoltà e interventi alternativi. *Proposte per la salute mentale, 5*: 55–59.

Ferruta, A. (2010). Il seminario clinico di gruppo come esperienza analitica, accanto all'analisi e alla supervisione. In G. Gabriellini (Ed.). *Giovanni Hautmann e il pensiero gruppale*. Pisa: Felici.

Foresti, G., & Rossi Monti, M. (2010). *Esercizi di visioning. Psicoanalisi, Psichiatria, Istituzioni*. Rome: Borla.

Freud S. (1900) *The interpretation of dreams*, Standard Edition.

Green, A. (2000). The central phobic position. *International Journal of Psycho-Analysis, 81*: 429–451.

Kaës, R. (2007). *Un singulier pluriel*. Paris: Dunod.

Hautmann, G. (2007). Il paziente tra dualità analitica e la molteplicità seminariale. *Rivista di Psicoanalisi, 4*: 1057–1064.

Ogden, T. H. (2004). On holding and containing, being and dreaming. *International Journal of Psycho-Analysis, 85*: 1349–1364.

Panksepp, J., & Biven, L. (2012). *The archaeology of mind*. New York: Norton.

Roussillon, R. (1995). *Primitive agony and symbolization*. London: Karnac.

Winnicott, D.W. (1971). *Playing and reality*. London: Tavistock Publications.

CHAPTER SIXTEEN

Teaching psychoanalytic psychotherapy to residents in psychiatry

Windows of friendship or animosity?[1]

Do-Un Jeong

> If you know the enemy and know yourself, you need not fear the result of a hundred battles. If you know yourself but not the enemy, for every victory gained you will also suffer a defeat. If you know neither the enemy nor yourself, you will succumb in every battle.
>
> (Sun Tzu, *The Art of War*)

Psychoanalytic communities, international and domestic, are concerned about the colonization of psychiatry by biological subspecialties and the consequent marginalization of psychoanalysis and psychoanalytic psychotherapy (PAP) (Kernberg & Michels, 2016; Wallerstein, 1991). In dealing with the concern, it is imperative to teach PAP to residents in psychiatry well enough (Goin, 2006). It will not only produce competent psychiatrists but also maintain PAP as the powerful therapeutic tool for psychiatric patients. Also, PAP training can supplement descriptively operative DSM-5 (Diagnostic and Statistical Manual of Mental Disorders, 5th Edition, American Psychiatric Association, 2013) system with psychoanalytically informed diagnoses in understanding patients. It may lead to an increase in the number of applicants to psychoanalytic training.

Teaching PAP is complex (Mellman & Beresin, 2003). No consensus appears to exist for what and how much we should teach residents. We do not know much about the current situation and the obstacles. We need data. In this paper, I aimed to explore the issues by collecting basic data, studying them, and arriving at suggestions.

Subjects and methods

I interviewed eight graduating PGY-4 (i.e., the fourth year of residency after one-year internship) residents (aged 29–34, seven males and one female) at the Seoul National University Hospital (SNUH) Department of Psychiatry, Seoul, Republic of Korea. I have been working at the hospital as a full-time faculty since 1985. The one-to-one interviews were conducted during their last working month (i.e., within a month after the national board-certification examination) and lasted about an hour, focusing on each resident's experience of PAP. After each interview, interviewees completed a survey that consisted of 15 questions such as initial motivation for choosing psychiatry, the distribution of interests among three areas of psychiatry (i.e., biological, psychoanalytic, and social) before, during, and after their residency, PAP experience and degree of satisfaction, and obstacles/suggestions for improvement. Lastly, I asked whether they would employ a psychoanalyst as a full-time faculty if they were the department chair.

As a comparison group, I also interviewed eight PGY-2 residents (aged 26–32, five males and three females). At the time of the interview, they had had no exposure to the formal PAP education/training such as individual supervision, group supervision, and book reading.

Results

All of the interviewed residents, eight PGY-4 and eight PGY-2, completed and returned the questionnaire.

Initial motivation for choosing psychiatry: When the PGY-4 residents were asked about their motivation for choosing psychiatry, no one reported that they had an exclusive interest in biological psychiatry among the three areas. In comparison, three PGY-2 residents responded that they chose psychiatry being only interested in biological psychiatry.

Distribution of interests: Five PGY-4 residents gave higher or equal scores of interest in psychoanalytic psychiatry around the time of graduation (indicated as "After" in Table 16.1), compared with those before residency (indicated as "Before" in Table 16.1). This result is clearly visible in Figure 16.1.

All PGY-2 residents except one reported that they had an even lower interest in psychoanalytic psychiatry, compared with their counterparts in PGY-4 before coming to the residency program.

Table 16.1 Distribution of interests in biological (B), psychoanalytic (P), and social (S) psychiatry among PGY-4 residents (N=8) before, during, and after training in psychiatry

PGY-4 Before B/P/S	During B/P/S	After B/P/S	PGY-2 Before B/P/S
50/**50**/0	90/10/0	20/**70**/10	30/50/20
45/45/10	75/20/5	50/40/10	40/**40**/20
50/**40**/10	85/10/5	30/**50**/20	50/30/20
40/**40**/20	60/20/20	40/**40**/20	60/**30**/10
50/**40**/10	70/20/10	50/35/15	50/**25**/25
50/**40**/10	80/10/10	60/30/10	70/**25**/5
40/30/30	60/20/20	50/**30**/20	70/**20**/10
70/**20**/10	85/10/5	65/25/10	80/**10**/10

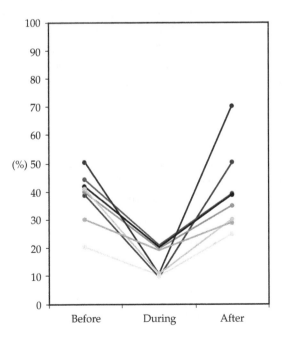

Figure 16.1 PGY-4 Residents' distribution of % interest in psychoanalytic psychiatry before, during, and after residency

About the hypothetical question: All 16 residents in two classes except one in PGY-4 responded that they would be willing to employ a psychoanalyst as a full-time faculty if they were the department chair.

PAP experience: During the four years of residency, four PGY-4 residents experienced a total of 3 to 5 PAP cases, three had 6 to 10 cases, and only one had more than 10 cases. A total number of individual supervision ranged from 20 to 90 sessions (median 40). An average number of supervisions per patient ranged from 3 to 20 sessions (median 9). All PGY-2 residents were in the starting phase of their PAP experience.

On the degree of satisfaction with PAP training, all PGY-4 residents reported 'unsatisfactory'. All of them agreed that their PAP training had been insufficient, despite half of them ranking within the top five in the national board-certification examination (PAP competency assessment is a significant mandatory part of it).

Obstacles to PAP training: Three major obstacles reported by the PGY-4 residents were educator/supervisor shortage, limited time allocation for PAP training, and unfavorable medical care environment. The three obstacles were followed by the issue of a government-controlled national health insurance system. Interestingly, the PGY-4 residents did not regard the progress of biological psychiatry as a signficiant obstacle to PAP training.

PGY-2 residents also mentioned educator/supervisor shortage and limited time allocation for PAP training. However, external factors such as medical care, environment/health insurance system did not seem to be of concern to them yet. PGY-2 residents also reported that the progress of biological psychiatry was the least significant obstacle to PAP training.

Table 16.2 Wish list about PAP training by psychiatry residents

#wished-for	PGY-4	PGY-2
More functional patient referral system	2	1
More time for PAP/more accessibility	1	2
More frequent case discussion	1	–
More systematic supervisor availability	1	1
More education on the theory/ psychodynamic formulation	2	1
More individual attention	2	–
Innovation in healthcare system/ insurance	1	–
Improvement in low fee structure	1	–

Residents' wish list for improving the PAP training: The PGY-4 residents suggested more diverse ways of improving the PAP training than PGY-2 residents (See Table 16.2). In comparison with PGY-2 residents, PGY-4 residents took account of external factors (the healthcare system/insurance/fee structure) in addition to internal educational/training factors.

Subjective experiences collected from interviews: Current patient referral system at the SNUH Department of Psychiatry was reported to be significantly dysfunctional. PGY-4 residents raised two most manifest issues. First, the majority of referrals for PAP were made by faculty members. This makes it difficult for residents to refuse the unsuitable cases. One PGY-4 resident recalled that one out of five referrals to him had not been suitable for PAP. Second, the majority of referred patients were on multiple medications. The patients made regular visits to the referring faculty for drug refills and supportive therapy.

One of the PGY-4 residents half-jokingly complained: in teaching PAP to them, they should have been treated like toddlers. He added that it was traumatic sometimes, knowing he was not good enough and not knowing what to do about it.

PGY-4 residents considered individual supervision as most helpful, followed by group supervisions and book reading.

Discussion

I have a strong feeling that I have rediscovered my residents in the process of going through this simple study. Despite having committed myself to teaching PAP for almost 30 years, I realize that I have not yet got to know them well enough. Interviewing the graduating PGY-4 residents enabled me to understand more who they are and what they want from PAP training. It was a big relief to note that they maintain and express a significant degree of interest in psychoanalytic psychiatry even after 'unsatisfactory' PAP training.

I am the only certified psychoanalyst faculty at the SNUH Department of Psychiatry. It has 31 full-time (17, 10, and 4 in three separate hospitals) and 22 clinical faculty members, 43 post-residency fellows, and 37 residents. All of them are loaded with inpatient/outpatient care, education/training of medical students/residents, clinical/basic research activities, and administrative responsibilities. The resident rotation schedule is always very tight and busy, covering the three main and one affiliated hospitals. Time always limits the consistency of training programs and PAP training is not an exception. Some residents are busier, being in graduate programs, Master's and PhDs.

At the time of this study, among the clinical faculty members, there were one Freudian psychoanalyst and a few Jungian analysts as well as various therapists covering from group to sex therapies. The diversity of the clinical faculty's expertise is designed to be helpful to residents. However, it could be a potential source of confusion and disintegration in PAP training.

Findings support that PAP training at the SNUH Department of Psychiatry needs significant improvement. It is far from meeting each resident's expectation to obtain quality PAP training and become a psychiatrist with competence in psychotherapy.

In 2014, one resident from my department shockingly failed the board-certification, due to the low score in PAP competency assessment. So, I introduced two solutions into the PAP training. First, quantitatively I maximized residents' exposure to it by opening up my teachings to all the residents, regardless of the PGY class, except the individual supervision sessions. This included book reading (one semester) and group supervisions for PGY-2 and PGY-4 residents (each, one semester). I also encouraged them to attend relevant extra-mural programs available to them. These included lectures, case discussions, and group supervision programs offered domestically by psychotherapeutic/psychoanalytic societies. Second, I chose a practical, manual-style book on PAP (Cabaniss, Cherry, Douglas, & Schwartz, 2011) for book reading and tried to stay away from theory-dominant books. I find it impractical for busy working and least experienced residents to read sophisticated books and papers on PAP. In the book reading and case discussions, I tried to attract their attention to several key concepts of PAP so that they could use them in the diagnostic and therapeutic encounters with patients. Simultaneously, I kept asking them open-ended questions to help them strengthen their capacity to think psychodynamically.

In 2015, one year after the failed resident case, all PGY-4 residents passed the national board-certification and four of them proudly ranked within the top five. Nevertheless, the relief seems to be very temporary, reflecting on the graduating PGY-4 residents' overall dissatisfaction with PAP training and the PGY-2 residents' low interest in psychoanalytic psychiatry, as revealed in this study.

I suppose that currently in Korea as well as in other countries, the relationship of PAP (and psychoanalysis) with University Departments of Psychiatry is facing the challenge of being chosen as a friend or a foe (Kernberg, 2011; Kernberg & Michels, 2016; Wallerstein, 2011). The external reality in Korea regarding the PAP service for patients is not friendly

at all, enforcing an unreasonably low-fee system. Financially and administratively, the healthcare delivery system and insurance system, both under
rigid control by government and health maintenance organizations, do
not and will not encourage residents to maintain sufficient interest in PAP
after graduation. Internally, the PAP training during residency even in my
department, which is considered to be most prestigious, seems to be dysfunctional. And they need significant improvement.

With all the external and internal obstacles to the quality PAP training for residents, it is highly likely that they develop confusion, frustra-
tion, and disappointment, resulting in a lack of confidence. It may lead
to distancing themselves from PAP and developing animosity against it.
Animosity may further spread out to psychoanalysis and psychoanalytic
communities.

What do we do about it then? Here are suggestions:

1   Since the PGY-4 residents consider the individual supervisions as
     most helpful, the training program should increase residents' acces-
     sibility to individual supervisions. Considering the shortage of intra-
     mural supervisors, the training director should encourage them to
     seek supervisions actively from outside resources. It is my strong
     argument that competent psychotherapists/psychoanalysts should
     initially provide supervisions of significant duration for resident psy-
     chotherapists in the beginning stage. In that way, supervisees could
     develop the solid foundation on which their therapeutic experience
     would pile up. The supervisions should offer practical solutions rather
     than teaching complex theories (Shanfield, Matthews, & Hetherly,
     1993). 'Fireman' supervisors should also be available to residents for
     crisis intervention in the psychotherapy process. It would be beneficial
     not only to resident therapists but also to their patients.
2   Book- and paper-readings work much better when they use a 'easy
     and quick' method (Ingram, 2006). Residents are busy, and attendance
     is inconsistent. Unsystematic, incoherent, and irrelevant education is
     the source of confusion, frustration, and possible animosity. Clinical
     vignettes are most helpful for them to understand the psychother-
     apy process. Identification with a competent psychotherapist as well
     as a good clinical case is not only educational but also emotionally
     supportive.
3   The PAP training program is recommended to establish a well-
     functioning patient referral system. First, it is advised to refer rela-
     tively uncomplicated patients ('neurotic,' without serious personality

issues) to the beginning residents, especially considering that once-a-week psychotherapy prevails among them. In that way, confusion might be lessened, and therapeutic confidence might be enhanced. Second, the referral should focus on patients free of psychiatric drugs, solely for PAP other than supplementing drug therapy. In case the referred patient also sees the referring faculty member clinically, there would be distorted working alliance/transference relationships.

4   Residents' experiences regarding supervision vary significantly depending on who the supervisor is, although they view individual supervision as the most valued. A significant number of intra-mural supervisors are neither psychotherapists nor psychoanalysts, while it is not always feasible for residents to obtain supervisions from the extra-mural supervisors because of time limitation and expenses. Minimal attention has been paid to enhance the PAP supervisory competency of the faculty members. My department used to pay careful attention to PAP teaching. However, with the retirements of psychoanalytically oriented professors and the emergence of biological psychiatry, interest in PAP became maximally diluted. Through the years, the number of faculty members with psychodynamic orientation has decreased greatly. Currently, I have reasonable suspicion that the nature of individual supervisions these days may not be sufficiently psychodynamic. I recommend that training hospitals should allocate to residents supervisors who are trained to be psychodynamically informed. To be more successful in training supervisors, a model of "teaching the teachers" could be developed (Riess & Herman, 2008) and they should also be taught on boundary violations (Heru, Strong, Price, & Recupero, 2004).

5   Peer group supervision among residents should be encouraged. It could function as a self-help group, increasing the knowledge/skills and boosting morale. It would be ideal to set up one group per PGY class. The training director is recommended to support the groups by arranging a faculty member to advise the activity.

6   PGY-1 residents' clinical experience is confined to inpatients care in closed and open wards, with the main training focus on psychopharmacology. The program should also provide them with basic training in the psychodynamic formulation and psychotherapeutic skills to be used in their first year of inpatient care. It is very important since inpatient wards are ideal for them to experience and follow up on the effects of psychotherapy. Particularly, open ward inpatient experience should include active PAP application to the inpatients.

Otherwise, they lose the very nurturing opportunity. It appears to be a major mistake in the resident training program of Korea since the PAP requirement begins in the PGY-2 (Korean Neuropsychiatric Association, 2016). The PGY-1 residents are recommended to learn how to think psychotherapeutically early enough in their professional development.

7   Psychoanalytic communities should actively invent feasible measures to attract biological psychiatry-dominant Departments of Psychiatry to recruit a psychoanalyst as a full-time faculty member, without waiting in vain. In this study, almost all the residents agreed to employ the full-time psychoanalyst faculty. However, there are practical issues. One is how to persuade the hospital administrators of its value (including the financial one). The other is how to devise the way for the psychoanalyst faculty to survive and succeed in promotion and acquisition of tenured position. I suggest that the most feasible strategy would be for a psychoanalyst to develop and maintain double specialties. This is true of my professional development, being a sleep medicine specialist as well as a psychoanalyst. And it has worked.

Considering the present and the near future, the political climate in psychiatry appears to be far from becoming friendly and receptive to psychoanalytic psychiatry. In spite of the concern, I suggest that the psychoanalytic community should stop worrying and complaining and focus on making small changes continuously, with the ultimate aim of making friends with more psychiatrists. The strategy is particularly for the residents. Once they become our friends, they would be good candidates for future generations of psychoanalysts.

In various aspects, it is essential and crucial for us to offer residents in psychiatry quality PAP training. It is reassuring that the residents in this study gave the least attribution to the progress of biological psychiatry as an obstacle to PAP training.

The twenty-first century could become a fertile ground for the integration of psychoanalysis with the expanding knowledge of neuroscience. Training emphasis on PAP does not rule out the training on psychopharmacological interventions. Rather, an integrative way of thinking for PAP and psychopharmacology should be promoted (Cabaniss, 1998).

I accept the limitation of this paper. It depended on interview/self-report, and the data was from one particular training program at a university hospital. It only had a small number of participants, not allowing serious statistical analyses. Therefore, the arguments made in this paper need further validation. A future study with expanded design remains to be done. For example, in addition to residents' subjective perception of PAP training, an objective measurement of major PAP skills such as therapeutic alliance (Summers & Barber, 2003) could be adopted to evaluate residents' PAP competency.

Note

1 This paper was partly presented at the IPA Boston 2015 Congress.

References

American Psychiatric Association (2013). *Diagnostic and statistical manual of mental disorders* (5th ed.). Washington, DC: American Psychiatric Association.

Cabaniss, D. L. (1998). Shifting gears: The challenge to teach students to think psychodynamically and psychopharmacologically at the same time. *Psychoanalytic Inquiry*, *18*: 639–656.

Cabaniss, D. L., Cherry, S., Douglas, C. J., & Schwartz, A. R. (2011). *Psychodynamic psychotherapy: A clinical manual*. New York: Wiley.

Goin, M. K. (2006). Teaching psychodynamic psychotherapy in the 21st century. *Journal of the American Academy of Psychoanalysis and Dynamic Psychiatry*, *34*: 117–126.

Heru, A. M., Strong, D. R., Price, M., & Recupero, P. R. (2004). Boundaries in psychotherapy supervision. *American Journal of Psychotherapy*, *58*(1): 76–89.

Ingram, D. H. (2006). Teaching psychodynamic therapy to hardworking psychiatric residents. *Journal of the American Academy of Psychoanalysis and Dynamic Psychiatry*, *34*: 173–188.

Kernberg, O. F. (2011). Psychoanalysis and the university: A difficult relationship. *International Journal of Psychoanalysis*, *92*(3): 609–622.

Kernberg, O. F., & Michels, R. (2016). Thoughts on the present and future of psychoanalytic education. *Journal of the American Psychoanalytic Association*, *64*(3): 477–493.

Korean Neuropsychiatric Association (2016). *Residents Training Program and Curriculum*. Seoul, Republic of Korea: Korean Neuropsychiatric Association.

Mellman, L. A., & Beresin, E. (2003). Psychotherapy competencies: Development and implementation. *Academic Psychiatry*, *27*(3): 149–153.

Riess, H., & Herman, J. B. (2008). Teaching the teachers: a model course for psychodynamic psychotherapy supervisors. *Academic Psychiatry*, *32*(3): 259–264.

Shanfield, S. B., Matthews, K. L., & Hetherly, V. (1993). What do excellent psychotherapy supervisors do? *American Journal of Psychiatry*, *150*: 1081–1084.

Summers, R. F., & Barber, J. P. (2003). Therapeutic alliance as a measurable psychotherapy skill. *Academic Psychiatry*, 27(3): 160–165.

Wallerstein, R. S. (1991). The future of psychotherapy. *Bulletin of the Menninger Clinic*, 55(4): 421–43.

Wallerstein, R. S. (2011). Psychoanalysis in the university: The natural home for education and research. *International Journal of Psychoanalysis*, 92(3): 623–639.

CHAPTER SEVENTEEN

Proving the impact of psychoanalysis on daily psychiatric practice

Structured programs and clinical guidance

Joachim Küchenhoff

Introduction

In the beginning I want to briefly outline my professional background so that the reader might be better able to follow my argument. I am a psychoanalyst, member of the German psychoanalytic association DPV and of the Swiss society of psychoanalysis SGPsa and, thus, member of the IPA. I am a psychiatrist as well and a university lecturer at Basel University. For over 8 years now, I have been the head of a psychiatric institution, the psychiatric in- and outpatient hospital of the Swiss county Baselland. The institution offers a comprehensive psychiatric service for 239 in-patients and around 50 patients at three day hospitals; in addition, there is a huge outpatient department. Previously, I worked full-time as a tenured professor for psychotherapy at Basel University. My motivation to leave the university and to take on the extra responsibility of such a large non-university unit was to find out how far I could go in applying psychoanalysis to ALL sectors of psychiatric care. For the last 20 years, I have also been in charge of the postgraduate teaching for psychiatric residents in the whole area of the north-west of Switzerland, which I have initiated and for which I have – together with many co-workers – developed a curriculum.

In the following paper, as the title suggests, two forms of teaching will be highlighted:

a) the formal teaching for residents and how psychoanalysis can be and should be implemented in it;
b) the informal and everyday (sort of) bedside teaching, the teaching that is implied in a psychoanalysis-based approach to psychiatric patients.

Part 1: Formal teaching

1.1 Training course Psychotherapeutic Basic Tools (PBT)

The PBT is a teaching program for residents at the beginning of their psychiatric career. In psychiatric postgraduate clinical training, residents work directly with patients from the first day onward; in medical school, they have gained a rough knowledge concerning psychiatric disorders generally – or at least they should have. Perhaps, they have had a few courses on doctor–patient relationship. Postgraduate education in Switzerland provides no instruction in specific psychotherapy before the third year of postgraduate training. Prior to that, residents will not have had any specific teaching in psychotherapeutic methods. But they will have to talk to patients although they haven't yet chosen the therapeutic approach they want to specialize in.

The training course on psychotherapeutic basic tools, the PBT, wants to alert residents to the concepts of working in and working with the therapeutic relationship. It is a supra-institutional training course. The participating residents come from psychiatric institutions that are members of the regional board of the network for advanced psychiatric education. Students are being taught in groups of 16–18 residents; there are two trainers in each group. Residents from the same hospital are mostly allotted to different groups. The classes are four hours long and the groups meet for one afternoon each month for a year. The timetable is divided into two parts: first, there is a theoretical input; after a short break, a practical exercise takes place. All residents have to bring a videotape of an interview with a patient, which they have personally led, to the class at least once. The interview should roughly correspond to the theoretical topic that has been introduced in the first part of the session. We have established didactical rules for how best to work with the interviews; at first, all participants watch the video sequence, which should not last too long. Then, alternatives to the interventions, which the presenting resident showed in the video, are deliberated. If the group decides that an alternative interpretation or commentary would have been more appropriate, a role-play will happen next. This allows the participants to get an impression of how the therapist's contribution may shape the interaction positively or negatively. Throughout the year, the participants follow the steps of an imaginary patient through the psychiatric institutions and treatment forms, starting with admission to the hospital, covering suicidal crises, interactions with partner or family of origin, to psychosocial reintegration and other issues. Whenever possible, the same group stays together for the duration of the course, so that residents who work in different institutions can come to know each other, and so that the tutors might be able to use the evolving group dynamics for didactical purposes.

The first three meetings introduce the participants to the concept of the therapeutic relationship including aspects of transference and countertransference. This will be the perspective from which all the steps in the therapy with the imaginary patient are evaluated. And this is also where psychoanalysis comes in, because it is psychoanalysis that allows best to reflect on the therapeutic relationship. In PBT, psychoanalysis is not taught directly, but it is used as an instrument to help the residents take their (countertransferential) affects seriously, to watch the patient carefully and to be open-minded, that is to use one's free floating attention, and in the end to be able to define the unconscious relational patterns connected to the patient's symptomatology. The residents that take part in the training course learn how important it is to reflect on the therapeutic relationship and how helpful psychodynamic concepts can be for becoming aware of the patient's verbal and non-verbal expressions and one's own affective and spontaneous reactions to the patient. Thereby, they learn that psychoanalytic concepts may be helpful for the encounter with a patient in a psychotic crisis or with a patient in an early stage of dementia, that is: in all circumstances of the day-to-day clinical business.

In 2005 and anew in 2009, we have written and edited textbooks that serve as a manual for the training course.[1] They cover all topics that should be treated throughout the course and describe to the tutors how to proceed didactically.

1.2 Operational Psychodynamic Diagnosis (OPD)

The next step towards introducing psychoanalysis into psychiatric care and to teach psychoanalysis to psychiatric residents is training through the OPD system. Operationalized Psychodynamic Diagnosis (OPD) is a multiaxial diagnostic and classification system that is based on psychodynamic principles.[2] It is analogous to those systems that are based on other principles such as DSM-IV and ICD-10. The OPD is based on five axes: I = experience of illness and prerequisites for treatment, II = interpersonal relations, III = conflict, IV = structure, and V = mental and psychosomatic disorders (in line with Chapter V (F) of the ICD-10). After an initial interview that lasts 1–2 hours, the clinician (or researcher) can evaluate the patient's psychodynamics according to these axes and enter them in the checklists and evaluation forms provided. The OPD-2 has been further developed from a purely diagnostic system into a system that includes a set of tools and procedures for treatment planning and for measuring change. It can be used to determine the appropriate main focuses of treatment and develop appropriate treatment strategies as well.

OPD is very useful for teaching psychodynamic principles to a resident. What he or she will find there is a complex but well-defined set of psychodynamic terms that have been found to be reliable and valid. Even though the majority of the terms are truly psychodynamic, they are operationalized, that is: made manageable for the beginner who is not – as yet – trained in psychoanalysis. The young doctor is well acquainted with operationalized diagnostic criteria; the methodology in which the OPD system proceeds is thus familiar to him or her. This makes it easier for him or her to access and then accept the system.

OPD is taught in specialized training seminars that have a specific structure, and all training centers exert identical standards. Compared to the PBT, OPD is far more advanced in psychodynamics; that is the reason OPD can serve as a second step. In my psychiatric center, I offer OPD seminars every six months; in between, small groups meet regularly under the supervision of an external OPD expert to discuss clinical cases through an OPD perspective.

All psychodynamic diagnostics have a severe disadvantage: they need time – and time is money when psychiatric hospitals are confronted with significant budgetary and monetary cuts – as they are in Switzerland and Germany. Hence, there might not be enough time in clinical practice for including these diagnostics, and using OPD might interfere with the necessities and pressures of daily practice in psychiatry, especially in acute situations. That is the reason we have tried to find a formula allowing OPD to be implemented step-by-step together with a group of OPD co-workers.[3] In many occasions, the resident might not need the whole array of diagnostic tools. On admission of a patient to the hospital, for instance, only axis I (one) might be needed. With the help of axis I, the resident can explore the accessibility of the patient to psychodynamic treatment, find out about the patient's therapeutic preferences and his or her personal illness concept and decide how to proceed with psychodynamic diagnostics. In other circumstances, it might be best to apply the axis IV structural diagnosis in order to define prominent structural deficiencies. This allows for an early intervention to help the patient improve their affect intolerance or control of impulses.

Part 2: Informal Training

So far, structured and formalized training tools have been highlighted. They are important, but they are not exhaustive. The vivid routine of integrating a psychodynamic approach into daily business is the most important. It is only then that psychodynamics are "normalized" and really a part of the psychiatric education. A few examples for how this integration can be achieved will now be presented.

2.1 Conjoint Therapy Planning

Most inpatient treatments are short-term therapies. The patients will stay in the hospital for no longer than a few weeks. It is thus advisable to limit the therapeutic aims and focus on the most urgent issues. These include psychopharmacological care, social rehabilitation, organization of after-care etc. From a psychodynamic point of view, the formulation of a focus can be helpful for defining and delineating the main psychotherapeutic aims. The focus serves as an integrating formula that links the different therapeutic approaches by defining a common and shared central aspect; as a result, the focus enables coordination of the team's work. What is needed then is a team conference on the patient's ward with all members of the staff where they can communicate the results of their individual assessments. These results can then be evaluated and, finally, used to attain a focus formulation that summarizes the patient's main object relations and their conflictual or structural concerns and helps to find the appropriate therapeutic approach.[4] Again, the OPD system may serve as a conceptual background for the focus formulation, but other psychodynamic approaches may be just as useful. Thus, the residents and the other team members become aware of the advantages of a psychodynamic approach: it guides them to a conjoint therapeutic team process; it helps them to better understand the patient's object relations, to define the central conflict or the personality organization of the patient, and to use the diagnostics as a starting point for the appropriate and fitting therapeutic measures.

Thus, using the psychoanalytic approach as an integrating formula is useful for a therapeutic team in conjoint therapy planning; but the integrative potential of psychoanalytic reasoning as an overarching framework can be used on a wider scale throughout the psychiatric institution. Staff members do have to apply all sorts of different therapeutic approaches every day; they need a binding framework holding them together, and psychoanalytic reasoning is well suited to provide it. It is only then that – to give an example – psychopharmacological treatment and psychotherapy are brought together; instead of applying drugs and psychotherapy side by side without mutual interference, a "psychodynamic psychopharmacology" allows to reflect the chances, limitations and adverse side effects of drug treatment in terms of the patient's subjective experience, to define the impact on the patient's personality and to decide whether this impact is helpful or detrimental here and now and thus to define specific pharmacological targets on psychodynamic terms.[5] If the resident who has been educated in narrow scientific and neurobiological terms has the chance to realize that pharmacological treatment improves by being integrated into a psychodynamic frame he or she may soon become interested in psychoanalysis.

2.2 Crisis conference

In the psychiatric hospital of which I am in charge, we have introduced a special conference in urgent crises, which we call "crisis conference." All partners involved in the inpatient's therapy are entitled to call for such a crisis conference. The conference must be established within 48 hours and it includes the resident, the senior psychiatrist, the consultant, members of the nursing team, the physiotherapist, maybe the sports therapist – whoever was involved in the patient's treatment. As the clinical director, I take part as well and chair the conference. The crisis conference is convened only in moments of a real crisis and imminent danger. Typical triggers are a permanent suicidal proneness that interferes with dismissal from the hospital, a homicide threat, an elderly patient's wish to be let go and allowed to die etc. In most instances, the team already knows the solution to their problem; they merely need someone to help straighten out their ideas, to contain their fears and countertransference blockades and to support their therapeutic plans emotionally but also legally – thus, they need help to establish or re-establish a symbolic order that was threatened to be disturbed by the patient's psychic disorder. I wouldn't be able to lead the crisis conference without my psychoanalytic abilities – by letting the members of the crisis conference take part in my psychodynamically guided considerations, I can serve as a teacher and therefore as a role model and a good guide to psychoanalysis.

2.3 Supervision of the team and of the institution as a whole

The best training in psychoanalysis for the resident is to sense – as it were – a psychodynamic atmosphere within the institution, to feel that the personal resonance, the affects in the therapist, the conflicts between members of the staff etc. all are seen as potentially relevant to the therapeutic outcome. To learn that these factors are not discarded as merely disturbing or private, but that they are taken in earnest so that time and money can be invested into the working-out of countertransference reactions either on an individual or on a team level, to understand mirroring phenomena where conflicts of the severely disturbed patient are projected onto the team members, to reflect on a team's working ability, e.g. on the formation of "basic assumptions" in the team due to institutional problems.

If psychoanalysis is allowed so far into the institution, there will have to be psychodynamic supervisions that can work with the dynamic factors mentioned above. This means that the teams need a psychodynamically trained supervisor who is able to work with the affective processes during therapies and in the team. Even as a unit, the institution itself may be submitted to an institutional supervision on a psychoanalytic basis – for many years, we had a group analyst and institutional counselor who came once every semester to moderate large groups consisting of all levels of the institutional hierarchy. Thus, in the end, the resident notices that psychoanalysis may be at the center of a psychiatric institution.

Concluding remarks

Instead of presenting a summary of the present paper, 12 rules for teaching psychoanalysis to psychiatric residents will be presented. These rules might sound basic and naïve at first; but I don't think they are – they help prevent mistakes in introducing psychoanalysis in psychiatric care:

1 Don't take too much for granted concerning residents' knowledge and experience – they have much less experience and knowledge than you might think!

2   Don't be too theoretical!

3   Don't expect that residents will greet quotations from Freud texts (or other psychoanalytic authors) with awe just because you think they are tremendous!

4   Don't try to lead residents to a new (and somewhat remote) area of psychiatry they are not acquainted with; rather help them to explore their own field of work and start from there!

5   Be useful for residents! Show them how useful psychoanalysis can be for solving their daily clinical problems.

6   Provide a "transitional supervisory space" from the start and encourage the trainees to present their cases with all affects and conflicts.

7   Don't devaluate the common psychiatric forms of treatment – and don't introduce psychoanalysis as a (superior) alternative! Rather connect your psychoanalytic approach with the usual psychiatric procedures!

8   Be – on the other hand – explicit in stating that you are convinced that psychoanalysis should not confine itself to the psychoanalytic cure proper but is very useful for application in psychiatry.

9   Let the residents have an idea about your therapeutic practice – show them self-made videos, let them be present when you interview patients.

10 Be careful in choosing your didactical approach; be modern, use modern media; let them participate actively!

11 Be credible by allowing psychoanalytic reasoning into all levels of the institution, including organizational matters. Don't relegate psychodynamics to a small and well fenced-off area but let it be an important factor throughout the entire organization.

12 Try to find psychoanalysts who are ready to serve as senior psychiatrists, consultants, clinical directors – this is the most difficult thing to do, in my experience: there are still not enough psychoanalysts ready to devote themselves to psychiatric care. But you'll never be able to establish psychoanalysis alone, you need a team!

Notes

1 Küchenhoff, Joachim, & Mahrer Klemperer, Regine (2009). *Psychotherapy in psychiatric daily care* [book in German]. Stuttgart: Schattauer.

2 OPD Task Force (Ed.) (2008). *Operationalized Psychodynamic Diagnosis OPD-2. Manual of diagnosis and treatment planning.* Cambridge, MA: Hogrefe & Huber.

3 Sammet, I., Himmighoffen, H., Brücker, J., Dreher, C., Olshausen Küchenhoff, C., Wilmers, F., Wolf, A., Zell, P., & Küchenhoff, J. (2012). OPD in the hospital: An algorithm for structuring the diagnostic process with the Operationalized Psychodynamic Diagnostics OPD-2. [Article in German]. *Zentralblatt für Psychosomatische Medizin und Psycotherapie, 58*(3): 282–298.

4 Küchenhoff, Joachim (2004) *Psychodynamic short term and focal psychotherapy* [book in German]. Stuttgart: Schattauer.

5 Küchenhoff, Joachim (Ed.) (2016) *Psychoanalysis and psychopharmacology* [book in german; in press]. Stuttgart: Kohlhammer.

CHAPTER EIGHTEEN

The white bicycle
How could general psychiatry benefit from psychoanalytic theories and practice?[1]

Levent Küey

Diagnosis and treatment in general psychiatry, as a formulation and as a joint reconstruction process between the clinician and the patient, is an ongoing process in clinical care. Accordingly, a twofold task is faced. On one hand, the clinician is in need of making a comprehensive diagnostic assessment to construct a valid and working formulation of the patient's situation and a treatment plan, and on the other hand, a solid ground for a psychotherapeutic alliance should be established.

Besides being one of the essential paradigms in psychiatry, the theory and practice of psychoanalysis offer remarkable contributions to the clinician in managing these tasks. Understanding the meaning of human suffering through empathy in a judgement-free milieu is essential in the establishment of rapport, compliance and for a better clinical outcome. Basic concepts of psychoanalysis, with particular attention to intrapsychic and interpersonal conflicts and the related psychodynamically oriented psychotherapeutic skills could be useful for psychiatrists and mental health professionals in various clinical settings, especially in an era of dehumanizing algorithmic diagnostic and treatment approaches.

In this chapter, the author revisits the possible contributions of psychoanalysis to general psychiatry, on the basis of his experience and relevant literature. In fact, all through this chapter questions as, "How could a general psychiatrist benefit from psychoanalytic theories and practice? What could a general psychiatrist expect from psychoanalytic theories and practice?" are kept at the back of the author's mind and are intended to be discussed. "The white bicycle", a brief vignette from the authors' clinical practice, will be presented to broaden the scope of discussion.

The clinical encounter in general psychiatry

Whatever the theoretical orientation of the psychiatrist is, the clinical encounter, where the clinician and the person seeking help meets, has some commonalities.

First, the relation between the clinician and the person is a human interpersonal interaction built by the demand of the patient with a specific reason, i.e., to diminish the suffering of the person. It is mainly a verbal and nonverbal communication relying on the impact of exchange of words and signs or behaviour. Clinician–patient communication during the clinical encounter is a multifaceted process. From a psychoanalytic point of view, the psychiatrist and the patient, besides interacting as two real persons, are also both acting and reacting to Each Other via the *imagined* and *internalized* Other. This creates *a virtual reality* right in the consulting room. On both sides, there is not only *one self*, but also *a perceived* and *an expressed self*. The interview room hosts a small group of real and virtual people, in this sense (Küey, 2013).

Second, in all clinical encounters, the person is consulting due to some emotional pain and suffering which he/she is experiencing. This experience and the expression of it by the person lead to a perception and experience in the clinician. The expression of the person and the impression and interpretation formed in the psyche of the clinician, together, built up the dynamics of this joint, ongoing interpersonal human interaction. Through this relation, i.e., a therapeutic process of restoration and reconstruction in the psyche of the person, it is expected that the person overcomes or decreases his/her suffering with the help of the clinician. Using the marathon as an analogy, and as the marathon runner novelist Murakami (Murakami, 2008) indicated,

> Pain is inevitable. Suffering is optional. Say you're running and you start to think, *Man this hurts, I can't take it anymore.* The *hurt* part is an unavoidable reality, but whether or not you can stand any more is up to the runner himself.

The therapeutic process aims to acknowledge and accept the pain caused by the various unavoidable human conditions in our life marathon (e.g., aging gradually every year, loosing beloved ones, or reality of mortality) and comfort and restore the integrity of the person working through and transforming suffering or at least living tolerably (Bolognini, 2006) with it (e.g., tolerating life stages, mourning the loss of a significant other).

A third common feature in all clinical encounters is the question in the mind of the clinician: How can I collaborate with this person to reduce his/her suffering and to reconstruct his/her integrity? At this point, we could emphasis that the theoretical orientation of the clinician will shape and accompany this process and set the context and the therapeutic techniques used.

Current practice of general psychiatry

A brief critical review of the current paradigms and practice of general clinical psychiatry and residency training programmes shows that it is profoundly shaped by the descriptive biological paradigms. This means the medical approach is the prevailing practice and there is little, if any, space for psychotherapies. The conventional medical approach works in three steps: diagnosis, explanation and treatment.

The descriptive diagnostic step is based on the widely used so-called atheoretical, pragmatic categorical classification systems. Although these systems helped to raise the reliability of clinical diagnosis to a certain extent, they ignore the intra-category heterogeneity, and the uniqueness of the person seeking help is offered as a sacrifice to the spirits of diagnostic categories. The assessment of the aetiology is done in the context of *explanation* not *understanding* and focuses on the biological variables and to some recent life events, at best. The richness of the theories of developmental psychopathology and psychiatry is ignored and reduced to cross-sectional assessments. Intervention and treatment is usually undertaken according to the evidence based practice guidelines and prescribing medications. The time strain that the clinicians face in many outpatient departments across the world reinforces this cross-sectional, reductionist medical exercise in the general practice of psychiatry.

We were warned by Weich and Aray (2004) a decade ago, "We may now be at the limits of what this approach of categorical systems of phenotypic classification is capable of achieving". Furthermore, Cloninger (1999) stated that "there is no empirical evidence" for "natural boundaries between major syndromes", that "no one has ever found a set of symptoms, signs, or tests that separate mental disorders fully into non-overlapping categories", and that "the categorical approach . . . is fundamentally flawed".

In fact, diagnosis and treatment in psychiatry, as a formulation and as a joint reconstruction process between the clinician and the patient, is an essential step in clinical care. Accordingly, a twofold task is faced. On one hand, the clinician is in need of making a comprehensive diagnostic assessment to construct a valid and working formulation of the patient's situation and a treatment plan, and on the other hand, a solid ground for a therapeutic alliance should be established. Whatever the treatment is, psychotherapy or pharmacotherapy or a combination of both, the establishment of the therapeutic alliance at first contact or interview is an essential priority as a starter.

As far as the current treatments are concerned in general practice of psychiatry a meta-analysis of randomized trials in which the effects of treatment with antidepressant medication were compared to the effects of combined pharmacotherapy and psychotherapy in adults with a diagnosed depressive or anxiety disorder will be mentioned here. This study has shown sufficient evidence that combined treatment is superior for major depression, panic disorder, and obsessive-compulsive disorder. The results also suggested that the effects of pharmacotherapy and those of psychotherapy are largely independent from each other, with both contributing about equally to the effects of combined treatment. It is concluded that combined treatment appears to be more effective than treatment with antidepressant medication alone. Additionally, these effects remained strong and significant up to two years after treatment. Briefly, this study highlighted that monotherapy with psychotropic medication may not constitute the optimal evidence based treatment for common mental disorders (Cuijpers et al., 2014).

Despite such strong evidences, an investigation of recent trends in the use of outpatient psychotherapy in the general population have revealed that, during the decade from 1998 to 2007 psychotherapy assumed a less prominent role in outpatient mental health care as a large and increasing proportion of mental health outpatients received psychotropic medication without psychotherapy (Olfson and Marcus 2010).

The practice of general psychiatry needs the contributions of psychoanalytic/psychodynamic theory and practice in improving it towards a more human based good clinical practice. We could mention some of the major contributions in this regard: on integrating psychodynamic psychiatry in the mainstream of general clinical practice in psychiatry (Schwartz et al., 1995), on integrating psychoanalytic conceptual and practical tools into clinical interview, into the work of the mental health team, and psychiatric inpatient treatment (Quartier, 2004; Quartier & Bartolomei, 2013);

on the psychological aspects of pharmacologic treatments from a psycho-analytic perspective (Busch & Sandberg, 2007); on integrating new neuro-scientific evidences with psychodynamic understanding so that clinicians can reach a real formulation of a bio-psychosocial approach in clinical practice (Gabbard, 2014) are current challenges. Also work on the poten-tials of what psychodynamic psychotherapy could offer clinicians in creat-ing new ways of practising in order to improve the quality of lives of their patients via a more comprehensive listening, reflecting and intervening (Cabaniss et al., 2011) and on how essential therapeutic principles could be incorporated into clinically relevant patient management (Bienenfeld, 2005) are some other studies of relevant importance. Furthermore, the current marginalization of psychodynamic work within the mental health field could be tackled with conducting empirical research. As emphasized by Levy and Ablon (2009), sound empirical research has the potential to affirm the important role that psychodynamic theory and treatment have in current psychiatry and psychology.

Nevertheless, the crucial question deserves to be elaborated further: How could psychoanalytic/psychodynamic theories and practice contrib-ute to the practice of general psychiatry?

Possible contributions of psychoanalytic/psychodynamic theories and practice to general psychiatry

Just because people ask you for something doesn't mean that that's what they really want you to give them

Lacan

In general clinical practice, from an epistemological point of view, the clinicians should be aware of that they can never be *objective observers*, since they are not free of their own observations. Hence, *the reality of the patient* is not independent from the conceptual and emotional constructs of the clinician (Jaspers, 1913[1997]). The *subjectivity of the clinician* is a part of the clinical work to be taken into consideration and managed by the clinician.

Besides evaluating the transference issues of the person, the clinician should also implement an insight oriented perspective to see his/her own feelings, reflections and countertransference issues. It is stated that the concept of countertransference has evolved and gained central impor-tance in current psychoanalytic theory and practice (Michels et al., 2002).

The *subjectivities of the person and the clinician* are to be taken as *the objective evidences emerged at the clinical setting*. In understanding and managing this complex process the clinician could use the theoretical and practical tools of psychoanalysis. Let us review some possibilities on such contributions at different levels of the clinical work step by step.

Interview and establishment of the rapport

Clinical encounter is a specific human encounter built by the demand and for the benefit of the person seeking help and this interaction is based on the communication between the two. The principles and dynamics of verbal and non-verbal communication (Küey, 2013) sets the context and framework of the interview. Psychiatric interview is shaped on principles of psychoanalytic psychotherapy, with special emphasis on empathy that requires a balance between fusion and separateness (Bolognini, 2004), and not only on what is expressed but also not expressed or latently or distortedly expressed and on non-verbal cues. A systematic way for listening, reflecting on what is heard and observed, and making choices about how and what to say during the interview are essential contributions of the psychodynamic theory (Cabannis, 2011).

Respect to the *suffering* and *subjectivity* of the person is a priority in establishing the rapport. A non-judgemental, containing, humane attitude is a must: not *objectifying* the person as a mere victim of psychopathology but *subjectifying* the person as an active co-agent of the development of psychopathology; besides, not *passivation* of the person as a mere *receiver* of treatment but *activation* of the person as an effective co-agent of the therapeutic relation and intervention.

Description of the problems, patterns and diagnosis

A detailed description of the current problems that lead the person to seek help at that time of his/her life, and of the behavioural and emotional patterns, is the first step in working with the complexity of diagnostic process in general psychiatry. This description also includes not only what is *said* but also what is *expressed* during the interview; behaviours (especially the non-verbal cues) and attitudes of the person at the clinical setting and towards the clinician are attentively recorded. The repetitive patterns of behaviour either expressed in the therapy office, or during daily life, or over a lifetime are searched as important gateways to develop further insight.

Clinical practice in psychiatry takes place in the context of language. Language is a means of expression and verbalization on one hand and reciprocally, a means for reconstructing the clinical practice, i.e., psyche of the patient. Language shapes the clinical practice and is shaped by it. In other words, the discourse of the patient not only reflects his/her intrapsychic reality but also reconstructs it. Paying attention to this interactional character of the discourse of the person opens the doors to further understanding. Diagnosis is not a mere categorization, made by the clinician, of putting symptoms into various clusters but is a joint, ongoing reconstruction process.

Diagnostic categories are not the reality itself but human made conceptual constructs to be used in helping the clinician to understand the internal reality of the person. Consequently, respect for the uniqueness of the person becomes a priority in describing the current problems and symptoms.

Reviewing the developmental history and rewriting
the unique life story of the patient

One of the major contributions of psychoanalysis is the emphasis on using the theories to find out causative links between the current problems and the past. It is not listing a chronology of life events but searching the developmental story for the *conflicts*, *knots* and *traumas*, covering prenatal development, the first years of life, early relationships, childhood, adolescence and adulthood periods. This approach gives the clinician the opportunity of evaluating the situation not only in a cross-sectional manner, but also in its historical and longitudinal context. Besides, it sets the basis for forming working hypotheses about what is happening now, and what might happen in the future. Understanding which patterns are resisting, which are remaining, which are fading, and which are emerging is possible via a historical psychodynamic perspective. The meanings of the patterns and symptoms in the person's concrete life story and emotional attributions and transferences could be questioned and revealed where possible.

Reconstructing and rewriting the unique life and illness story of the patient, compared to taking a mere cross-sectional snapshot, helps the clinician to integrate the disease perspective with a life story perspective. Such an approach constructs the ground for not only assessing the present and the past but also for developing hypotheses about the possibilities of the future.

Formulation

An often neglected exercise in general practice of psychiatry is making a comprehensive and integrative formulation (Sperry et al., 1992). Such a formulation assists the clinician to find the best ways in helping the person and includes the biological, socio-cultural and cognitive–behavioural perspectives, where the psychodynamic perspective should be an essential part. The formulation includes the hypotheses of the clinician which cannot be proven directly. These working hypotheses based on the clinical facts, are generated to help the clinician through the clinical work and are tested, disregarded, confirmed or replaced with alternative ones.

A psychodynamic formulation embraces the early cognitive and emotional difficulties, ego and ego functions, the drives, unconscious and subconscious elements of conflicts and defence mechanisms, object relations along with interpersonal dynamics, issues of self and existence and attachment styles. Besides, problems with self-esteem, relationships with others, characteristic ways of adapting (Cabannis et al., 2013) are covered in a psychodynamic formulation.

Another essential part of a comprehensive formulation includes the strengths of the person, e.g., more adaptive ego functions and more mature defence mechanisms, conscious coping styles and psychosocial support systems.

A differential feature of a psychodynamic formulation is the focus on how the person thinks, feels and behaves considering the impact and development of unconscious thoughts and feelings. Constructing a psychodynamic formulation is not only necessary for short- or long-term psychotherapy but also for psychopharmacologic treatment alone (Cabannis et al., 2013). Evaluating the attitudes of the patient towards medication is a first step in such a formulation. When undertaking psychopharmacologic treatment, information about some pre-existing opinions, feelings and attributions of the patient about medication should be revealed (Cabannis et al., 2013). In line with this information, the styles of management and adaptation of the patient to stress are invaluable for psychopharmacological treatment. Medication may have specific meanings for patients which need to be included in such a formulation. These meanings attributed to medication may include a variety of relevant clinical material. The patient may attribute the prescription of medication to a biological causation of his/her problems; to a deficiency in his/her self-esteem or failure of resilience that needs to be supported by an external agent (i.e., medication); similarly, to an external control over his/her body and free will (Busch &

Auchincloss, 1995), or to problems with basic trust and dependency. The psychodynamic formulation in the service of a pharmacologic treatment enables the clinician to predict and manage the reactions of the patient to this treatment in the context of his/her patterns of object relations, i.e., relating to self and others.

Formulation is not a *fait accompli* or *done-and-all-done* type of exercise; it is an ongoing process. Re-formulation wherever *new–old* material arises, or re-formulation wherever *new–new* material arises or re-formulation regarding the treatment responses become a necessity to keep up with the dynamic nature of the clinical work.

Besides, self-formulation of the patient should be an integrative part of a comprehensive formulation. The person's answers to questions as, "What are his/her own explanations and interpretations of the situation? What are his/her emotional and cognitive attributions to the problems and patterns? What are his/her preferences and hypotheses in terms of intervention/treatment?" must be incorporated in the formulation.

The interventions and treatment

The clinician, after describing the current patterns and understanding the developmental and historical links, aims to set specific treatment goals, choose therapeutic strategies, construct meaningful interventions and conduct the process. Psychoanalytic/psychodynamic therapy provides a solid ground to the essentials for beginning the treatment, including fostering the therapeutic alliance, setting the frame and setting goals. Furthermore, whatever the treatment chosen and agreed by the clinician and the patient is, either psychotherapy or pharmacotherapy alone, or a combination of both, the assets of a broader range of insight oriented psychotherapeutic interventions have many new routes to offer the clinicians.

The intervention and treatment plans should not be built merely on the treatment algorithms developed for diagnostic categories but on the unique life story of that specific individual.

The current practice of general psychiatry is traumatized with a reductionist approach where *the patient complains, the clinician diagnoses and treats, and the patient drops out*! Indeed, reductionist practice in general psychiatry decreases the compliance rates. As an example, in the course of treatment with antidepressants, between 30% and 60% of patients do not take their medications as prescribed, hence non-adherence to antidepressant medication is a significant clinical issue in the management of many patients with depressive disorders (Demyttenaere, 1997; Demyttenaere & Haddad, 2000). Among the reasons for patient non-compliance, along with the side effects and stigma and attitudes toward drugs, another important factor is the patient–doctor communication failure (Johnson, 1981); i.e., a relation focused on *explaining* rather than *understanding*. This problem shows the need for transforming the clinical work, covering diagnostic assessment, formulation and treatment, to a collaborative, joint, ongoing, reconstruction process, by incorporating the contributions of psychoanalytic/psychodynamic theories and psychotherapeutic tools into the general practice of psychiatry.

As a conclusion, the theory and practice of psychoanalysis, besides being one of the essential paradigms in psychiatry, offer remarkable contributions to the clinician in managing the clinical work. Understanding the meaning of the human pain and suffering through empathy in a judgement-free milieu is essential in the establishment of rapport, and for a better compliance and clinical outcome. Basic concepts of psychoanalysis, with particular attention to intrapsychic and interpersonal conflicts, and to the potential of enabling the clinician and the patient "to distinguish more clearly internal reality from external reality, and the past from the present, thereby minimizing the confusion and the transfer-interferences in our contact with the world" (Bolognini, 2013), and the related psychodynamic oriented psychotherapeutic skills could be useful for mental health professionals in various clinical settings, especially in an era dominated by dehumanizing algorithmic diagnostic and treatment approaches.

At this point, a brief vignette from my clinical practice, 'the white bicycle', will be presented to broaden the scope of discussion.

The white bicycle

Time, place, context

It was early autumn of 1996; after the summer holidays and just before the fall term of the school starts. A clear day, in İzmir (Symrna), on the Aegean coast of Anatolia; time for late summer sun and the early chilly evenings of the Mediterranean climate. İzmir does not only have a soft climate but also a relaxing psycho-social life and milieu and is considered as the most *Westernized* city of Turkey, welcoming vast immigration for the last two centuries (Küey, 2014).

The person seeking help

A lady of 38 dropped herself into the chair of a psychiatric consultation room of an outpatient department of a general hospital, certainly not offering an intimate milieu. Consultation rooms of different medical branches, including psychiatry, located side by side along a long corridor. People seeking help would come to a general registration desk, ask for a place in a line and wait in the hall until called to enter the psychiatrist's office.

She came as the first afternoon patient and was complaining of "total sleeplessness" and asking for "a strong medication". The clinician's first impression confirmed the complaint; she really looked as if she had not slept at all; with full red eyes circled with dark shadows, along with a deep, sad expression, as if frozen on her face since time immemorial.

She is an elementary school teacher, and has been married to a man of the same profession for 14 years. They had migrated to İzmir, from the far Eastern Anatolian city of Kars, two months ago. Kars is one of the cities with the most migration in the country, described by Pamuk (2000) as: "It wasn't the poverty or the helplessness that disturbed him (in Kars); it was the thing he would see again and again during the days to come in", "These sights spoke of a strange and powerful loneliness. It was as if he were in a place that the whole world had forgotten, as if it were snowing at the end of the world."

In early July, a month after the spring term was finished, they happily moved to İzmir, with their 12-year-old daughter. In fact, they had been hoping to make this move for the last couple of years. Just the day after they had moved to İzmir, the daughter and the father went to buy a bicycle for her. The parents had promised this as a gift for her graduation from elementary school, 5th grade. Actually, she had graduated two months ago, while they were still living in Kars, but she had to wait for a white bicycle until they had moved to İzmir. The parents had thought that it would not be socially acceptable for the young daughter of teachers to be running around on a bicycle in that small conservative community. Most of the families of the girls of that age were arranging marriages for their daughters in the region. So, she was very much looking forward to moving to İzmir and her freedom to ride a most highly desired white bicycle; this time, not only in her dreams but also in her daily life!

The clinician

In this nice weather, during the lunch break, the clinician, aged 36, went out for a light lunch, with his close friend, a neurosurgeon. While, they were enjoying their after-lunch coffees and playing backgammon, they were also chatting about their summer holidays and beloved daughters and sharing the challenges of fatherhood.

The daughter of the neurosurgeon, aged 7, had nocturnal enuresis, and the clinician was helping her to overcome this problem; now, the fathers were discussing what could be the proper parental attitudes and behaviour in this situation. The neurosurgeon also revealed his own problems of enuresis in his childhood, and his parents' threats of planting him on the toilet all night long. Issues of trans-generational transmission went far beyond the end of the backgammon game.

On the other hand, the clinician's daughter, aged 3, had also some health problems lately. She had an infection of the upper respiratory tract a couple of weeks ago, with a high fever. She developed a febrile convulsion, while her father was trying to cool her down under the shower, in the middle of the night. It was a really hard and traumatizing time for both of them.

After the convulsion was over, her father took her to the hospital and with his fellow neurosurgeon they both did their best to help her compassionately. When taken back home that evening, she was feeling better and slept peacefully at first. But, her body temperature was fluctuating and the parents followed up and continued cooling her in case of need, in rotations, all through the night.

During that long day and night, at one break, the father had a chance at last to hide himself in a room for a while, where he welcomed his tears and cried. His sorrow and tears made him recollect an old childhood memory.

He was around six, by then, and just after a febrile sickness of about a week, his father had gifted him with a red football. He was allowed to go out to play with friends on the streets, happily again. He had missed kicking a ball for so long! One hard kick made the ball fly over the backyard wall of a house nearby and the kids started screaming for the ball to be thrown back. The wall was too high for the kids to see the inside the garden. They shouted at the top of their voices: "We want our ball back, please throw it back!"

After a while, which felt like a year for the kids, someone started shouting from behind the wall.

It was the angry voice of the neighbour: "Didn't I tell you not to play in front of my house, you are making so much noise, I am tired of you. Here is your ball, get your ball and your ass out of here. Go to hell!" Yes, the ball was thrown back, but with a big knife cut on it.

The kid, later to become the clinician, gave a hug to the torn ball and ran to his 'hell'. Entering home and without saying a word to anyone, he found a room for himself under the sofa to cry and welcome his tears. Yes, the later clinician remembered this memory of his red ball while struggling to help his daughter with her fever.

Well, in a week, the daughter recovered and the clinician also; but, of course, with the painful prints of this experience in their own emotional library archives, written on the clay tablets where experiences of loss and threats of loss were imprinted.

Back to the clinical setting and encounter

The lady put her documents on the clinician's desk and with an angry voice, and exclaimed:

"I cannot sleep at all, I want sleeping pills."

First words of the clinician, rather spontaneously, came out to be as,

"What happened, did you lose your sleep?"

Her answer was striking:

"NO, NO, I did not LOSE anything, I want to sleep, give me MY pills."

After a short hesitation, the clinician asked, "YOUR pills?"
A tough confused rejection came from her again:

"NO, NO . . . but yes. I want pills! I meant a strong medication to make me sleep forever!"
"Well, OK, I will certainly help you to restore your sleep. But, please tell me, what is this 'MY pills' issue?" insisted the clinician.

The lady went into an outbreak and crying out, shouted:

"I want MY daughter back!"

During the interview, in due course, it is revealed that, three weeks ago, her daughter while riding her bicycle near their home, was hit and killed by a car, the driver of which was an unlicensed young boy!

The clinician hardly managed to remain focused and carried on the interview. She was in tears while giving the details of their long awaited dream of moving to İzmir, and her daughter's desire for a white bicycle. At the same time, she was experiencing and expressing her absolute disbelief in what had happened. "What was my sin to deserve this punishment!" she frequently proclaimed without asking for a reply. Eventually, they were able to reach a compromise – that she would come to see the clinician again the next day. The clinician, quite contrary to his usual practice in bereavement situations, also advised her to take 10 mg of Amitriptiline, at nights.

While, he was writing down the prescription and explaining the effects/side effects of the medication, she interrupted with a shy low tone of voice:

"What colour are these pills?"
"White"
"Good, I will take them . . ."

After the patient had left, the clinician locked the door, took a deep breath and, holding his head in his hands, let his tears pour forth, crying out all his emotional pain, re-reading and reconstructing his clay tablets of suffering once more, where experiences and traces of loss and threats of loss had been imprinted.

This case vignette, summarizing a consultation in a crisis situation very briefly, also emphasizes the complexities of emotional interactions of the clinician with their patients. Moreover, the importance of paying attention to the emotional experiences, not only the patient's but also one's own, and how to become more attuned to one's own experience of a patient (Maroda, 2012), is elaborated.

The person expressed her need in an indirect and concealed way: talking about 'a loss'; not the loss of her daughter but her sleep. The clinician's mind, on the other hand, was full of the issues of parenthood and the health problems of his and his friend's daughter. Triggered by these fearful phantasies of loss in his internal reality and his observation of her sad looking funereal gaze, he made an exclamation as, "did you lose your sleep?" instead of asking, "what kind of sleep problems do you have?", as he would usually do. He had partially passed over the conventional discourse of a medical interview, revealing some of his own subconscious. This made the internal realities of both get in contact. The clinical encounter became a setting where both met not only the Other but also Each Other. This link between the internal realities of both, even very fragile at the beginning, set the basis for a therapeutic alliance. A genuine channel for a humane touching of two psyches became possible.

Promising some medication (but not sleeping pills) was kind of a reward presented to the person. The *meaning* of reward for her was to be revealed in the due course of the treatment, which lasted about two years with sessions once every two/three weeks. A process of bereavement and mourning was complicated by deep depression and her personal history. She had struggled all through her life, aiming at independent personal, economic and social well-being; becoming a teacher; marrying a well-respected colleague; educating children of low economic classes (similar to her family origins) were her major life tasks and accomplishments. Her heartfelt desire of migrating to İzmir was meant to be the concrete reward for her life struggle, comforting sufferings of the past. The meaning attributed to migration turned into a deep tragedy instead of a reward. Her profound self-guilt, leading to clinical depression soon after the first stroke had passed, was accessible in this context.

Another important point deserving to be emphasized in this vignette is the strong rejection of the patient when questioned about any loss. Only knowing the basics of psychoanalytic concepts and defence mechanisms (e.g., reaction formation) could help the clinician to see the *yes* in a *no*; i.e., which "no" means in fact a "yes".

Although there are various psychoanalytic oriented psychodynamic schools and therapies, some core common issues that may be relevant to any daily clinical practice of psychiatry and mental health and also general medicine needs further elaboration.

Conclusions

In search of a remedy for my malady I realized, the malady itself was the real remedy for me.

In search of an evidence for myself I realized, my ownself was an evidence for me.

Mısri (1618–1694)

Not only does the praxis of general psychiatry but also that of general medicine and the training of psychiatry residents and medical students need to be enriched by the contributions of psychoanalytic/psychodynamic theories. Why?

First, multi-morbidity of physical and mental disorders seems a rule rather than an exception (Goodell et al., 2011). A significant portion of the adult population has co-occurring physical and mental disorders. In the 2003 National Comorbidity Survey Replication (NCS-R), more than 68% of adults with a mental disorder had at least one medical condition, and 29% of those with a medical disorder had a comorbid mental health condition (Alegria et al., 2003). Mental health workers should keep in mind that the reasons of multi-morbidity are complex and bidirectional. Medical disorders may lead to mental disorders, mental conditions may increase the vulnerability for specific medical disorders, and mental and medical disorders may share common predisposing and triggering factors (Goodell et al., 2011). This high multi-morbidity demands an integrative understanding and management of all illnesses, including their psycho-analytic/psychodynamic aspects.

Second, all illnesses and their treatment processes, including the ones classified as *pure* medical disorders, have psychological/emotional aspects that need careful attention of the health workers. These emotional aspects, contributing to the development of the medical disease or having an impact on the treatment process or both, need the clinician to have competency in understanding and managing them; e.g., at least, the emotional meanings attributed to the symptoms or formulation of the primary and secondary gains.

Third, any medical treatment should be undertaken in collaboration with the person as a *subject*; hence, the clinician should be aware of the conscious and unconscious worlds of the person, for a better rapport, compliance and outcome. Psychoanalytic/psychodynamic concepts with their potential for deepening such an integrative understanding of human beings in health and ill health should be a part of medical training and practice of general medicine and psychiatry.

Fourth, at any clinical setting, the main focus of the person seeking help from health workers is on pain and suffering. Any illness either classified as physical and/or mental disorder causes emotional pain and suffering. The term *patient* itself is a derivative of the adjective *patientem* (in Latin) defined as "bearing, supporting, suffering, enduring, permitting", and of the noun *pacient* (late fourteenth century, from Old French) defined as "suffering or sick person under medical treatment" (Harper, 2011–2014). Life is obviously a very rich but difficult and demanding process, and psyche is constructed and reconstructed in the struggle to deal with it. The dynamic turbulence created in the currents of mental life by these struggles lead people to develop means of avoiding pain: various ways of seeing, thinking, feeling and behaving can all serve this purpose. Much of this activity takes place out of awareness (Johnstone & Dallos, 2006). Psychoanalytic/psychodynamic theory and practice provides the health and mental health workers the perspective that there is an *internal world* (subjectivity) constituted differently from *external reality* (objectivity). It emphasizes the fundamental influence of the unconscious elements of this internal world on people's lifestyles in health and illness. Furthermore, it stresses the repetitive character of these unconscious attempts to avoid pain since the awareness is limited. Failing defences or these repetitive patterns give form to maintain patterns of mental disorders (Johnstone & Dallos, 2006). Mental health workers, only via a psychoanalytic perspective, could formulate the role of the unconscious in the development of the *malady* and the process of *remedy*.

Fifth, suffering forces the person to confront the thoughts and feelings that were previously put in the archives of clay tablets and mostly kept hidden from the conscious mind because they seemed to be too much to deal with. Mental health workers, via psychoanalytic/psychodynamic formulation, could help the patients to *reformulate* or to *reconstruct* what they are experiencing in a more inclusive way, and to confront, accept and tolerate the pain and find ways to decrease the suffering.

Sixth, the ongoing joint *understanding and reconstructing processes* that the clinician and the person develop about these difficulties expand the person's awareness. They are focused on broadening the scope of *insight* compared to more behaviour management oriented psychotherapies. So, through the therapy process they are expected to open up new options for recovery, resilience and conflict management. The person's capacity to bear emotional pain and cope constructively with dissatisfaction and suffering is enhanced, and the ability to reflect on and be curious about their own experiences is developed. Furthermore, as stated by Busch (2013), the person with the development of a psychoanalytic mind, "can acquire the capacity to shift the inevitability of action to the possibility of reflection". Busch illustrates that while the analyst's expertise is crucial to the process, the analyst's stance, rather than mainly being an expert in the content of the patient's mind, is primarily one of helping the patient to find his own mind.

Consequently, this understanding of psychoanalytic/psychodynamic perspectives may be helpful in our daily practice of general psychiatry, where we try to find answers to that fundamental question of "how can we collaborate with this unique person to diminish his/her suffering and to reconstruct his/her integrity?" At this clinical encounter, where *the personal archives of emotional tablets* of the two meet, a challenge for the clinician is to harmonize the current available scientific universal knowledge and the uniqueness of that person.

Today, in general psychiatry, there is no meta-theory to help us to understand and explain *the clinical truth*. In fact, we do not need such a meta-theory, but we need multilevel/multidimensional approaches. We should be modest, honest and respectful towards *the clinical truth*. The clinicians need different perspectives and paradigms at different levels. Psychoanalytic/psychodynamic schools and therapies are valuable for practitioners of general medicine, psychiatry and mental health in confronting these challenges.

Note

1 Some of the opinions written in this chapter were presented at the various sessions of the International Psychoanalytic Association 49th Congress, Boston, 2015. This text does not contain any sensitive clinical confidential material; they have been either removed or comprehensively anonymized.

References

Alegria, M., Jackson, J. S., Kessler, R. C., & Takeuchi, D. (2003). *National Comorbidity Survey Replication (NCS-R), 2001–2003*. Ann Arbor, MI: Interuniversity Consortium for Political and Social Research. *American Journal of Psychiatry, 167* (2010): 1456–1463.

Bienenfeld, D. (2005). *Psychodynamic theory for clinicians* (Psychotherapy in clinical practice series). Philadelphia, PA: Lippincott, Williams & Wilkins.

Bolognini, S. (2004). *Psychoanalytic empathy*. London: Free Association Books.

Bolognini, S. (2006). *Like wind, like wave*. M. Garfield (transl.). New York: Other Press.

Bolognini, S. (2013). The institutional and fantasy family of the analyst. An informal talk translated and adapted from Italian by Susanna Bonetti and Dawn Farber. Available at https://xa.yimg.com/kq/groups/4531804/473710094/name/The+Institutional+and+Fantasy+Family+of+the+Analyst.docx (in English) [accessed 3 March 2015] or (in German) Die institutionelle und die innere Familie des Analytikers. *Forum der Psychoanalyse, 29*(3): 357–372.

Busch, F. (2013). *Creating a psychoanalytic mind: A psychoanalytic method and theory*. New York: Routledge.

Busch, F. N. & Auchincloss, E. L. (1995). The psychology of prescribing and taking medication. In H. Schwartz, E. Bleiberg, & S. Weissman (Eds.). *Psychodynamic concepts in general psychiatry*. Arlington, VA: American Psychiatric Press.

Busch, F. N., & Sanberg, L. S. (2007). *Psychotherapy and medication: The challenge of integration* (Psychoanalytic Inquiry Book Series). New York: The Analytic Press.

Cabaniss, D. L., Cherry, S., Douglas, C. J., & Schwartz, A. R. (2011). *Psychodynamic Psychotherapy: A clinical manual*. Oxford: Wiley-Blackwell.

Cabannis, D. L., Cherry, S., Douglas, C. J., Graver, R., & Schwartz, A. R. (2013). *Psychodynamic formulation*. Oxford, UK: Wiley.

Cloninger, C. R. (1999). A new conceptual paradigm from genetics and psychobiology for the science of mental health. *Australian and New Zealand Journal of Psychiatry*, *33*: 174–186.

Cuijpers, P., Sijbrandij, M., Koole, S. I., Andersson, G., Beekman, A. T., & Reynolds C. F. (2014). Adding psychotherapy to antidepressant medication in depression and anxiety disorders: A meta-analysis. *World Psychiatry*, *13*(1): 56–67.

Demyttenaere, K., & Haddad, P. (2000). Compliance with antidepressant therapy and antidepressant discontinuation symptoms. *Acta Psychiatrica Scandinavica Supplement*, *403*: 50–56.

Demyttenaere, K. (1997). Compliance during treatment with antidepressants. *Journal of Affective Disorders*, *43*(1): 27–39.

Gabbard, G. O. (2014). *Psychodynamic psychiatry in clinical practice*. Washington, DC: American Psychiatric Publishing.

Goodell, S., Druss, B. G., & Walker, E. R. (2011). Based on a research synthesis by Druss and Reisinger Walker. Mental disorders and medical comorbidity. The Robert Wood Johnson Foundation: the Synthesis Project, Policy brief no: 21. Available at www.rwjf.org/content/dam/farm/reports/issue_briefs/2011/rwjf69438 [accessed 3 March 2015].

Harper, D. (2011–2014). *Online Etymology Dictionary*. Available at www.etymonline.com/index.php?term=patient [accessed 27 February 2015].

International Psychoanalytical Association 49th Congress (Changing World: the shape and use of psychoanalytic tools today) 22–25 July 2015, Boston, MA. Available at www.ipa.org.uk/Congress/Congress_Programme/Congress_Themes/Programme.asp [accessed 3 March 2015].

Jaspers, K. (1913). *General psychopathology*. J. Hoenig, & M. W. Hamilton (1997, transl.). Baltimore, MD: Johns Hopkins University Press.

Johnson, D. A. (1981). Depression: Treatment compliance in general practice. Acta *Psychiatrica Scandinavica Supplement*, *290*: 447–453.

Johnstone, L., & Dallos, R. (2006). *Formulation in psychology and psychotherapy-making sense of people's problems*. New York: Routledge.

Küey, L. (2013). Communication. In D. Bhugra, P. Ruiz, & S. Gupta (Eds.) *Leadership in psychiatry*. Oxford, UK: Wiley-Blackwell.

Küey, L. (2014). Sürgün ve hüzün: Izmir'in amane şarkıları (Refugee and grief: "the amane songs" of Izmir). In A. G. Küey (Ed.) *Psychoanalytic encounters-8*. Istanbul: Bağlam Publishers (in Turkish).

Lacan, J. Seminar XXIII, March 23, 1966, quoted by, Fink, B. (1999). *A clinical introduction to Lacanian psychoanalysis: Theory and technique*. Cambridge, MA: Harvard University Press.

Levy, R. A., & Ablon, J. S. (2009). *Handbook of evidence based psychodynamic psychotherapy: Bridging the gap between science and practice* (Current Clinical Psychiatry). New York: Humana Press.

Maroda, K. J. (2012). *Psychodynamic techniques: Working with Emotion in the therapeutic relationship*. New York: The Guilford Press.

Michels, R., Abensour, L., Eizirik, C. L., & Rusbridger, R. (2002). *Key Papers on Countertransference: IJP Education Section* (The IJPA Key Papers Series). London: Karnac Books.

Misri, Mehmet Niyazi (1618–1694), a hymn by a Turkish soufi poet, translated into English from Turkish by L. Küey. Available at http://niyaziimisri. blogspot.com.tr/2012/10/derman-arardm-derdime-derdim-bana.html (in Turkish) [accessed 25 February 2015].

Murakami, H. (2008). *What I talk about when I talk about running*. New York: Vintage International.

Olfson, M., & Marcus, S. C. (2010). National trends in outpatient psychotherapy. *American Journal of Psychiatry, 167*: 1456–1463).

Pamuk, O. (2005). *Snow*. New York: Vintage International.

Quartier, F. (2004). Bir Klinisyen olarak Freud. Aliefendioğlu B (2005) (transl.). "Freud clinicien": pratiques cliniques contemporaines en psychiatrie et en médecine, coll. thématiques en santé mentale. Paris: Doin, Küey A. G. (Ed.). Istanbul: Bağlam Publishers (in Turkish).

Quartier, F., & Bartolomei, J. (2013). *Psychiatrie: mode d'emploi. Théorie, démarche clinique, expériences*. Paris: Doin.

Schwartz, H., Bleiberg, E., & Weissman, S. (1995). *Psychodynamic concepts in general psychiatry*. Arlington, VA: American Psychiatric Publishing.

Sperry, L., Gudeman, J. E., Blackwell, B., & Faulkner, L. R. (1992). *Psychiatric Case formulations*. Washington, DC: American Psychiatric Publishing.

Weich, S., & Aray, R. (2004). International and regional variation in the prevalence of common mental disorders: do we need more surveys? *The British Journal of Psychiatry, 184*: 289–290.

CHAPTER NINETEEN

"What shall we do?"
Bridging psychoanalysis and non-analysts[1]

Susana Muszkat

This short paper reflects on the existing paradox of psychoanalysis: if on the one hand it has become a cultural heritage to the Western world, on the other, it has been distancing itself from the contemporary world and other theories of knowledge. In order to address this matter, I describe a three-party initiative that has resulted in a book series directed to the lay public and written by psychoanalysts in accessible language.

The book series was born with a double purpose: (1) to allow the lay public to have access to consistent psychoanalytic knowledge in a colloquial and simple language, beyond its most common use restricted to the private clinical sphere, and (2) to share reliable information passed on by qualified psychoanalysts in areas such as mental health, education, family dynamics and others. Each author, writing in simple but consistent language, will deal with a specific problematic.

The series *What shall we do?* aims to bridge psychoanalytic knowledge and psychoanalysts' expertise with the everyday needs and suffering of the non-psychoanalytic community.[2]

Psychoanalysis, as we all know, has become a relevant part of human history and heritage. Widespread initially throughout the Western world, it has, in the last 15 or so years, gained spaces and an increase in interest in what were previously unthinkable regions for psychoanalysis. These, range from Eastern Europe to Asia, including countries such as Latvia, Serbia, Montenegro, Kazakhstan, China, Russia, India and so many others.

Psychoanalysis is undoubtedly part of the way we currently understand and explain social configurations, historical conflicts, social movements, human relations in general and family relations in particular.

It is at the basis of any educational project as it is part of the curriculum in most medical schools. Furthermore, it is part of the program of most undergraduate and post-graduation courses of Economics, Communication, Marketing, Law, Pedagogy, Social Work, Sports, Arts, History, the list goes on! Wherever human beings are involved, there is room – and often the need – for a psychoanalytic perspective.

There is no doubt as to the importance of psychoanalytic knowledge and its relevance in understanding the world today. As much as that is true, it is also true that psychoanalysis as science and as a clinical resource for human suffering has been significantly losing ground as other fields and methodologies gain the forefront.

Back in 2009, Elisabeth Roudinesco gave an interview to an important Brazilian newspaper (*O Estado de São Paulo*, 09/20/2009), where she affirmed that "Freud's legacy is, in one way or another, behind all forms of emancipation experienced by the twentieth century society, of which feminism and women's liberation are just two of such examples" (p. D6, free translation by author).

It would be safe to state that, since its founding by Freud, up to current days, the psychoanalytic movement has always been split in at least two contradictory directions: the wish to expand and be included as a trustworthy theoretical body to as many people and parts of the world as possible on the one hand. On the other, it is marked by an elitist position of inclusion of the alike and exclusion of the different. Naturally, along the way, many of the alike become different, thus excluded.

In fact, psychoanalysis as a theory of knowledge moves in the opposite direction of that of its institutionalization, where the latter, represented by its societies and study groups carry strict and selective standards for new members. The same is true of its often-rigid hierarchical forms of organization.

In the interesting book, *The Freudians* (1998), Edith Kurzweil discusses what she calls the *different psychoanalyses* as a result of the different cultural groupings where each of them was developed. She describes how analysts themselves have often had a hard time finding a common ground of agreement, such are the controversies of the various interpretations regarding the *real* psychoanalysis. Consequently, many times analysts could not agree as to whether their disagreements had to do with true the-oretical differences or if they were the product of subjective unconscious factors (p. 3).

Have we been arguing among ourselves and in the process forgotten to include others? Have we forgotten to integrate with other mental health fields? Have we failed in making our specificity and expertise known to non-psychoanalysts – regular people who may benefit from what we can offer but have no accessible links with us?

To expand but not include: a psychoanalytical paradox, still true to a greater or lesser degree in the various training institutes of the IPA societies, in the different scientific fields and among the lay public.

Psychoanalysis as well as psychoanalysts, often times are portrayed by the media or by general public opinion in a caricatured manner: the mute, distant, all too-serious analyst. The couch, the long years, the high frequency, and the connection mistakably made of analysis as exclusive of highly disturbed patients have become iconic as some of the psychoanalytic 'strangenesses'.

What might be the reasons for such distancing of the psychoanalytic language from the people? Aren't people those that psychoanalysis is meant for? And should people who suffer and need us as professionals adapt to psychoanalysis in order to benefit from its methodology or should we learn to listen to people in their singularities and find ways to communicate with others outside the psychoanalytic community? Roudinesco, again, says: "Psychoanalysts, in their majority, have become conservatives" (p. D6).

This is quite an intriguing observation, especially when referring to a field of knowledge that came to life as an extremely revolutionary and groundbreaking theoretical body. She explains: "Psychoanalysts have become uninterested in what regards social matters. In this way they have become conservatives" (p. D6).

What shall we do? is an initiative that intends to convey in simple and accessible non-psychoanalytic language, psychoanalytic knowledge that may be of service to people outside the clinic.

It is not a self-help book, as it does not offer prescriptions, define norms or prescribe formulas of how to solve human difficulties, but rather acknowledges them and opens up channels to think and provide understanding regarding the multiplicity of human experience.

The reader of these books may be someone who is actually going through the problem him/herself, some family member or friend who is also living the problem closely and wishes to gain more information and helpful resources, or professionals of diverse fields who encounter themselves with such problematics in their work space.

The fact that each of these books is written by psychoanalysts who are acknowledged specialists and researchers on each of the areas being discussed, may be a reliable source of information, a scientific guide to approach lay people with the problems faced.

It is a form of practicing psychoanalysis beyond the walls of the traditional clinical space; thus, allowing the reader to demystify and shed a light on issues that may be a cause of great pain and anxiety when clouded by lack of information, shame, fear, or merely not knowing how to access professional information.

The books will cover topics such as health, psychology, education, family issues, gender issues, psychic disorders, addictions and many others.

The first three numbers have been launched in 2016, and three more will have been launched by the end of 2018, discussing the following topics: Alcoholism, Family Violence, Shame, Professional Orientation, Self Esteem and Eating Disorders. Some other titles under way are: Aging, Adolescence, Depression, Compulsion, Passion, Homosexuality, Marijuana, Adoption and many others.

What shall we do? (O que fazer?) will initially be published in Portuguese in both paper and e-book formats.

Notes

1 This paper continues a discussion of a previous paper I wrote, published in the *Brazilian Journal of Psychoanalysis*, 43(4) (2009). Reprinted by kind permission of the journal.
2 This book series developed and coordinated by Luciana Saddi, Sonia Terepins, Thais Blucher and Susana Muszkat, of the Brazilian Psychoanalytic Society of São Paulo, had its first volume supported by the IPA through the *Psychoanalysis and Mental Health Field* committee, chaired by Claudio Eizirik, and is published by Blucher Publishing House, of São Paulo, Brazil.

References

Kurzweil, E. (1998). *The Freudians, a comparative perspective*. New Brunswick, NJ and London: Transaction Publishers.

Muszkat, S. (2009). *Os Paradoxos da Psicanálise* (Paradoxes of Psychoanalysis). *Revista Brasileira de Psicanálise*, 43(4). São Paulo, Brazil.

Roudinesco, E. (2009). Interview. *O Estado de São Paulo*, 20 September, p. D6. São Paulo, Brazil.

CHAPTER TWENTY

A "bridge" between psychoanalysis and psychiatry

Andrea Narracci

This essay is a tribute to the work of Jorge Garcìa Badaracco.

Towards the end of the 1960s, Garcìa Badaracco began treating the patients of Borda Psychiatric Hospital in Buenos Aires using the knowledge he gained during the previous years in Argentina and Europe, especially in France, both in Psychiatry and Psychoanalysis.

Garcia Badaracco reorganized Borda's ward in order to make it more human, giving patients back areas that had originally been dedicated to them and creating better conditions for many of the new patients. With the help of his coworkers, he invited patients' relatives in to discuss the discharge from the Psychiatric Hospital. The relatives found Garcìa Badaracco's behavior somewhat bizarre, since the patients he intended to discharge had been hospitalized for years. However, they continued taking part in the meetings.

Garcìa Badaracco then began holding these meetings on a regular basis and invited all interested patients to join, along with their relatives and those working in the ward. Such meetings were later named Multi-family Psychoanalysis Groups (MFPG).

Through empirical observation of the participants, Garcia Badaracco and his co-workers sensed that even though the patients' parents often considered their children as very different from themselves, patients were actually very similar to the parent they had a closer relationship to. This led them to the idea that patients were like "caricatures" of their own parents.

Garcìa Badaracco thought that this very element could be considered the empirical acknowledgement of a symbiotic bond between parent and son, as Psychoanalysis already assumed. The failure of this bond to evolve could then account for the rise of the pathology, as it had prevented the development of the autonomous functioning of the child's mind and prevents the development of the child's autonomous functioning.

Garcìa Badaracco named this kind of bond "pathologic and pathogenic interdependence" and believed that its cure is about being able to loosen it, in order for both parent and child to discover their own independent "healthy virtuality".

The Multifamily Psychoanalysis Group (MFPG) is a large group made up of several family units, including patients. One or more members of each family unit can attend it.

The MFPG has some basic rules:

1   Each participant has the right to talk.
2   Speakers and speeches are equally important.
3   Those who prefer to remain silent must listen carefully and respectfully, without interrupting.
4   The order of speakers is decided by a show of hands.
5   If possible, direct dialogues should not be encouraged: up to four operators will assist in order to facilitate the starting of the "conversation" and ensure that the rules and speakers order are respected. Operators themselves also have the right to talk.

The specific features of the MFPG are:

1   The metaphoric mirroring between members belonging to different family units. Such phenomena can only happen in this type of group: observing what happens in other families, every participant can rethink of what happens in his or her own home.
2   Multiple transferences. Every participant's transference can be compared to all kinds of similar relationships within the group. For instance, a father could believe that he's not able to talk with his or any other child anymore. By attending the group, he finds out that he's able to talk with a child from another family unit; building on this, he can start to realize that he'd actually be able to talk to his own child too.

3   Being involved in the unfolding of these two phenomena (metaphoric mirroring and multiple transferences) can allow family members to resume their ability to represent. Such ability was not lost, they were just unable to use it as they were involved in pathological interactions, as could happen in any family.

When the basic rules of the MFPG are respected and all the mechanisms mentioned before are adopted, the participants' minds can start to function based also on the "primary process" and not only on the "secondary process". Each mind will then start functioning as part of a "widened mind" (mente ampliada). The mente ampliada originates a thought composed of all participants' speeches and thoughts.

This will make it possible for dissociated elements in the mind of each participant to resurface. Such elements, as we know, can be very useful in "giving meaning" to mental suffering, both psychotic and otherwise.

Our work in the Institution has been inspired by this vision.

In 1997, I opened my first group in a residential treatment centre for psychotic and borderline patients. At that time, I thought the group might help the families to welcome their relatives back after the discharge from the centre. The aim was to raise a higher level of awareness about the future development of their relationships. Such development had to be seen as the outcome of hard work that had to keep on going, involving all the family members.

After a few years, I founded two other groups in two community mental health facilities in the health district of Rome where I was working at the time. Since then, with the help of many other talented colleagues, I've been able to start groups in all other facilities within the area I was in charge of coordinating (outpatient mental health facility, psychiatric service for diagnosis and therapy, therapeutic residential care). The area was, at that time, made up of four health districts, assisting a community of patients counting more than 500,000 people.

The presence of a group in each facility did change the relationship with patients and their close relatives, and also among operators, both in each service and from different services.

Multifamily Psychoanalysis influences operators, patients and their relatives, as it sets a mood that facilitates self-observation in each participant.

Self-observation helps to focus on what anyone can do in order to improve he/she's current situation, and helps operators to stop feeling alone when they face mental illness. Rather, operators can learn or relearn to face it all together, side by side, one with another.

The deep emotional and intellectual bond that developed among operators was the impulse to design an intervention's plan where each facility would represent a fundamental stage of a comprehensive therapeutic path: the so called "Quadrilateral".

The stages of this therapeutic path are the Psychiatric Service for Diagnosis and Therapy in the hospital, the Intensive Therapeutic Residential Care, the Unit for Youth Psychotherapy and the Outpatient Mental Health Facility. These facilities are all part of the Community Mental Health Facility and should develop a shared intervention's plan shortly after the admittance of a patient in any of them, making sure that operators from all of the four stages are involved in the plan.

Indeed, Multi-family Psychoanalysis has deeply changed the way of thinking about psychiatric intervention and its realization. Psychiatric issues can now be addressed along a path through the different facilities of a health department, framed in the psychoanalytic thought.

Bibliography

Garcia Badaracco, Jorge, *Demonios de la mente. Biografia de una esquizofrenia*, Buenos Aires, Eudeba, 2005.

Garcia Badaracco, Jorge, *Comunidad terapeutica psicoanalitica de estructura multifamiliar*, Madrid, Tecnipublicaciones, 1989.

Garcia Badaracco, *Jorge, Psicoanalisis Multifamiliar. Los otros en nosotros y el descubrimiento del sì mismo*, Buenos Aires, Paidòs Psicologia Profunda, 2000.

Garcia Badaracco, Jorge and Andrea Narracci, *La Psicoanalisi Multifamiliare in Italia*, Antigone Edizioni, Torino, 2011.

Mitre Maria, Elisa, *Las voces del silencio*, Ciudad Autonoma de Buenos Aires: Sudamericana, 2016.

Narracci, Andrea (ed.), Psicoanalisi Multifamiliare come esperanto, Antigone Edizioni, Torino, 2015.

CHAPTER TWENTY ONE

Psychoanalysis and psychiatry

Florence Quartier

The field of health has massively changed over the last few decades, and treatment in psychiatry has greatly evolved: the patient can often be treated as an out-patient without disrupting his or her social and family life. Then the interest in relational problems has also greatly evolved. Treatment can continue over a long period and thus become an interesting and intimate element in the history of the patient and his or her family circle. Also, medication, although not always having fulfilled its early promise, is useful and can be even more so if it is possible to prescribe it sparingly. To this I would add that, in many countries, patients and their entourage have become true partners and make an active contribution to the evolution of the institutions.

* * *

What this means is that many psychiatric care providers wish to include the relational theme in their training. They clearly feel the need to talk about their clinical practice and to discuss relational problems so as to have a better understanding of what is at stake in the context of the treatment. In fact, it is the doctors and nurses as well as other care providers who feel so strongly about how complicated and at the same time interesting it is, working with people suffering from serious psychiatric problems. And they express how tiring and disconcerting it is to do this work hour after hour and day after day. Over and above the highly diversified approaches offered today, beyond the contribution made by medication, beyond neurobiological research, the evidence is clear: it is the relationship established with the patient that remains the main working tool in psychiatry.

Specifics of the relationship between care worker and patient

One could call psychiatry "the art of meeting" (paraphrased from Shea, 1998). It is therefore clear that an analyst can very usefully work in psychiatry and, today, can collaborate with all the other care providers. He also needs to take account of certain factors specific to in-patient care: the relationship in psychiatry is often accompanied by certain constraints (in an emergency room or within the hospital with a patient in crisis, unwilling to be treated). Right away this relationship holds surprises, both pleasant and unpleasant, disappointments or too great a sense of satisfaction. This is often clearly recognized, but is still poorly defined. The analyst may also transmit certain notions, enabling every care provider to understand the origin of a provocative, childish manner. He can explain what contributes to arrogant, even violent behaviour and help to understand the strength of repetition.

To be able to call on a general understanding of psychiatric functioning, for example the evolution of the child into the adult, often enables care providers to benefit more from a delicate situation in which they find themselves: they are able to see that the limits imposed by ethics can cause difficulties and they well realize that they are involved in a more personal sense than they would wish. For psychiatric care providers there is a risk of error (misplaced or untimely activism, an unwelcome or abusive influence or even seduction, all of which are traumatic for the patient) and there is also the possibility of bringing to light the signs, the elements that only appear in the daily routine during a hospital stay or a privileged link with a particular care provider (a nurse, an occupational therapist in a workshop, etc.). For his part, the analyst can learn a lot from his contacts with the psychiatric care providers. For him, it is the equivalent of a real life situation, a contact with the *reality principle*. He has to contend with certain difficulties that he has not faced or no longer faces; he can discover the constraints that weigh on psychiatry and from that point, become a member of the team in the vast field of mental health. He can of course stay in his specific role which is also helpful. This is evident in the contribution from Professor Levent Küey who works in tandem with analysts, calling on them to participate in the psychiatric service that he heads in Istanbul.

The issue is to work with all these elements. That is what enriches communication and provides an opportunity of setting up a partially new clinic. This work can take account of changes occurring in psychiatry, development of psychoanalysis, and links that today can be (re)created between psychoanalysis and psychiatry.

Transmission, opening, exchange

Up to now, in Western Switzerland we have had the luck to maintain a dialogue between psychiatry and psychoanalysis. Psychoanalysis in the curriculum for trainee psychiatrists is still taught today. Admittedly the context is now more challenging and, indeed, nothing can be taken for granted. But, as in other countries, there is also opposition. It is not always easy to develop reciprocal links; some institutions are reticent or even hostile to the idea of a psychoanalytic contribution. Indeed, certain psychoanalysts are against the idea of contact with institutions. We set out here what it is possible to achieve when the context is suitable. Professor Küchenhoff announced clearly in his introduction that he had left the university milieu and it is in his role as an analyst that he runs a psychiatric institution. In this context, he has developed an important and fruitful dialogue between psychoanalysis and psychiatry. Another example is that offered by Professor Küey, a psychiatrist who requires his analysts to run supervision sessions for his teams.

Psychiatric institutions today are subject to heavy constraints which force them to explain themselves when a contribution is not being made to social order. So? From the point of view of the care providers the continuing demand for quality clinical work is there and it is at this level that it is possible to establish links between psychiatry and psychoanalysis in the field.

It involves, and the same situation applies to us as to our predecessors, helping care providers discover the clinical riches contained in the relations established in psychiatry and to respond in a manner relevant to their desire to enhance the effect of the psychotherapeutic aspects of the treatment. It involves transmitting certain psychoanalytic ideas in a form that is clearly understood by everyone and, above all, useful in the specialized context of psychiatry. We propose a theoretical–practical approach that enables every care provider to stay on course in a relationship with every patient even when the latter is difficult to tolerate, destructive, or extremely odd. This approach enables care providers to keep their motivation throughout and to avoid de-motivation or even burn out, to discover the depth of clinical work and to avoid falling into a routine. Another distinct aspect of this work which we feel is extremely important to emphasize: each care provider must realize that all patients, without exception and whatever the gravity of their problem, can benefit from specific relational care. We can work with teams dealing with agitated and serious borderline patients as well as teams treating prisoners who have committed serious crimes. We can also help to discover the richness in clinics for elderly people and move away from a reasoning where we limit ourselves to evaluating their deficiencies. The same applies to the person with a mental handicap where we can emphasize the positive elements brought out by the care providers, those that can best take account of the person and of his history. We have always emphasized that there is no reason to deprive someone of the riches of his unconscious.

Work in multidisciplinary groups, (re)discovering psychoanalysis

For many years I have been working with multidisciplinary groups in institutions, psychiatric centres for adults or the elderly, and psychiatric services in the prison sector. It is very important to emphasize that the "I" here represents what an analyst can do. We shouldn't think that it is about me (Florence Quartier). The participants are doctors, nurses, social workers, psychologists and other care providers. In psychiatry, many teams are worried about having to complete questionnaires when they need to work rapidly. Also, the push for results prevents the team from establishing a personal dialogue with each patient. This is one of the current major concerns in psychiatry. I would like to insist on how we can contribute to the protection of clinical practice. The transmission of psychoanalysis, showing the richness of the clinical practice experience is at the heart of these present concerns.

The method we have used has a long history. Already in the 1970s we studied with analysts who worked with us in psychiatry. All of them were full members of the IPA (Diatkine, Quartier, & Andreoli, 1991; Racamier et al., 1973).

The working groups are set up on clear guidelines. These are the more important elements:

First, our method is to encourage an open discussion. It is up to the group participants to decide who will introduce a difficult situation: it is often a doctor and a nurse. They don't give a classical medical presentation. I suggest they outline the patient's current situation and explain why they need or want to discuss this specific case at this specific time. The patient's history will probably come out during the discussion, although it isn't immediately necessary to delve into the past. It is surprising to observe how often the group participants start the debate before the introduction of the case has been completed. It does not matter: the questions come up and I take them. Everyone has the right to participate. Part of my role in the group is to point out the rich complexity of the points being made. Otherwise, such points may have been missed by the participants, who are perhaps too close to a relationship with a patient, which they find too difficult or too repetitive.

Second, the work is always carried out within the framework of ongoing training programmes set up by the institution. I do not want to run the risk of being an analyst parachuted into an institution without any knowledge of how it functions. That's why I always co-host the session with one of the institution's senior doctors. He or she is there to put the debate in context and remind the group about the general policy of the institution.

Taking account of the present difficult climate for institutions, and also for psychoanalysis, albeit in a different way, it seems important to establish a constructive link with the heads of institutions before starting to work with the care providers. It is not a case of forcing the door, nor of imposing the analyst's presence. It is far better to work with the heads of institutions to reflect on the subject of clinical work and to take account of the context of each individual institution (Gravier, 2015).

The group discussion is focused exclusively on clinical work. Our method is on work done in the group but not as a group dynamic: it stays in a clinical context. It is important to emphasize this aspect, because it is here that the work of the group, the work of the doctor, and my own work converge: we all have a common interest in defending clinical practice. In my view, this way of working is very suitable for integrating analytical ideas into the institutional context.

What happens during the open discussion? Little by little we can:

- bring out the richness of clinical practice, and this applies to every single patient whatever his or her situation or pathology (prisoners, senior citizens, serious psychosis in the adult);
- give to each participant the desire and the courage to enter into the relationship with the patient;

- suggest useful links between practice and theory. This is an aspect I greatly enjoy. If the group wishes, I take the time to develop any point in a more theoretical manner. I provide a wide variety of references, from different eras and from different analytical schools of thought. I want to help the participants to discover texts that provide a precise answer to their questions. In my opinion, the transmission of our rich and dynamic clinical heritage is a very important part of our work today.

At this point in the work and the debate, I always come back to the patient whose case has been discussed by the group, so that everyone can leave the meeting with renewed interest and motivation.

From our side, what can we think about such a discussion with the participants? An aspect that I wish to emphasize is that we very often feel the need to rebuild the foundations of psychoanalysis. Today we work a lot with doctors, nurses and psychologists, who know nothing or very little about analysis. They may know it exists but in their view it's often an outdated way of working. At the same time, these colleagues are faced with the difficult problems imposed by the clinic: it is hard and sometimes very painful to meet a patient who is referred to as "borderline". Doctors and nurses today have their interview techniques and they are certainly highly useful techniques. But when I propose in parallel to (re)discover psychoanalysis, they are very interested. For example when I make clear:

- the complexity of the links with the past;
- the complexity of the continuity between normal and pathological;
- the complexity of the link that the patient constructs with each care provider.

In this case I don't necessarily use the term "transference". For example when the group is worried about a *young adult*, I prefer to emphasize certain subtle elements picked up during the group discussion on the patient, which are similar to the elements that "normally" appear in adolescence: aspects of narcissism, megalomania and so on. By doing this I can develop a certain way of seeing that includes different movements of mental functioning at different moments of development. A young "psychotic" adult has a pathological functioning and at the same time he has "normal" functioning. We rarely go beyond adolescence with adult patients in psychiatry because it is often their adolescence that is more relevant than the rest of their childhood. But of course I draw attention as to how childhood experiences permeate the adult psyche. I do not interpret the patient's case from the material presented or, if I do "interpret", it's only in general terms, to give an idea of what constitutes narcissism or Oedipal movements.

My desire is for the participants to have some sort of proof through clinical facts. In this way, they are faced with these elements of adolescence which continue to contribute to the problems of the adult but which they could not see before our discussion. Naturally I tell them that adolescence is the result of what went before. The aim is to offer the patient the possibility of obtaining a psychotherapeutic effect during the psychiatric treatment.

Before I conclude, let us take a look into the past. As I mention above, we learnt this way of working many years ago, at the start of our training in the 1970s.

At that time, psychiatry and psychoanalysis were connected in a way that seemed totally natural to us. For example, René Diatkine came to Geneva regularly, and we were able to observe him working as a psychoanalyst in psychiatry. Diatkine was familiar with our institutions in Geneva and we saw him as a close and approachable colleague. With Diatkine, the work was focused on the interview with the patient and on the discussion with the whole team. We therefore "touched" the transference, we "felt" the unconscious, and we understood the relevance of the psychoanalytical approach.

Twice a month he would spend an entire day with us, working with the whole team and giving everyone a chance to express his/her ideas. We started our training in psychoanalysis in parallel. I'm not sure whether we really appreciated the opportunity we were given at that time to construct a professional identity in such a privileged setting.

When René Diatkine stopped coming to Switzerland, the work between psychoanalysis and psychiatry was maintained, and this link is still alive. There are some multidisciplinary groups working in several institutions in Switzerland and France: we have found examples in Greece and, several years ago, also in Turkey with Ayça Gurdal-Küey and Professeur Levent Küey.

And now it has become clear that we can create or recreate the links between psychiatry and psychoanalysis. The time is right because we are able to develop our practice with many different patients. And I emphasize once more that the aim is to offer the patient the possibility of obtaining a psychotherapeutic effect during the psychiatric treatment. It is important because psychiatric patients are still often neglected. Today, everyone working in the field of mental health and wishing to maintain a vibrant clinical practice can combine psychiatry and psychoanalysis. It is an interesting and important challenge, as much for psychiatry as for psychoanalysis.

References

Diatkine, R., Quartier-Frings, Fl., & Andreoli, A. (1991). *Psychose et changement.* Paris: PUF.

Gravier, B. (2015). Quand la psychanalyse nous aide à accompagner les sujets violents. A partir de quelques concepts clés de l'œuvre de Cl. Balier. *CarnetPSY, 191,* July–August.

Racamier, P-Cl., Diatkine, R., Lebovici, S., & Paumelle, P. (1973). *Le psychana-lyste sans divan,* Coll. Science de l'homme. Paris: Payot.

Shea, S. Ch. (1998). *Psychiatric interviewing: The art of understanding.* Ed. Saunders Company. New York: Elsevier.

CHAPTER TWENTY TWO

The movement of therapeutic communities in Italy
Myth and reality

Marta Vigorelli

The movement of therapeutic communities in Italy has had, as its precursors, some brave psychoanalysts who, since the end of the 1960s, have created innovative experiences and more humanising units within traditional psychiatric hospitals outside the cities where numerous inpatients were living in alienated conditions and cut off from civil society.

The Italian Mental Health Act of 1978 (Basaglia Law or Law no. 180) brought reform to the psychiatric system in Italy which led to the closure of all the asylums. This led to a gradual replacement of psychiatric hospitals with a range of community-based services, some run by the public and others by private sectors. The decision to close the asylums was a necessary one in order to renew an interest in patients as human beings and in their treatment. It was designed to alleviate their suffering. The psychiatric reform law allowed for the best form of psychiatry to be developed. These conditions have promoted inclusion. On one hand, those in the acute phases of mental illness are now admitted to general hospitals, and on the other hand local services have set up community services. Both of these are geographically close to the place where patients live. In this historical and institutional framework thousands of therapeutic residences have flourished in Italy, 1,730 in 2000 alone and more than twice that number today. As well as this, educational rehabilitation programmes have been established for severely ill psychiatric patients, only some of which follow a therapeutic community methodology. The cultural climate of democratic renewal has been fuelled by the commitment of many pioneering psychoanalysts and phenomenologists united by a bio-psychosocial model. This has encouraged the emergence of several scientific societies including Mito & Realtà, an association for therapeutic communities and residential establishments founded in 1996. It brings together a group of professionals from a psychodynamic background, who are passionate about education and research, from a network of about a hundred therapeutic community centres scattered in the north, centre and south of Italy.

This paper is the outcome of the reflections of our association and will focus on the dynamics of the therapeutic community as an evolutionary path (Ferruta, Foresti & Vigorelli, 2012). This is different from other forms of care, and is suitable for specific types of residents (adults, adolescents and children), with different psychopathologies (psychosis, borderline or antisocial personality disorders, dual diagnosis, etc.). Inspired mostly by the British movement initiated by Tom Main, R. D. Hinshelwood and M. Johnes, by the French movement under the aegis of Racamier and Sassolas and by the Philosophy of Recovery, Mito & Realtà has formulated some key factors to construct an "Italian model" of a Therapeutic community. Notwithstanding the diversity in the types of foundation, statutes and organisation (private, accredited or public), the first core feature common to all therapeutic communities is a democratic approach with a distinct yet constantly dialogic clinical and organisational leadership, a staff group that operates as followers and promoters and supports the multiple activities with group co-responsibility oriented to integration and maintenance of a safe and protective emotionally nurturing climate both for the residents and the staff.

The common factors are as follows:

- A focus on the construction of the subject and his/her relationships with the group on the basis of the psychoanalytic theory of the unconscious and the therapeutic relationship following Bion's work in groups and Infant research theory.
- The main therapeutic factor is sharing the everyday life and the quality of interpersonal relationships.
- The therapeutic community is a global therapeutic resource that treats through its integrated functioning (bio-psychosocial levels): the group of patients and the group of care-givers, in partnership with

the families and the social network, form the treating device without privileging any aspect of community life more than others.

- The therapeutic community offers a developmental process defined in time where it is possible to develop potentials that are realistically assessed and with personalised treatment plans.
- The therapeutic community offers to the patients an environmental dimension with a specific architecture that differs from the hospital and the family. It is a place where there is a sensory and emotional climate that nourishes and sustains fragile subjectivity, gradually creating a secure base. It is a place for meeting and discussing predisposing conditions, favourable affective experiences of transition between isolated individual subjectivity and sharing with others, as well as the possibility to have consultancies and individual and group psychotherapies to allow psychic growth and subjectivisation processes.
- This organisational approach is based on the collaboration and participation of its members, staff and patients, and the functional nature of large and small groups. Goals: sense of belonging and responsibility.
- Individual–group dialectics: the treatment plan is formulated differently for each patient, with specific timing and characteristics that can foster personal expression. However, individualised treatment plans are challenged by the community approach, as it seeks to construct subjectivity at a group level.
- The TC has defined yet permeable boundaries which are open to inclusion (both subjective and professional) in the local social fabric and to a constant theoretical–clinical exchange with other therapeutic communities regionally, nationally and internationally.
- Maintenance and evaluation: a prerequisite for the effective functioning of a community is the ongoing training of its staff to overcome the risks of recurrent crises and destructive dynamics. The therapeutic communities also tend to suffer from isolation and self-reference with a great danger of going back to the institutionalisation typical of the asylums. Therefore, the complexity of this method requires constant maintenance of the institutional group and its leadership, through different tools. These function as a culture of inquiry. The tools commonly used are: clinical and staff supervision, consultancy and training – in particular through experiential workshops: "Learning from action", "Living Learning", "Authority Leadership Innovation (ALI)".

In this context, Mito & Realtà has established a peer review and accreditation project of self-assessment and assessment based on action research.

This has linked clinical assessment and training, which aims to monitor community groups, and develop and share strengths and skills. Taking a cue from the experience of the UK-based Community of Communities programme at the Royal College of Psychiatrists, the Italian model begins with a self-assessment of each community to which follow-up meetings provide external feedback. The emphasis is on participation and experiential encounter, on reflection on clinical and organisational aspects of the community, and on dialogue among peers aimed at quality improvement and change. To this end, the research team of Mito & Realtà, in conjunction with the DTC and Group Analysis Laboratory, in collaboration with the Faculty of Psychology at the Universities of Milano-Bicocca and Palermo, have developed a number of tools for different therapeutic community groups. Specifically, the manual VIVACOM and UTEFAM (for patients and families) includes the following areas: general organisation, healing climate and environmental comfort, general characteristics of care, activities aimed at families, the safety of patients and staff, personnel management and training, clinical documentation and information systems, quality and research. These areas are considered the fundamental aspects of community life. The communities included in the project are divided into triads, each of which produces a written report on the basis of the manual for self-assessment (VIVACOM and UTEFAM). Subsequently, on the basis of a timetable agreed in advance, in turn, each of the triad communities welcomes the representatives of the other two for discussion and reflection on the findings. The basic goals of visiting are: reflect on the strengths and weaknesses of each community, define shared quality standards, exchange procedures, tools and experiences, enable a qualitative and quantitative research, set targets for annual improvement, transfer of best practices, creating a network of communities with a common culture. This assessment process has highlighted so far great potential for transformation involving all the TC components: staff members, residents, families and leadership. This is being achieved through self-help, as we are increasingly operating in the context of depleted funding for services.

Reference

Ferruta, A., Foresti, G., & Vigorelli, M. (Eds.) (2012). *Le comunità terapeutiche: Psicotici, borderline, adolescenti, minori*. Milan: Raffaello Cortina Editore.

INDEX